K·I·S·S

DK

The Only Guides You'll Ever Need!

THIS SERIES IS YOUR TRUSTED GUIDE through all of life's stages and situations. Want to learn how to surf the Internet or care for your new dog? Or maybe you'd like to become a wine connoisseur or an expert gardener? The solution is simple: Just pick up a K.I.S.S. Guide and turn to the first page.

Expert authors will walk you through the subject from start to finish, using simple blocks of knowledge to build your skills one step at a time. Build upon these learning blocks and by the end of the book, you'll be an expert yourself! Or, if you are familiar with the topic but want to learn more, it's easy to dive in and pick up where you left off.

The K.I.S.S. Guides deliver what they promise: simple access to all the information you'll need on one subject. Other titles you might want to check out include: Playing Guitar, Living With a Dog, the Internet, Microsoft Windows, Astrology, and many more to come.

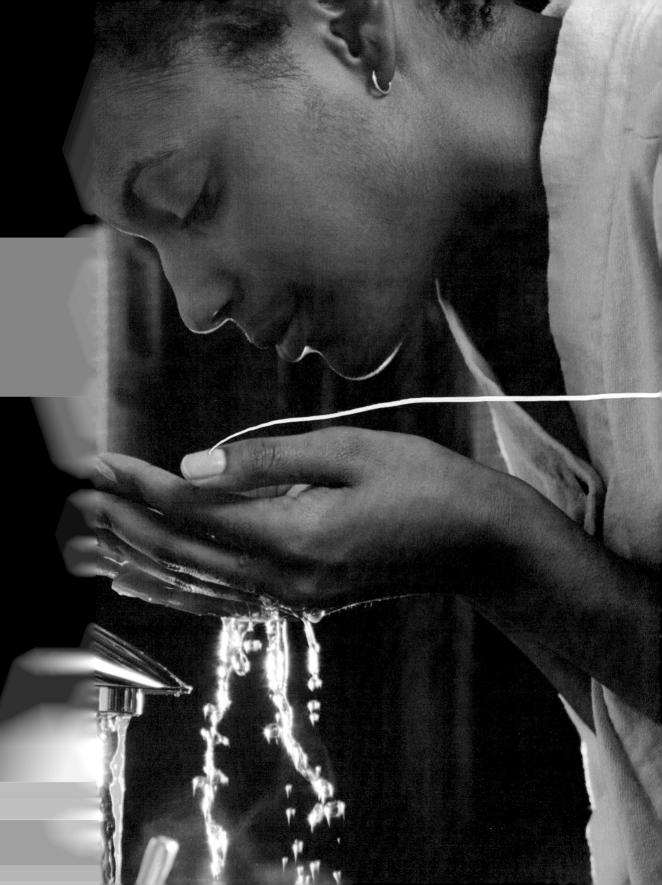

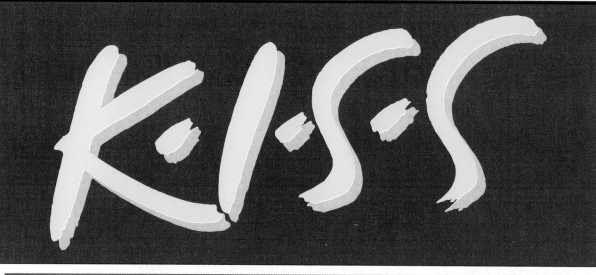

Beauty

STEPHANIE PEDERSEN

Foreword by Victoria Moran

Acclaimed author and advocate of women's wellness

A Dorling Kindersley Book

LONDON, NEW YORK,
MUNICH, MELBOURNE, DELHI

DK Publishing, Inc.
Senior Editor Jennifer Williams
Line Editor Lisa Lenard
Copy Editor Joy Dickinson
Category Publisher LaVonne Carlson

Dorling Kindersley Limited
Project Editor Caroline Hunt
Project Art Editor Simon Murrell

Managing Editor Maxine Lewis
Managing Art Editor Heather McCarry

Production Heather Hughes
Category Publisher Mary Thompson

Produced for Dorling Kindersley by

studio cactus Ⓒ

13 SOUTHGATE STREET WINCHESTER HAMPSHIRE SO23 9DZ

Project Editor Kate Hayward
Project Art Editor Laura Watson
Editorial Assistance Jane Baldock
Design Assistance Sharon Moore

Library of Congress Cataloging-in-Publication data

Pedersen, Stephanie.
KISS guide to beauty / Stephanie Pedersen.
    p. cm. -- (Keep It Simple Series)
"A Dorling Kindersley Book."
ISBN 0-7894-8146-4
1. Beauty, Personal. I. Title. II. Series.
RA776.98 .P43 2001
646.7'042--dc21

                                                    2001002551
                                                    CIP

DK Publishing, Inc. offers special discounts for bulk purchases for sales promotions or premiums. Specific, large-
quantity needs can be met with special editions, including personalized covers, excerpts of existing guides, and
corporate imprints. For more information, contact Special Markets Department,
DK Publishing, Inc., 95 Madison Avenue, New York, NY 10016 Fax: 800-600-9098.

Color reproduction by Colourscan, Singapore
Printed and bound by Printer Industria Grafica, S.A., Barcelona, Spain

See our complete catalog at

www.dk.com

Contents at a Glance

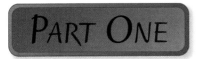

PART ONE

The Basics

Real Beauty
About Skin
Complexion Care
What's Your Problem?
Beyond the Basics

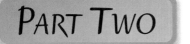

PART TWO

Hair Care

All About Hair
Caring For Hair
Hairstyle Essentials
Color You Beautiful
A Change in Texture

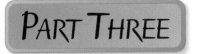

PART THREE

Makeup

Makeup Fundamentals
Giving Good Face
Brow Know-How

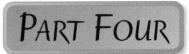

PART FOUR

Nail Care

About Nails
Caring For Your Nails

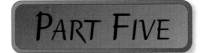

PART FIVE

Beauty and Beyond

Body Care
Considering Cosmetic Surgery
Creating a Beautiful Life
Bringing It All Home

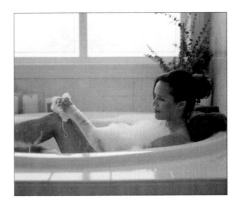

CONTENTS

PART ONE The Basics

CHAPTER 1   Real Beauty   22

CHAPTER 2   About Skin   30

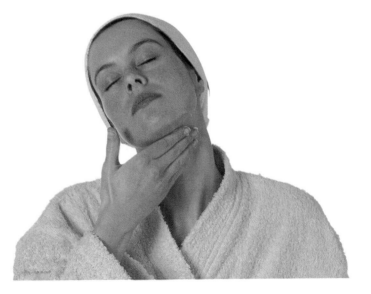

PART TWO Hair Care

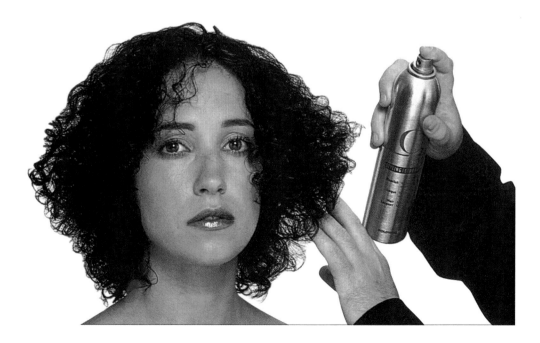

PART THREE Makeup

PART FOUR Nail Care

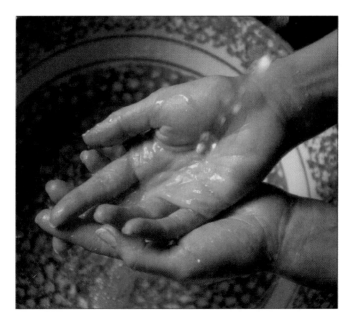

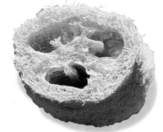

Appendices

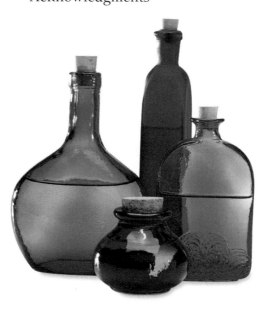

Foreword

ENHANCING THE WAY WE LOOK *ought to be a joy. Ideally, we would cherish the raw materials – our faces, bodies, and personalities – and have fun pampering ourselves and playing up our best features. Unfortunately, we all too often take a derogatory view of the way we look and expect miracles from diets, make-up, and hair styles.*

This is a reasonable attitude given the unreasonableness of our culture when it comes to the way women are supposed to look. The majority of magazines, television commercials, and movies imply that we should all be tall, thin, have an ample bosom, thick hair, full lips, perfect teeth, and never age a day beyond 25. Such expectations are not only unrealistic; they're depressing. Inability to reach this impossible perfection can lead to giving up entirely, deciding that beauty is the province of those born beautiful, out of the reach of mere mortals like the rest of us. This is unfortunate, because every woman alive has a well of inner beauty that can show on the outside, too. This ageless, dauntless beauty is the combination of heart, soul, talent, passion, energy, and confidence that makes each of us unique. The more we develop these qualities, the richer the radiance we can expect to see in our eyes, our smiles, the way we move, and the way people perceive us.

Once we realize that we are exquisite by virtue of our individuality, we can appreciate our physical selves as the outward manifestation of our one-of-a-kind essence. It took me years of trial, error, self-searching, and self-discovery to realize this truth: each one of us was born beautiful, and maintaining this state is not a matter of slavish devotion to the cosmetic counter. It is rather a process of self-acceptance, self-regard, and self-care – the kind of self-care so eloquently detailed in this book.

The fundamentals of looking terrific are, well, fundamental. Start with good health, good grooming, and good humor. Add awareness – and acceptance – of your physical assets and liabilities. Finish with enough knowledge about diet, exercise, hair-care, skin-care, and the like so your physical self can reach its highest potential.

In the K.I.S.S. Guide to Beauty, Stephanie Pederson gives us a head start on all of those fundamentals. You'll find here a wealth of valuable information and useful instruction, clearly presented and with an understanding of the time constraints under which all of us live. The author cuts through the silliness of "the latest beauty secrets" to reveal the practical and the proven: necessary knowledge about our bodies and minds, attitude adjustments so we'll be on the right track from the outset, and tricks of the trade that can help any one of us look splendid.

A true resource, the K.I.S.S. Guide to Beauty is a pleasure to read from start to finish, and refer back to again and again. You'll be invited to return to these pages by the warm writing style, the brilliant illustrations, and information so abundant you can feast on it now and nibble more later. As a welcome change of pace in the world of beauty guides, this one comes from the vantage point of compassion – whether the topic is cruelty-free cosmetics or "the beauty of self-esteem." You will feel better about yourself just by reading the K.I.S.S. Guide to Beauty. And by putting even some of its wisdom into practice, you will find that the person who looks back at you from the mirror is getting more attractive all the time.

VICTORIA MORAN

Introduction

ANYONE CAN BE BEAUTIFUL. *Really. It just takes a little know-how. Fortunately, the K.I.S.S. Guide to Beauty offers this know-how in generous amounts. Designed to show you exactly how to be beautiful, this book challenges the conventional belief that good looks are something you are born with.*

Written from an insider's point of view, this friendly guide helps you look better than you ever thought possible. Just what makes me qualified to write about beauty? Let me say right off that I am not a supermodel, top makeup artist, hairstylist, or personal trainer. What I am is a beauty and health journalist who has spent the last 12 years researching and writing about ways to look and feel your best. Like many of you, I have a husband, family, pets, a nine-to-five job, friends – and a shortage of time to do all the things I'd like to. Also like many of you, I do not have flawless skin, well-behaved hair, perfectly symmetrical features, fat-free thighs, or a makeup artist and hairstylist on call for when I go out, nor do I have thousands – or even hundreds – of dollars to spend on my looks. I am an everyday woman who enjoys her looks, and who wants you to enjoy yours as well.

Just how do I plan on helping you reach your beauty potential? The same way I was helped: by being shown that beauty is about life, fun, energy, pleasure, sensuality, intelligence, and individuality. Being beautiful has more to do with attitude and self-care than the rigid definitions of beauty we find at the movies, on television, and in magazines. When you begin exploring what beauty is, you'll find that it is an intensely personal quality. To some people beauty is voluptuous, while to others it is angular; some people see beauty in freckles, others see it in an olive complexion; beauty can be eyes like pools or a happy squint, a wide mouth or a cherubic pucker. No matter what your features, there are individuals who will find them beautiful, and I want one of those individuals to be you. A happy consequence of this is that when you relax and enjoy your own looks, others will be encouraged to enjoy your looks, too.

To help you play up your gorgeousness, the K.I.S.S. Guide to Beauty *offers practical, how-to advice on every aspect of beauty, starting with the complexion and moving outward. Learn the role that health plays in achieving flawless skin. Discover cutting edge age-reversal treatments. Find out how to care for your hair the right way. Find the secret to discovering a hairstylist you trust. Learn how to use makeup to make your pretty features prettier and to diminish those you are less fond of. Determine whether salon manicures are a worthwhile beauty booster. In addition, should you still decide there is a feature you can't live with, the K.I.S.S. Guide to Beauty discusses cosmetic surgery.*

Models and other "professional beauties" know the enormous role the body plays in total beauty; for any of you who need to be reminded of this, there is a chapter on body care. Lastly, read about wellness techniques that will help you create a beautiful persona – or aura, if you will. Of all your features, this may be the strongest determiner of personal beauty. For those of you who'd like further guidance, you'll find numerous beauty resources, from must-read books to must-visit web sites. It is my hope that by the time you've finished the K.I.S.S. Guide to Beauty, you'll look and feel better than you ever have. Ready to be beautiful? Relax and enjoy the book.

Happy reading!

STEPHANIE PEDERSEN
NEW YORK CITY

What's Inside?

THE INFORMATION in the K.I.S.S Guide to Beauty *is arranged so that you can learn how to take care of your skin, hair, makeup, and nails, and find out about cosmetic surgery and lifestyle issues.*

PART ONE

Part One contains a thought-provoking discussion of beauty, as well as information on the historical and cultural aspects of attractiveness. Because healthy skin is considered essential to good looks, we'll look at how to care for and improve the state of your skin.

PART TWO

In Part Two, I'll tell you all about gorgeous hair – and how to go about looking after and styling your own locks. Everyone's hair has different needs, so we'll look at styles, cuts, and salon services best suited to your individual tresses, tastes, and lifestyle.

PART THREE

Part Three delivers an item-by-item look at the many types of cosmetics available, what makeup works best for whom, and the best places to buy cosmetics, plus advice in applying makeup to enhance your natural gorgeousness.

PART FOUR

In Part Four, I touch on ways to keep nails healthy, offer descriptions of popular nail grooming tools, show you how to perform home manicures and pedicures, and discuss the pros and cons of salon nail services.

PART FIVE

Part Five is where I address all those beauty extras – such as body care, health, cosmetic surgery, emotional state, and mindful living – that can help you feel better about yourself and look even more beautiful.

The Extras

THROUGHOUT THE BOOK, you'll notice a number of boxes and symbols. They emphasize the information provided, giving you an insight into the world of beauty, and helping you become more beautiful than you already are. You'll find:

Very Important Point

Some information you simply must know. If a topic deserves special attention, I'll alert you.

Complete No-No

This warning alerts you to products or practices that can cause you harm, embarrassment, expense, or needless toil.

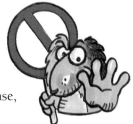

Getting Technical

Beauty can get technical. When it does, I'll let you know so that you can read more carefully.

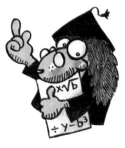

Inside Scoop

Throughout the years I've picked up a plethora of insider beauty tips. I share them with you here.

You'll also find some little boxes that include information I think is important, useful, or just plain fun.

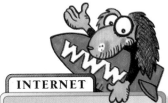

Trivia...

These are entertaining, thought-provoking facts that will give you in-depth knowledge of beauty and beauty culture.

DEFINITION

Here I'll define words and terms for you in easy-to-understand language. You'll also find a glossary at the back of the book with beauty-related lingo.

INTERNET

www.dk.com

The Internet is a fantastic place to research cosmetics, conditions that affect your looks, beauty trends, and beauty lore. I've included some of my favorite web sites.

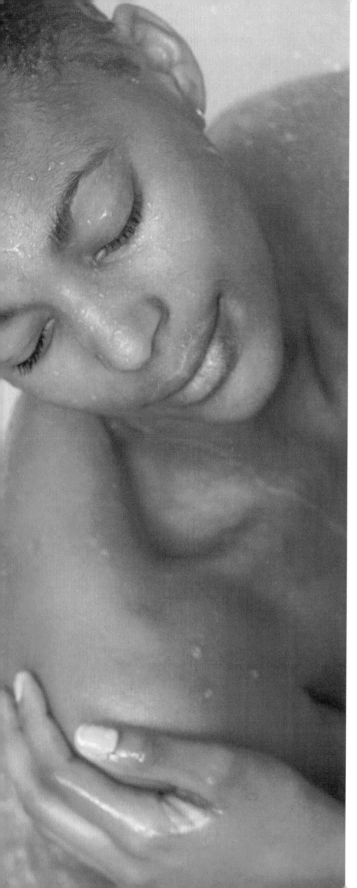

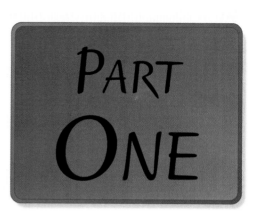

PART ONE

LEARN TO RESPECT AND CARE FOR YOUR SKIN

THE BASICS

Each one of us is beautiful. Some of us already know this. The rest of us, however, are so fixated on what we dislike about ourselves that we're unable to see our *gorgeousness*. This book will help the rest of us recognize and celebrate the *lovely* things about ourselves while simultaneously improving, diminishing, or erasing elements that affect our *self-esteem*.

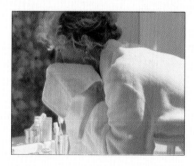

This section places beauty in perspective, with information about its history, the scientific theories surrounding it, and the cultural elements that influence it. As you'll see, there are numerous contrasting opinions about what makes a person attractive. Interestingly, the one component that all eras and cultures agree upon is healthy-looking skin. For that reason, Part 1 also focuses on skin care – the absolute foundation for unselfconscious loveliness.

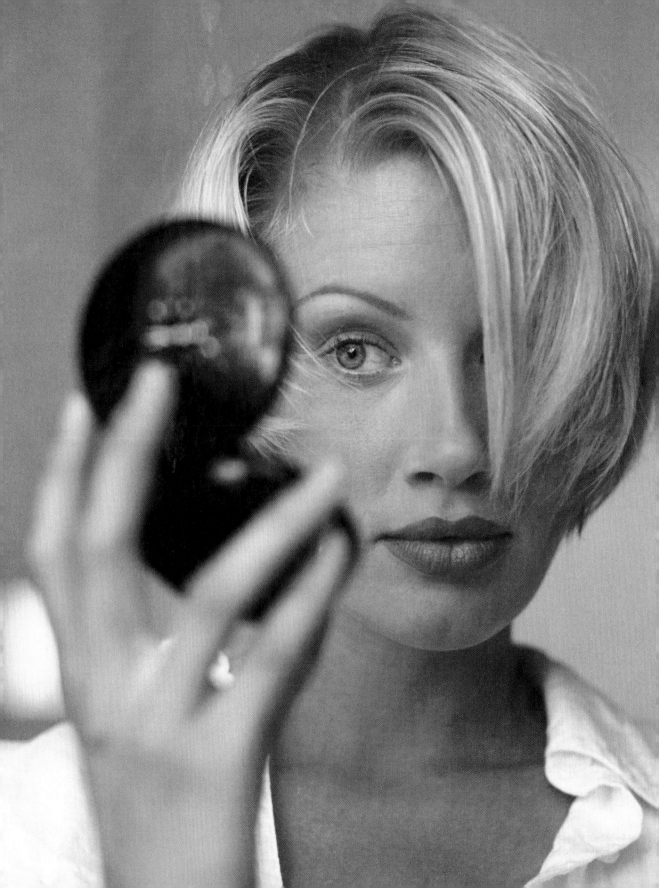

Chapter 1

Real Beauty

IN THE 19TH CENTURY, pale skin was such an important beauty ideal that middle- and upper-class women avoided the sun. This changed during the 1920s; as more people made their livings indoors, suntans became a sign that the wearer could afford leisure time. Similarly, throughout early history, body fat was appealing because it showed that a person was prosperous. Today, when high body-fat levels are more the norm, thinness turn heads. Why? Because slimness indicates that a person has the time and income to spend on gym workouts. What does all this mean? Simply that beauty is not a fixed ideal.

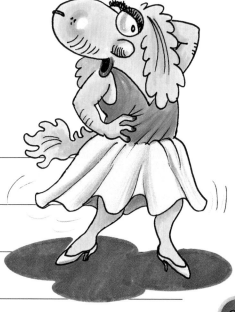

In this chapter...

✔ Beauty: A definition

✔ The importance of beauty

✔ Beauty timeline

✔ The beauty of self-esteem

THE WAY WE LOOK IS VERY IMPORTANT TO US

Beauty: A definition

WHAT IS BEAUTY? Webster's Collegiate Dictionary *says it is "the quality or aggregate of qualities in a person or thing that gives pleasure to the senses or pleasurably exalts the mind or spirit" – a definition that portrays beauty as an incredibly subjective quality. To a certain extent, it is. For instance, to you beauty may be large eyes, an aquiline nose, and a regal bearing, while a friend might see beauty as flawless skin and a bold jaw line. Equally, a co-worker could insist that a smooth forehead, a rosebud mouth, and impeccable taste in pantsuits are the pinnacle of beauty.*

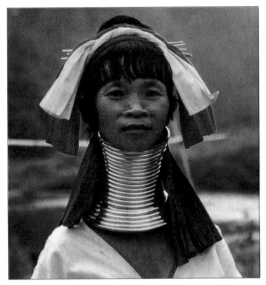

■ **What is considered** *beautiful to one culture can be baffling to another. For the Padaung women of Thailand, long necks are considered an ideal.*

Ask a scientist what beauty is and *symmetry* is the answer you'll probably get. Even though there are many cultural and personal preferences – such as hairless or natural legs; blue or brown eyes; large, pendulous breasts or high, firm breasts – the one trait appreciated in every culture is symmetry. Scientists reason that insects, animals, and humans favor the regular over the irregular. This is because when something – whether it be a flower, a landscape, or a face – has a recognizable pattern, it is easier to spot the out-of-place, the possibly weak, the unhealthy, or the dangerous. Interestingly, research has found that babies, too, prefer looking at both symmetrical patterns and symmetrical faces over asymmetrical ones.

DEFINITION

The word symmetry *originates from the Greek sum* metria *which means "same measure."*

The preferred type of symmetry in humans, animals, and insects is bilateral symmetry, which is of a left-to-right nature rather than up-to-down.

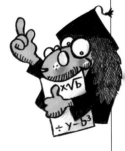

The importance of beauty

WESTERN CULTURE *seems so obsessed with beauty that a pertinent question might not be what it is, but why it is so important to us. Scientists believe that beauty serves a biological purpose: To ensure the continuation of the species by highlighting an individual's "mateability." Deep in our evolutionary past, before the invention of blood tests and medical exams, observation was the only way to determine whether a woman or man would be a capable bearer or guardian of offspring.*

Women with unblemished skin, symmetrical features, lush hair, good posture, and a *waist-to-hip ratio* of between .67–.80 were seen as disease-free, strong, and reproductively capable. Men with above-average height, good posture, and well-developed muscles were seen as powerful, fierce, and able to protect their family.

> **DEFINITION**
>
> *To find your waist-to-hip ratio, stand with your stomach relaxed. Find the narrowest point of your waist and measure. Record the measurement. Next, find the widest part of your hips and buttocks, then measure. Write down this measurement. Divide the waist measurement by the hip measurement. This is your waist-to-hip ratio.*

Early humans cared less about overall female weight than they did about a woman's waist-to-hip ratio, which many medical experts believe is a better visual indicator of health and the capacity for successful child-bearing.

Modern ideals

Today, as Earth becomes more and more overpopulated, continuation of the species is no longer a concern. We have in vitro fertilization, fertility drugs, and other medical ways to boost a woman's fertility, and it is rare that a man must physically protect his family from menacing marauders. So why do we still hold fast to earlier physical ideals? Because that's the way we evolved, say scientists. In other words, old ways die hard.

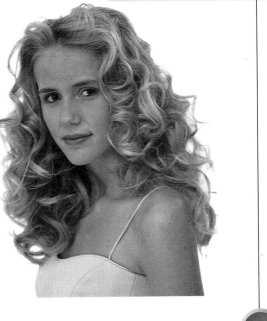

■ **A stereotypical Western** *ideal of beauty includes flawless skin, shiny, healthy hair, big eyes, even features, a full mouth, and a well-proportioned body shape. This ideal has remained true throughout Western history.*

THERE'S SOMETHING ABOUT THAT BABY FACE

In a study of Caucasian and Japanese women, researchers found that attractive female faces had a thinner lower jaw, shorter lower facial height, higher forehead, and relatively larger eyes than women who were considered average-looking or unattractive. These characteristics are what scientists call neotenous: infant-like features that are retained past sexual maturity. Neotenous facial features have been found to elicit protective and nurturing behavior in human care givers.

■ **The characteristics that determine** *female beauty may reflect a general preference for youthful-looking, "baby" faces.*

Beauty timeline

HUMANS HAVE ALWAYS PLAYED WITH their appearance. Throughout history, men and women have drawn attention to certain features, changed the look of some, and played down others for the sake of the current beauty ideal.

Cranial molding was popular among Egyptians in the 14th century BC and Mayans during the 3rd through 1st century BC. Other much-discussed permanent alterations include foot-binding in pre-Communist China, teeth-sculpting in pre-20th-century Bali, the extraction of lower teeth among the early cattle-herding Toposa people in Africa, and the face and body tattoos of Mayans and South Pacific Islanders. Below are some examples of beauty care techniques, trends, and issues found in various cultures throughout history.

1 Mud, ground plants, crushed insects, and animal excrement were used by early humans to safeguard skin from unattractive and unhealthy sunburns, dehydration, and insect bites.

2 In the centuries before Christ, the Egyptians developed elaborate bathing rituals to lighten and soften skin. They used perfumed oils to scent the body and ward

> **DEFINITION**
>
> Cranial molding, *also known as head-binding or cranial disfigurement, was performed by binding a newborn's head between two boards. The pressure permanently changed the shape of the skull, creating a profile in which the nose and front of the face formed a 180° angle.*

off wrinkles; hair extensions for thicker, longer hair; dyes for shinier, more eye-catching locks; and makeup made of kohl and mineral powders to accentuate features and trace blue veins on the skin, in an effort to mimic the translucence of fair skin. Early Greeks, Romans, and Chinese also enjoyed elaborate bathing, practiced skin care, and used skin-whitening makeup.

3 Early Persians, Indians, and Africans favored henna for skin-softening baths, hair dye, nail color, and facial cosmetics.

4 During Europe's Middle Ages, women wore decorative fabric patches shaped as stars, hearts, moons, or crosses on their faces to draw attention to certain features or to hide scars. A patch to the right of the mouth was called a "coquette mark" and indicated that the wearer was a flirt. A mark on the right cheek said a woman was married, while a patch on the left cheek meant that a woman was engaged. A patch at the corner of the eye advertised the wearer's life-loving nature.

5 During the late 18th century, the English parliament passed a law making it illegal for women to wear cosmetics, citing makeup as a form of trickery and witchcraft. It was during this time that British men stopped using cosmetics and cologne.

HENNA

6 In America and Europe, World War I is credited with women's interest in beauty. With men at war, women had the chance to work and play outside the home. Using their newly disposable income, many bought commercially made makeup for the first time. Hollywood screen stars and the creation of five-and-dime stores furthered the mainstream appeal of cosmetics.

7 During the 1920s, tanning became fashionable among the middle and upper classes. Designer Coco Chanel is credited with starting the trend.

8 During the 1990s, an increasing number of female celebrities began sporting the telltale, globe-like appendages known as breast implants. Ordinary American women quickly followed suit: According to the American Society of Plastic and Reconstructive Surgery, 32,607 women underwent breast augmentation in 1992; 39,247 in 1994; 87,704 in 1996; and 132,378 in 1998.

9 By the year 2000, the North American cosmetic and beauty industry totaled more than $20 billion in sales.

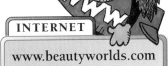

INTERNET

www.beautyworlds.com

At this smart web site, you can investigate such relevant topics as historical beauty icons, beauty in the animal kingdom, scientific studies on beauty, and information about how beauty affects self-esteem.

The beauty of self-esteem

THE FRENCH HAVE A SAYING, *"confortable dans votre peau,"* *which means looking and feeling comfortable in your skin. Science can unveil its latest beauty theory, Hollywood can showcase its dewiest starlets, fashion magazines can parade their stable of underweight models, your mother can criticize your hairstyle, cosmetic companies can display their latest colors specially designed for complexions different to yours, and some random guy on the street may inform you he'd like your breasts better if they were a different size. When it comes down to it, however, you are the only person who can make others see you as beautiful. No, this doesn't require magic, spell-casting, or mind control; it takes self-esteem.*

> ## Trivia...
> In one study, women who had intercourse with highly symmetrical men had orgasms 75 percent of the time, while women who had sex with asymmetrical men experienced orgasm only 30 percent of the time. The results also showed that symmetrical men were more likely to have an orgasm at the same time as their partner!

Humans not only perceive, but are also influenced by, each other's feelings. If people sense your self-hatred, there's a good chance they'll see you the way you subconsciously tell them to see you. In other words, you've got to believe you are attractive before other people will believe it. Throughout history, there have been beauties who could have been deemed too unusual, too plain, too ugly, too something, to be beautiful. Yet these smart ladies have ignored what society says is beautiful. They realize that to stand apart they must celebrate their own unique looks. We react to their self-comfort and are as comfortable with their beauty as they are.

Learning to appreciate yourself

Instead of worrying about what you look like, realize that your looks are only a small portion of what makes you unique. Take your mind off this small component and focus on your other characteristics, such as your spirituality, your generosity, your career, and your relationships with others. Always be aware that your body and face were created first and foremost to be functional.

Next time you compare yourself to a cover model, bring yourself back to reality with this tidbit: the average fashion model in 1968 weighed 8 percent less than the average woman; a model today weighs 23 percent less.

Celebrate your eyes, nose, mouth, and ears by bird-watching, smelling roses, enjoying a terrific meal, going to the symphony. Learning to appreciate your body and face for what they can do – instead of how they look – helps boost your self-esteem. If you are comfortable and relaxed about the way you look, you will have a natural radiance and elegance about you.

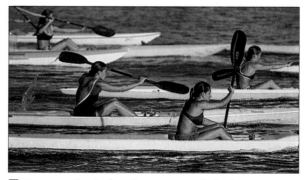

■ **Use your body** *for what it was made for by enjoying sports, exercise, sex, and other physical pursuits.*

Be happy being you

Celebrate the looks you were born with and play to your strong points. This may mean ignoring current fashion and wearing something that makes you feel good, whether that something be purple eye shadow that makes your green eyes shine like jade or an outdated hairstyle that plays up your bold profile.

When you are confronted with a media image of unrealistic beauty, ask yourself what it is about the image that is unnatural. You could write to or phone the television station or magazine responsible and let them know your thoughts. If your self-esteem is low, try reading confidence-boosting books, associating with positive people, or even visiting a therapist for professional help.

Don't dwell on airbrushed images of underweight models. Eleanor Roosevelt knew what she was talking about when she said no one (or no thing) can make us feel inferior without our permission.

A simple summary

✔ Symmetry is the scientific definition of beauty.

✔ Throughout history, humans have altered their appearance in the name of beauty.

✔ Self-esteem is the keystone to looking good.

✔ What is deemed beautiful differs according to era, culture, and even the individual.

29

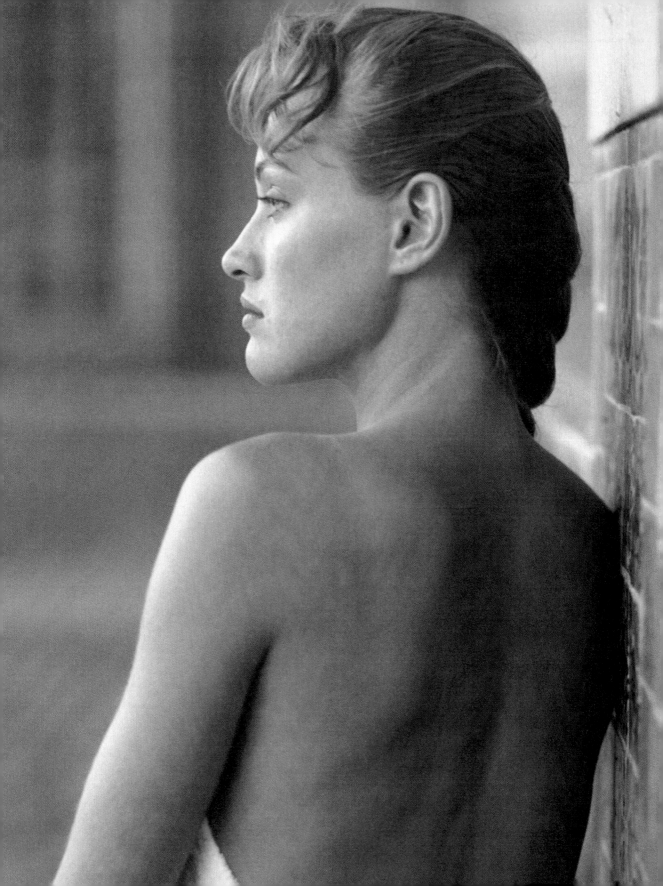

Chapter 2

About Skin

SKIN IS OFTEN THE FIRST THING WE NOTICE about each other. From it we can tell a person's health, age, background, and ethnic makeup. For instance, sallowness suggests anemia; wrinkles generally place the wearer's age at 40-plus; sunspots tell a story of adolescent tanning; and pitted scars suggest past acne. A fair, ruddy complexion may betray Celtic blood, an olive complexion points at Mediterranean ancestry, while a deep coffee says Africa. But how much do you really know about this amazing organ? Keep reading and learn more.

In this chapter...

✓ **What is skin?**

✓ **How skin ages**

✓ **Enemies of good skin**

✓ **Through the years: complexion behavior**

PERFECT, FLAWLESS SKIN IS SOMETHING THAT WE ALL ASPIRE TO HAVE

What is skin?

STRETCHING FROM 16 TO 20 SQUARE FEET *(1.5–1.9 m²) and comprising 15 to 20 percent of a person's body weight, skin is the body's largest organ. This protective covering acts as a barrier against pollution, radiation, the elements, harmful microorganisms, and physical trauma.*

But that's not all it does: Skin locks in the body's moisture, which keeps inner organs and muscles from drying out. To ensure that the body doesn't develop vitamin D-deficiency diseases such as rickets, the skin manufactures vitamin D from sunlight. Skin also helps regulate body temperature by sweating to cool things off and conserving heat when the air grows chilly. And, thanks to its many nerve endings, skin is responsible for our sense of touch, which allows us to sense pain, pressure, temperature, and pleasure.

Skin guards against heat loss in an ingenious way: by constricting its blood vessels. This conserves heat-giving energy, which is needed by the vital inner organs.

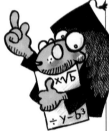

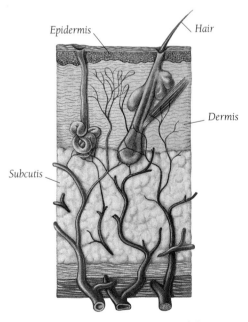

Epidermis — *Hair*

Dermis

Subcutis

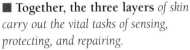

■ **Together, the three layers** *of skin carry out the vital tasks of sensing, protecting, and repairing.*

Taking a closer look at skin

Skin is composed of three layers. The top layer is called the epidermis. It measures less than 1 millimeter in thickness everywhere except on the palms and soles (where it is thicker) and the eyelids and inner elbows (where it is thinner). It is in the epidermis that new skin cells are created and melanin – the pigment that gives your skin its unique color – is produced. The dermis is skin's middle layer. It lies under the epidermis and is where skin's collagen and elastin fibers are located. These fibers give the skin structure. However, they lose their resilience as we age, causing skin to grow slack and creased. Blood vessels, oil or sebum glands, nerve fibers, hair follicles, and muscle cells are also found in the dermis. Skin's bottom layer is the subcutis. It acts as a reservoir for water and fat cells, and serves as a cushion between the upper layers of skin and the body's bones and muscles.

How skin ages

DEEP WRINKLES, LINES, *discolorations, rough texture, dryness, slackness – if you haven't already guessed, I'm describing the changes you may see as your skin ages. Why does skin change at all? As we mature, the cells that make up our bodies replace themselves more slowly. In skin's case, epidermal cells that once took 28 days to replace themselves may now take 30 or 32 days, leaving skin with a dull finish and rough texture. The shape of these cells also changes, which makes them less able to form the flat, unbroken layer necessary to protect against water loss. This leads to the dryness associated with age. Furthermore, the epidermis grows thinner – in some people it may become almost transparent.*

Your skin may appear more wrinkled when it is dehydrated, but you'll be glad to know that dry skin does not lead to permanent wrinkles.

In our older years, sun exposure may manifest itself in surprising ways: as dark tan or brown age spots on the arms, hands, neck, or face. This is because the cells that create melanin do not function efficiently with age. In addition, older skin is more subject to allergic reactions and sensitivities than younger skin because it is less capable of defending itself against irritants, so pink blotches and rashes may also appear.

Aging skin

Changes in skin's dermis contribute to much of the slackness that accompanies our golden years. Collagen and elastin fibers – skin's structural support – degenerate, leaving behind weakened reinforcement for skin's upper layer. This is responsible for loose skin and those deep folds you may notice between your nose and mouth or mouth and chin. Even skin's bottom layer, the subcutis, is at fault; it produces fewer fat cells, and it is fat cells that give younger skin its plumpness. And lastly, there's gravity, which – let's face it – can make a droopy situation even droopier.

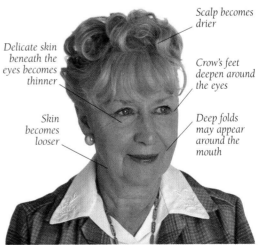

Delicate skin beneath the eyes becomes thinner

Skin becomes looser

Scalp becomes drier

Crow's feet deepen around the eyes

Deep folds may appear around the mouth

■ **During the aging process,** *fine lines, wrinkles, loose skin, and folds become more accentuated and more difficult to disguise.*

Enemies of good skin

PICTURE SOMEONE WHO has a seemingly flawless complexion: their skin boasts a healthy glow, firmness, regular-sized pores, and an absence of splotches or broken veins. If you don't have one of these people in your life, perhaps you've seen one or two on the street, on the subway, or in a grocery store. It seems that, if you want skin like that, you've got to pick your parents.

You've probably heard that the best defense against aging is good genetics. Perhaps this accounts for why stars such as Katharine Hepburn and Paul Newman have enviably slow-aging faces. While there is a great deal to be said about DNA, there is hope for the rest of us who were born to average-complexioned parents. Depending on the dermatologist asked, 75 to 90 percent of our skin's damage is caused by us. More specifically, it is caused by the choices we make every day.

THERE'S NO SUCH THING AS A GOOD TAN

Most people know that sunburns are dangerous and can increase one's future risk of skin cancer. Yet many people believe that tans are okay. Terms like "base tan," "mid-level base," "tanning plateau," and "breakthrough tan" are common among avid tanners. These folks may go to a tanning salon to get a "bit of color" before a tropical vacation, thinking that a man-made "starter tan" will act as a base that will allow them to tan, not burn, once they hit the beach. Well, in case you haven't heard this from your dermatologist, let me be the first to tell you: There is no such thing as a healthy tan. A tan – no matter how light or deep, no matter where it came from – is your skin's response to ultraviolet injury. Any time you tan, you damage your skin and increase your chances of premature aging and skin cancer.

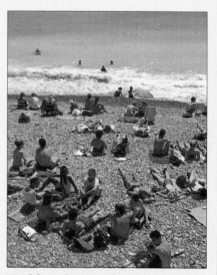

■ **Although it is relaxing** *to sit on a beach soaking up the sun's rays, a suntan can permanently damage your skin.*

Sun damage

According to dermatologists, the sun's ultraviolet rays are accountable for more skin damage than any other factor. These rays come in two main types: UVA and UVB. UVA rays, which can penetrate cloud cover and glass, are often referred to as long-length waves. They are present in the same intensity throughout the day, remain strong even in winter, and are responsible for skin cancer and creating skin changes such as blotchiness and collagen breakdown often associated with aging skin. How do UVA rays do this? By penetrating skin to create *free radicals*. It is these free radicals that wreak havoc on melanin-making cells and degrade the skin's collagen and elastin.

UVB rays are sometimes called short-length waves and are responsible for tanning, burning, and skin cancer. They are at their strongest during late spring, summer, and early fall, at locations near the equator and at higher altitudes. UVB rays are most intense from the hours of 10 a.m. to 3 p.m.

Avoid indoor tanning! Not only is the ultraviolet light used by indoor tanning as dangerous as the sun's version, recent studies suggest that your chances of getting skin cancer are higher if you expose yourself to both sunlamps and the sun than if you expose yourself to the sun only.

The effects of pollution

We know pollution is bad for the lungs, can cause teary eyes, and may contribute to birth defects. But how does pollution affect your complexion? Most dermatologists believe the answer is "adversely." That's because pollution is comprised of chemicals, such as carbon monoxide, oxides of nitrogen, lead, and chlorofluorocarbons, which set off free radicals in the skin. These free radicals lead to collagen and elastin breakdown, which in turn leads to slackness. Especially sensitive faces may find that pollution causes rashes and other allergic reactions, while oily skin may suffer from blocked pores and increased greasiness in a polluted environment.

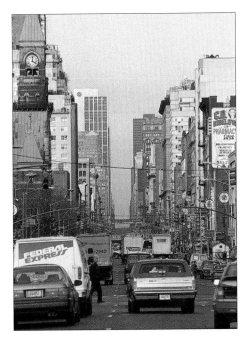

■ **In a busy city,** *pollution and grime collect on your skin, clogging pores and sometimes causing allergies.*

Recognizing a smoker's face

We are all familiar with what some doctors call "smoker's face": fine lines around the mouth from puckering lips; lines near the eyes from squinting through smoke; a gray-tinged complexion caused by nicotine-slowed blood circulation; thin skin, slackness, and dryness. But did you know that smokers also have higher rates of skin cancers and slower wound-healing rates than non-smokers, and are less able to utilize skin-friendly, antioxidant vitamins such as vitamin C? Moreover, cigarette smoke contains high concentrations of nitrogen dioxide ozone, a compound that damages the DNA your skin cells need to efficiently create new cells.

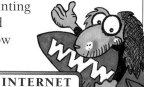

INTERNET

www.skinpatient.com

This site focuses on skin – as well as nail and hair – conditions. It features an on-line patient support group, and information on a wide range of cosmetics and their ingredients.

With so much going on in one face, a smoker can appear up to 20 years older than her nonsmoking counterparts. For instance, it is common for smokers in their 40s to resemble nonsmokers in their 60s. It's no wonder that, after sun exposure, dermatologists list smoking as one of the biggest causes of skin damage.

Several studies have shown that smokers' skin is an average of 40 percent thinner than nonsmokers' skin. Researchers say that this is due to restricted blood supply and the deterioration of collagen and elastin in the skin – both caused by cigarette smoke.

Heavy drinking

If you're at all health conscious, you know you should go easy on the alcohol – a few two-drink nights each week is plenty. That's because long-term alcohol abuse has been associated with liver disease and breast cancer. Yet the effects of a single night's binge can appear on your skin as early as the morning after, in the form of dehydration, or water retention under the eyes.

In addition, heavy drinking saps B vitamins from the body – especially folic acid and thiamine. Skin needs these B vitamins to

■ **If you want to enjoy** *healthy-looking skin, moderate your alcohol intake. If you have a glass of wine, make sure you drink plenty of water too.*

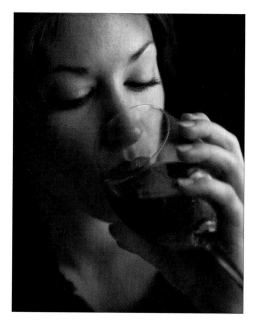

maintain health, so a deficiency can cause a pale, sallow complexion, dryness, slackness, and unexplained breakouts. Because alcohol dilates the blood vessels nearest your skin, heavy drinking can stress and weaken small blood vessels to the point that some may break, causing visible and unsightly broken veins on your face.

Lastly, a few too many drinks can cause neglect. After all, who feels like taking off makeup, washing the face, and putting on skin-care products when the room is spinning?

Stress

You've had a bad week – or maybe a bad month. You've been working overtime, your child is going through a difficult phase, your boyfriend's eyes have started wandering, your boss seems to hate you, and you have insomnia. In other words, nothing in your life is going smoothly and you are feeling more stressed than ever. Chances are a few obvious pimples have sprung up since your life got so hectic. How do I know that? What do you think my face does when I'm feeling frazzled?

BEAUTY SLEEP

Skin makes new cells twice as fast during sleep-time as during waking hours. Furthermore, several studies have found that sleep-deprived humans have lower levels of a growth hormone the skin needs to repair environmental damage and produce new skin cells. When cell replacement falls behind, wrinkles and slackness result. While individual sleep requirements vary, between 7 and 9 hours is average. As you get your beauty rest, avoid creating "bed wrinkles" by sleeping on your back; lying on your side or stomach means squashing your face into a pillow and then waking up with crazy crease marks. When we're young, these folds smooth out almost instantly. But as we age our collagen and elastin grow less resilient, meaning those creases can stay for hours – or even permanently.

■ **Plenty of nourishing sleep** *is one of the secrets of a good complexion and a healthy body. Try to maintain regular sleep patterns.*

The reason for a spotty complexion is simple: When the body is under stress, it releases adrenal hormones, which are known generally as "stress hormones." These hormones generate a number of changes in skin, including breakouts, oily patches, dry patches, sallowness, dark circles under the eyes, and rashes. Obviously, you can't avoid all forms of stress, but you can learn how to deal with them. Deep breathing, visualization, a professional or at-home massage, or even a spa-night at home can help relieve some of the tension. We'll talk more about these last two in Chapter 19.

Exercise boosts circulation, which in turn delivers oxygen-rich blood to the skin's surface. The short-term result is a beautiful glow. According to some skin-care experts, the long-term benefit of exercise is improved skin elasticity and more efficient new cell growth.

Rough treatment

As resilient as skin is, it also has a delicate side. Aggressive handling can make skin appear worn, abused, and just plain old. What qualifies as rough treatment? Picking pimples, which can cause scars; using overly hot water, which can break small capillaries and make skin dry; tugging at skin, which can break down collagen and elastin fibers and lead to slackness; and using harsh skin-care products, which can cause sensitivities and redness.

Skin and your diet

Severe diets that skimp on calories and on one or more nutrients are detrimental to your skin, and so are eating habits that include plenty of complexion-spoiling fast food. Here's a rundown of common nutrient deficiencies and how they affect your complexion:

- A lack of protein can lead to a dull, dry complexion and poor wound-healing.
- A shortage of iron can result in a pale complexion.
- A lack of vitamin A can produce dry skin or unexplained breakouts.
- A deficiency in vitamin B Complex can result in cracks at the corners of the mouth, unexplained breakouts, impaired wound-healing, and pallor.
- A lack of vitamin C can cause poor wound-healing, dullness, and easy bruising.
- A shortage of vitamin E can lead to poor wound-healing and dry skin.
- A lack of vitamin K can result in weak, broken, or distended facial capillaries.

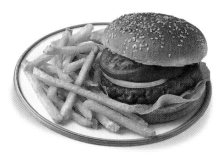

■ **By avoiding junk food** *and sticking to a diet containing all the necessary nutrients, you'll notice the difference in your complexion.*

Through the years: complexion behavior

I PROBABLY DON'T HAVE TO tell you that *skin changes as we age. After all, we look at people every day – we know that a teen's complexion is different from a 25-year-old's, which is different still from a 35-year-old's and so on. Although everyone's skin changes differently according to genetics, exposure to harmful substances such as ultraviolet light, lifestyle choices, and just plain luck, we can usually accurately guess a person's age within a decade simply by noting some of the signs talked about here.*

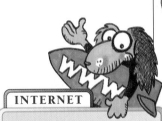

INTERNET

www.aad.org
www.dermatology.ca

At the web sites of the American Academy of Dermatology and the Canadian Dermatology Association, you can find out more about skin problems.

DEFINITION

Sebum is dermatologist-speak for oil, which is created in the skin and secreted through the pores. Its purpose? To keep skin moist and supple.

Your teens

Some teens are lucky: Their skin stays smooth, blemish-free, small-pored, and without a slick of oil anywhere. I have yet to meet one of these fortunate creatures, yet I am told by dermatologists that they do exist. For most people, however, the teen years are about breakouts. Blame it on puberty, which causes the body's sex hormones to go wild, creating body hair, deeper voices, breasts, larger hips, ovulation, and other signs of maturity. Of course, some of these mature things happen to boys, some to girls. At the same time, sex hormones also cause skin to pump out more *sebum*. Produced by the sebaceous glands surrounding the hair follicles, the sebum travels to the skin's surface via the pores. This sebum, combined with the dead skin cells that the epidermis is constantly shedding, clogs pores, creating blackheads, whiteheads, and pimples.

■ **During the teenage years,** *the body goes through many confusing changes and teenagers can become very self-conscious about their looks and their complexions.*

SKIN DURING PREGNANCY

Pregnancy not only affects a woman's figure, it can also affect her skin. Whether you're pregnant or just thinking about it, here's what your skin can expect:

 1 During the first trimester, you may get "the glow" associated with early pregnancy. This radiance comes from newly created blood vessels just under the skin that carry an abundant supply of rosy-making oxygen to the skin.

2 Sensitivities manifesting themselves as rashes or dry patches on your skin may develop. Just as you may become nauseated by certain foods or odors, your skin may develop sensitivities to any or all of the ingredients in your normal skin-care products.

3 Acne commonly occurs any time there is hormonal upheaval – puberty, menstruation, and yes, pregnancy. Ask your dermatologist and pregnancy-care provider about treating acne; many commonly prescribed antibiotics, such as tetracycline and *Accutane®*, cause birth defects. Trentoinin may also be linked to birth defects, making it smart to skip products containing this vitamin A derivative. Formulas with salicylic acid, a skin-care ingredient related to aspirin, is another no-no. However, some doctors say the topical antibiotic erythromycin is safe, as are alpha hydroxy acids.

4 Melasma – the "mask of pregnancy" – commonly occurs during the second trimester. Caused by hormone activity, the condition consists of brown patches on the forehead, cheeks, or above the lip. The hormonal changes of pregnancy make your skin more likely to develop dark pigment when exposed to sunlight. The common dermatologic prescription is sun-avoidance and use of hydroquinone bleaching creams once the baby is born and breast-feeding has stopped.

5 Broken blood vessels are common during pregnancy; they are caused by an increase in the body's blood volume, which puts pressure on small facial capillaries. Some of these veins will disappear after pregnancy. Others can be treated by a laser-wielding dermatologist.

■ **During pregnancy,** *gentle exercise keeps you healthy and promotes skin-nourishing circulation.*

Your 20s

The 20s are a transitional period for skin. Some people continue suffering the breakouts that marked their teen years. Other people's skin becomes normal, for the most part: not too oily, not too dry, with only an occasional breakout. You may find you need a light eye cream or even an occasional moisturizer, but your skin is still taut and dewy-fresh. For those prone to them, new moles may begin appearing.

The most surprising changes that may occur during this time are signs of childhood and teen tanning, such as freckles, maybe a few small broken capillaries, fine lines around the eyes and even faint discolored patches. Those of you who avoided the sun – lucky you – will probably see none of these signs.

Your 30s

The 30s are a funny time for skin. The complexion still looks firm and youthful, but as you move further into this decade, you'll notice "things" which seem to show up out of nowhere. I'm referring to fine lines around the eyes, maybe a furrow between the brows, the beginning of lines between the nose and mouth, or a subtle looseness under the jaw. More evidence of past sun damage may appear – such as freckles and tan patches – even though you've worn sunscreen religiously and kept out of the sun since your 20s.

You may have some oversized pores left over from your teen years or 20s, but you will notice that your skin doesn't produce the same volume of oil it once did. In fact, your complexion may range from slightly to very dry.

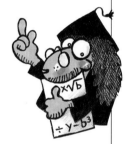

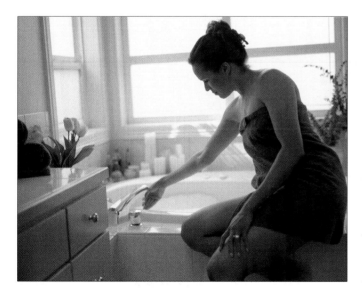

■ **In your 30s,** *sensitivities you never knew you had may manifest themselves as small rashes when you try a new skin-care product, and your skin, now drier, may need more moisturizing after a soak in the tub.*

Your 40s

If you've taken good care of yourself and your skin (or if you come from youthful genetic stock), now's the time your conscientiousness (or luck) will show. Your contemporaries may have the beginnings of under-eye bags, deep folds between the nose and mouth, looseness in the cheeks and jaw, slackness at the upper eyelids, furrows between the brows, not to mention possible mottled patches from past sun damage. You, however, may have only a few of these things, and none as severe as your friends.

Your 50s and 60s

As you move into your 50s, the skin glitches that appeared during your 40s grow more exaggerated. Your skin is thinner and less pliable than it once was. This makes it easier for deep folds to settle into those mobile areas of your face, such as the corners of your mouth, between the nose and mouth, and between the brows.

If you quickly pinch and release skin on your cheek or under your eye, it takes a while for the skin to return to its original position. Also normal for these two decades: discolored patches and an unevenly colored, mottled skin.

■ **If you have spent** *a lifetime resting a cheek on a hand, pulling at skin as you apply makeup, rubbing your forehead, or engaging in some other habit or mannerism, the results will appear as creases and webs of fine wrinkles when you reach your 50s and 60s.*

MENOPAUSAL SKIN

The hormone estrogen stimulates the production of collagen, a material that provides structural support for the skin. During menopause, decreasing estrogen levels cause a breakdown of this collagen, resulting in slackness and wrinkles. Skin also becomes more fragile and the top layers (epidermis and dermis) separate more easily. This results in slow-healing cuts or bruises from what seems like relatively minor rough handling. For this reason, it is important to treat your complexion with a gentle touch. Apply skin-care products and makeup by patting them gently into the skin; do not pull, rub, or stretch the skin! Furthermore, keep skin moist and pliable with morning and night applications of your favorite moisturizer.

No matter how you're aging, expect an increase in that soft, fine facial hair most older ladies have.

Your 70s and beyond

In your 70s, all the folds, slackness, wrinkles, thinness, and discoloration you noticed in your 50s and 60s grow more exaggerated. Though gravity has been in effect throughout your lifetime, you'll notice its consequences most strongly in your 70s. As a result, your facial and neck skin will have a looseness about them. Your skin will be dry and have a rough texture. Sensitivities are common during this time, and you may find products you used only a decade earlier may now cause a rash or itchiness.

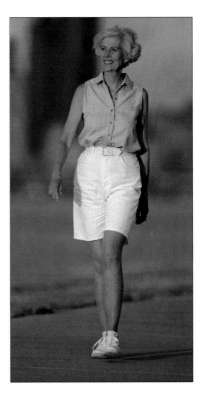

■ **If you have been** *careful throughout your life about sun exposure and skin care, it'll come as no surprise if people mistake you for a 60-year-old when you are well into your 70s.*

A simple summary

✓ Skin is the largest organ in the human body.

✓ Skin acts as a barrier, protecting our muscles and inner organs from dehydration, harmful microorganisms, the elements, and physical trauma.

✓ Skin has three layers: the epidermis, dermis, and subcutis, each with important functions.

✓ The sun is skin's number one enemy. Smoking comes second.

✓ Adequate sleep is the key to helping skin renew itself and for maintaining a good complexion.

✓ What you put – and don't put – in your body affects your skin.

✓ Each decade has its own complexion quirks.

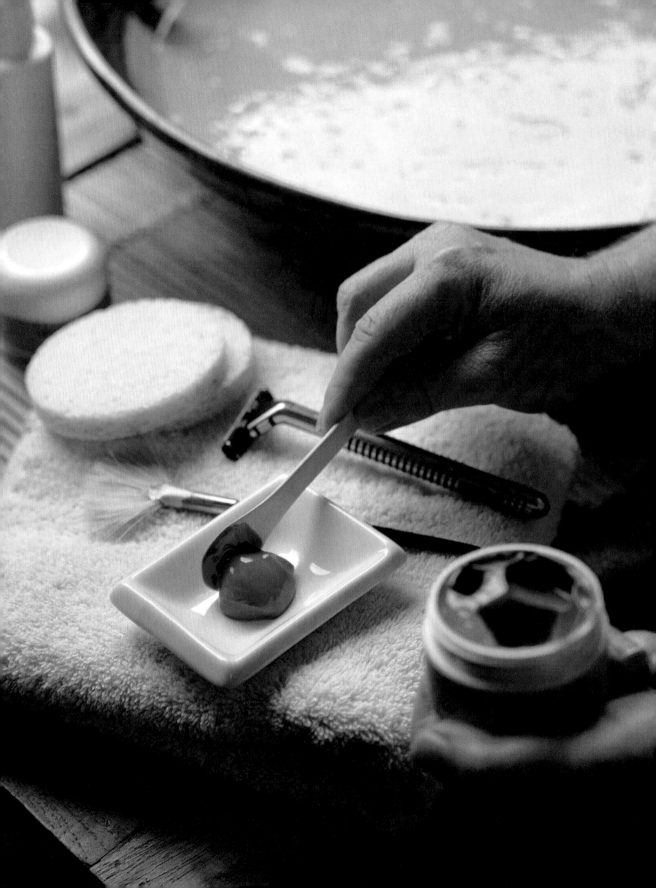

Chapter 3

Complexion Care

SMOOTH, PORELESS, AND FREE FROM SLACKNESS and deep lines, a flawless complexion has long been considered a mark of youth and beauty. But for some of us, achieving perfect skin seems impossible. Fortunately, good skin is do-able. It simply takes work. With a bit of knowledge, your skin will look better – and be healthier – than you ever thought possible.

In this chapter...

✓ What is my skin type?

✓ Cleansing your skin

✓ Moisturizers

✓ Zit zappers

✓ Exfoliation and masks

✓ Intensive facial treatments

✓ Sunscreens for the face

YOUR BEAUTY-CARE ROUTINE MAY INCLUDE EVERYTHING FROM MOISTURIZING TO MUD MASKS

What is my skin type?

THE TERM "SKIN TYPE" REFERS to two things: *how much sebum your skin produces, and where this sebum is most heavily produced. To find out your skin's type, you can do the tissue test: Simply wash your face with a gentle cleanser, wait 15 to 30 minutes, and then hold a facial tissue against your face for 5 seconds.*

Different skin types

If you have oily skin, you're probably aware of it already, but if you need confirmation, do the tissue test. Oily skin will cause obvious oil stains on most of the tissue. This type of skin is the result of too much sebum being produced. The constant flow of sebum stretches pores, so the skin may also have large pores. The complexion often looks shiny, and because excess sebum can mix with makeup and dirt to clog pores, oily skin is vulnerable to breakouts.

Normal skin is the ideal. It produces enough sebum to keep skin supple, but not so much that skin looks slick. If you have normal skin, the tissue test may produce light oil stains, but nothing more.

As we get older, our skin naturally produces less sebum, which is why more mature skin is so often dry. Yet young skin can also be dry if it doesn't produce enough oil to keep the epidermis moist. Depending on how dry the skin is, it may have a rough texture or be prone to flaking. And because not a lot of sebum travels through pores, the pores will probably be small. If you have dry skin, the tissue test will show no oily stains.

Combination skin

Quite a few of us have large pores and lots of oil around the nose, chin, and perhaps forehead. But we also have normal or dry skin under the eyes and on the cheeks. This is known as combination skin. If you have it, the tissue test will show oil stains in your oily areas, but will remain dry elsewhere. To treat combination skin, address the two zones separately, giving the oily bits the sebum-absorbing care they need, and moisturizing the dry or normal bits.

> ### Trivia...
> *While sensitive skin isn't considered a skin type, it is true that some skin – regardless of whether it is oily, normal, or dry – reacts to more factors than others. To ensure your skin remains reaction-free, you might want to avoid beauty products that contain these common irritants: preservatives, fragrance, dyes, oxybenzone, PABA, vitamin E, lanolin, and alpha hydroxy acids.*

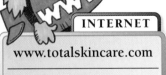

INTERNET

www.totalskincare.com

This comprehensive e-commerce site features an alphabetical listing of skin-care concerns, ingredients, treatments, and products.

Cleansing your skin

NO MATTER *what your skin type, excess sebum, grime, makeup, sunscreen, and other impurities can become imbedded in skin, clogging your pores and dulling your complexion. For this reason, it's important to wash your face at least twice a day.*

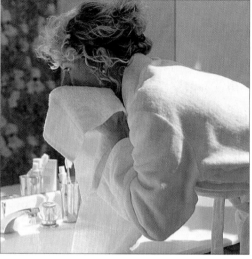

Look for a cleanser that suits your skin type. Check a product's label for descriptive terms: Words such as "strong" and "potent" indicate a high-powered formula good for oilier skins, while words such as "gentle" and "mild" hint at products suitable for drier complexions.

■ **Get into a daily routine** *of washing your face at night to cleanse your skin of the impurities that have built up during the day.*

Looking at soaps

Many skin-care experts claim you must never use soap on your face, while many dermatologists routinely tell their patients that soap is fine. I'm caught in the middle here. I personally think soap is a great, inexpensive option for blemished or oily skin, and I know more than one dermatologist who has prescribed antibacterial soap such as Dial® to their acne-ravaged patients. However, soap is drying; if you have a normal or a dry complexion you're better off with something else.

Complexion bars look like soap, but they are actually mild cleansers in bar form. Look for individual formulas targeting oily, normal, or dry complexions.

Liquid and cream cleansers

Liquid cleansers – sometimes called cleansing milks, cleansing lotions, or cleansing gels – have the consistency of thin to moderately thick body lotion. To use, spread a quarter-sized amount over dry or damp skin, then wipe off with a damp washcloth or rinse off with lukewarm water.

Depending on your age, you probably remember seeing your mother or grandmother use cold cream. This thick, luxurious cream is rubbed into the skin, where it melts makeup, excess sebum, and dirt. It is then wiped off with dry tissues or a slightly damp washcloth. Because of its heavy, oily nature, cold cream is always best-suited to dry skin.

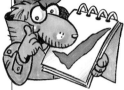

Sebum production speeds up in the summer, which contributes to grimy "summer skin." You may want to sneak in an extra daily cleansing during warm weather.

Makeup remover

This creamy product is designed to break down makeup for easy removal. It is not a substitute for a regular facial cleanser, which is specially formulated to sweep away excess sebum and impurities from the skin.

Not everyone needs makeup remover, nor does everyone need it all the time. Personally, the only time I use it is when I want to remove a thick layer of makeup.

Eye makeup remover is a special type of makeup remover made to melt budge-proof eye cosmetics such as waterproof mascara and false eyelash glue.

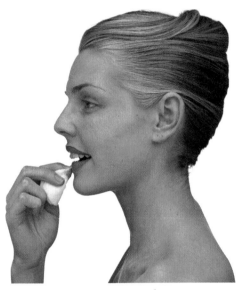

■ **You may want to use** *makeup remover to wipe off long-wearing lipstick or stubborn mascaras and eyeliners.*

Cleansing foams, wipes, and mitts

Cleansing foams are one of the newest types of cleansers. A liquid cleanser is taken up through a special pump, which converts the cleanser to foam. Generally, one "pouf" is more than enough to cleanse your face.

Cleansing wipes in zit-zapping formulas have long been popular with teenagers. It hasn't been until recently, however, that skin-care companies have created cleansing pads for normal and dry skins – something I am particularly grateful for. Not only are these pads great for gym and travel bags, they're a godsend for those of us who would rather crawl under the covers with makeup on than stand half-asleep at a bathroom sink slapping on and rinsing off cleanser.

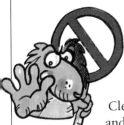

Don't spend money on expensive cleansers, because a cleanser is going to be on your skin for only a few seconds before being rinsed away. Save your beauty bucks for moisturizers, sunscreens, intensive treatments, and other products that will sit on your skin a while.

Cleansing mitts are an oddity. You simply don a mitt, moisten it with water, and rub it over your face. Yes, I was skeptical too, but I tried it and it pulled off all my makeup. The mitt's cleaning ability comes from a special weave of fibers.

When to use toner

There are people who claim toning is a vital part of good skin care, but the only time I use a toner is to degrease my skin on a grimy Manhattan summer afternoon.

TONING THE HOMEMADE WAY

Here are two recipes you could try making yourself:

Chamomile toner

This is a gentle toner for dry, normal, or sensitive skin. Use after cleansing, or whenever you need to freshen your skin.

- ½ cup of distilled witch hazel
- 1 cup strongly prepared chamomile tea

Combine the two ingredients in a glass jar or plastic container and store in the refrigerator for up to 2 days.

WITCH HAZEL

Sage-vodka astringent

This sage-vodka astringent is for oily or acne-prone skin. Use after cleansing, or when you need to freshen your skin.

- ⅓ cup dried sage leaves
- 1 cup water
- ½ cup unflavored vodka

SAGE LEAVES

In a small pot, mix the water and dried sage leaves. Bring the mixture to a rolling boil and boil for 5 minutes. Allow it to cool. Strain out the sage leaves and combine the liquid and the vodka in a glass jar or plastic container.

I may also use a toner if I need help in removing the oily residue left by a particularly heavy cleanser. That said, toners are purported to remove traces of cleanser and prepare the skin for moisturizer – not bad concepts at all.

Toners and astringents

Some of you may be confused about the difference between a toner and an astringent. So here it is. The word toner is used in two ways: as a general term for the product you use between cleansing and moisturizing, and as a particular kind of toner formulated without alcohol and used by those with normal to dry skin. Astringent is a word that means to draw out. It also refers to a type of toner – usually formulated with alcohol or some equally drying substance – used on oily complexions to draw out and remove excess sebum.

Moisturizers

MOISTURIZERS DO TWO THINGS: trap moisture below your skin's outer layer and soften skin's outer layer. This moisture and added softness makes dry – or just dehydrated – skin temporarily feel better, look better, and behave better. Like other skin-care products, however, there is no such thing as a one-formula-fits-all moisturizer. Here, we offer you a moisturizing primer.

Trivia...
If you read beauty magazines, you're sure to come across the word "crepey." This commonly used term refers to under-eye or other skin that has the texture of crumpled crepe.

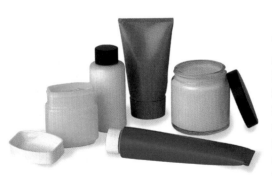

■ **Take the time to choose** *the moisturizer that is right for your skin type. There is an enormous array of products to suit your unique needs.*

Facial moisturizers

There is a dizzying array of facial moisturizers out there: gels, serums, lotions, creams, and balms. Some come in tubes, others in pump bottles, jars, or tubs. There are lightweight formulas for skin that doesn't need a lot of hydration and heavy-duty formulas for severely dehydrated skins. And there are moisturizers at all points between, some even with treatment ingredients designed to temporarily repair damaged skin. For the consumer, the choice can be confusing.

Unlike cleanser, which doesn't spend a lot of time on skin, moisturizer remains on skin all day. For that reason, it's important to research and experiment until you find one your skin responds well to. Keep in mind, however, that not everyone needs moisturizer. (I realize this is not what the lady at the cosmetics counter told you.) Oily and even some normal complexions have enough sebum – the body's own natural moisturizer – to trap moisture and soften skin; for these skins, adding something from a jar is overkill.

If you live in a humid area and have a dry or normal complexion, your skin may turn slick and greasy in the summer. If this sounds familiar, try going without moisturizer during the hotter months of summer.

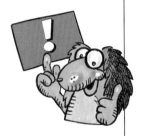

Eye creams

Eye creams are typically lighter in texture than most facial moisturizers and are formulated not to harm the eye's delicate tissues. I was a loyal eye-cream user during my young adult years, when my face was too oily for a moisturizer yet I needed something to address the slight dryness under my eyes. I am no longer an eye-cream user. The moisturizer I use on my face is the same one that gets patted under my eyes.

I realize that not everyone agrees with this. Many cosmetic-company salespeople and aestheticians – including my own facialist – strongly believe in using a separate cream for the eye area. Yet I know just as many dermatologists – including my own doctor – who think it's fine to use one moisturizer on all parts of your face. As long as, may I add, that moisturizer doesn't contain treatment ingredients that can irritate the delicate skin around the eye.

Throat creams

Throat creams are a bit like eye creams – some people find them helpful, but they're not necessary. Because the neck has fewer oil glands than the face, it is frequently drier. To help combat this drier texture, throat creams are often heavier than facial creams. Many also contain ingredients to temporarily firm skin, creating a tighter, younger look. If you consider your neck a problem area, go ahead and try a throat cream. However, if your medicine cabinet is already packed with skin-care products you don't use, a throat cream might become one more product to gather dust.

■ **When you apply a moisturizer** *to your neck, massage it into skin with an upward motion. Some experts claim this boosts circulation and promotes tautness.*

Zit zappers

IF YOU'RE LIKE ME, *the very sight of a new blemish has you searching for your cover-up. A better approach, however, is to make sure zits never show up – or at least, never grow very big – in the first place. Whether pimples are a daily battle for you, or a once-in-a-while occurrence, over-the-counter help is available.*

Easy spot treatments

Do not pick at your zits – you can cause nasty scars! If you positively cannot leave a blackhead or whitehead alone, try placing a clean forefinger on each side of the clogged pore and spread the skin taut. Often, you'll find the stuff in the pore pops out on its own.

For mild to moderate acne and occasional blemishes, over-the-counter products are effective. Benzoyl peroxide is the best spot-stopper around. It unblocks pores, dries up excess sebum, exfoliates the area, and kills the bacteria that cause pimples. Sulfur has long been used in zit medications – either alone, or with benzoyl peroxide – to dry excess sebum, lightly exfoliate the area, and kill bacteria before it can cause a pimple.

A dermatologist may prescribe a topical antibiotic, Retin-A, or azelaic acid, which is a grain-derivative that unblocks pores, exfoliates, and kills bacteria.

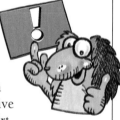

Salicylic acid (also known as beta hydroxy acid) is a popular ingredient in zit creams and is found in some cleansers, astringents, and masks. A relative of aspirin, it works by penetrating pores to loosen impacted sebum and dirt, which cause blackheads and can lead to whiteheads and cystic pimples.

RECIPES FOR HOME BLEMISH TREATMENTS

- Mix ½ teaspoon of yeast with a few drops of warm water to make a paste. Smooth over the pimple and rinse off after 20 to 60 minutes. Use once a day.
- Mix ½ teaspoon of baking soda with a few drops of warm water to form a paste. Smooth over the pimple and rinse off after 20 to 60 minutes. Use once a day.
- A drop of tea-tree oil can be dabbed on pimples up to twice a day. Test a tiny patch on your forearm 48 hours before using it to ensure it does not irritate your skin.

Exfoliation and masks

A QUICK AND EASY WAY *to keep skin healthy and improve its appearance is through* exfoliation. *The premise behind exfoliation is this: The dead skin cells and dirt that sit on your skin's surface make the complexion look dull and clog pores. Remove these and you reveal your skin's brighter, clearer, and fresher finish.*

DEFINITION

To exfoliate *means to remove the surface – in this case, the skin's surface layer where dead skin cells and dirt reside.*

Washcloths, facial brushes, and loofahs

If you use a washcloth, you've probably been exfoliating your skin for years without knowing it. The cloth's rough surface buffs away debris, yet is gentle enough for most people to use daily. Complexion brushes and loofahs are also exfoliators. However, because their surfaces can scratch, brushes and loofahs shouldn't be used more than two or three times a week. If your skin is easily irritated, avoid them completely.

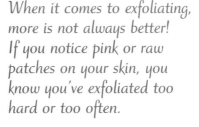

When it comes to exfoliating, more is not always better! If you notice pink or raw patches on your skin, you know you've exfoliated too hard or too often.

Mechanical exfoliants

Mechanical exfoliants are exfoliators that are driven by you, such as apricot-kernel scrubs, buffing beads, and pumice-based cleansers. These scrape away dead skin cells to make skin look fresher and encourage clear pores. Use one to three times a week; if your skin is particularly sensitive or you are using skin-thinning medication, limit use to once weekly. An easy way to convert your favorite cleanser to a mechanical exfoliant is to mix a half-tablespoon with a tablespoon of coarse-grind cornmeal, coarse sea salt, or coarsely ground almonds. After scrubbing, rinse well with lukewarm water.

■ **Use a loofah** *to exfoliate your skin when you are having a shower, and enjoy fresh, revitalized, healthy-looking skin.*

Chemical exfoliants

Chemical exfoliants take no physical work on your part – no rubbing, and no rinsing. These are chemical ingredients – such as enzymes or alpha hydroxy acids – that are added to moisturizers and treatment creams. They loosen and slough off dead skin cells, debris, and excess sebum.

Unlike manual exfoliators, chemical exfoliators are not instant brighteners; their effects are subtle and continual.

One of nature's most effective chemical exfoliants is papaya, which contains a strong enzyme called papain that dissolves excess sebum as well as dead skin cells. To try, smooth mashed papaya onto your face and leave it on for up to 5 minutes. You can remove it with a damp washcloth and a few splashes of water.

Using masks

Facial masks have a reputation as a luxury item, hence their fancy alternate spelling: "masque." Sure, masks are pampering, but they are much more than that: They are a way to infuse skin with beneficial ingredients and a quick, effective (albeit temporary) means of addressing skin issues such as flakiness, slackness, or excess oil. If you've never tried one, treat yourself.

Clay and mud masks

Anthropologists claim that clay and mud masks have been used since before the time of written language. With their superior oil-sopping, pore-clearing, and skin-tightening abilities, these masks continue to be popular among those with oily and normal skins.

Clay and mud masks can generally be used once or twice a week. They are applied to clean skin and allowed to harden for 15 to 40 minutes, before they are rubbed off with a wet cloth and the face splashed until remnants are removed. While many of these masks contain only a special type of purified mud or clay, many also contain added extras such as sulfur, alpha hydroxy acids, herbs, or botanical extracts.

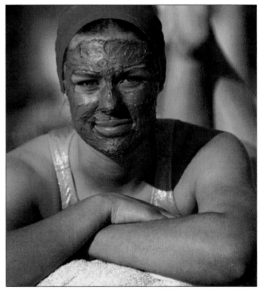

■ **While waiting for a clay or mud** *mask to harden, use the time to relax or pamper yourself, instead of treating it as a chore.*

54

Peel-off masks

Peel-off masks emerge from the bottle as a gel. To use, spread a moderate amount of the cool-feeling mask evenly over your face. Do not miss any spots! When the mask has dried, start at the forehead and peel it off; dead skin cells, pore-clogging gunk, and other debris are removed with the mask. Peel-off masks can be used by people with oily, normal, and dry skins, depending on the mask's individual ingredient list; its bottle should mention what types of skin the product works best for. These masks can severely irritate sensitive or thin skin, and skin being treated with alpha hydroxy acids or trentinoin products.

MAKE-AT-HOME MASKS

Here are some face masks you can try making at home:

Oatmeal mask

This purifying oatmeal mask is for normal to oily skin.

- ½ cup water
- 1 teaspoon dried rosemary or sage
- 1 ½ tablespoons oatmeal
- 10 raw almonds

OATMEAL

In a small pot, mix water and dried rosemary or sage leaves. Bring the mixture to a rolling boil and then boil for 5 minutes. Allow the mixture to cool to lukewarm. In the meantime, add the oatmeal and almonds to the bowl of a food processor or blender, and grind until they are a fine powder. Add enough of the herb liquid to create a thick paste. Gently spread the paste onto clean skin, avoiding eyes and mouth, and allow the mask to dry completely. Leave on for 15 to 30 minutes and then remove with a damp washcloth and warm water.

Avocado mask

This hydrating mask is ideal for normal or dry skin.

- ½ avocado, mashed
- 2 tablespoons plain yogurt

In a bowl, combine avocado pulp with plain yogurt. Apply it generously to your clean face and neck and leave it on for 20 to 30 minutes. Wipe the mask off with dry tissues – no rinsing is necessary.

AVOCADO

Epidermal treatment masks

For a strong dose of therapeutic ingredients, your best bet is an epidermal treatment mask. These masks are packaged in face-shaped sheets that have been infused with active ingredients such as antioxidants, moisturizers, or alpha hydroxy acids. They are modeled after medical epidermal patches, such as the ones used to deliver nicotine to smokers. Epidermal treatment masks can be used up to three times weekly.

Studies have shown epidermal delivery sends active ingredients deep into the skin without causing irritation. For smaller areas, some companies make epidermal patches designed to treat specific problem areas.

Suffer from blackheads? Don't have time for an all-out mask treatment? Smooth a pore strip over the infected area and wait 15 minutes. Pull off the strip and voilà – the sebum and dirt that were in your pores will be stuck to the strip. Pore strips are most popular for the nose, but some companies make versions for the chin, cheeks, and forehead as well.

Non-hardening masks

Soft and soothing, non-hardening masks are applied thickly to clean skin and allowed to sit for 15 to 40 minutes before being tissued or rinsed off. Popular non-hardening masks include calming gel-style versions, which are often formulated to pamper sensitive or irritated skins, and creamy moisturizing formulas designed to hydrate normal to dry complexions.

Try keeping your favorite non-hardening mask on in the shower. After cleansing your face, apply the mask and allow it to sit as you shave your legs, loofah your elbows, and shampoo and condition your hair. After 5 minutes, rinse the mask off. The steam will open your skin's pores and help the mask penetrate faster, giving you results in a short amount of time.

■ **Non-hardening masks** *are generally gentle and well-suited to sensitive skin. They can be used daily, if needed.*

Intensive facial treatments

IF YOU HAVE SUN DAMAGE, mature skin,
discoloration, or fine lines, your complexion may need more
than a cleanser, toner, and moisturizer to look its best. Enter
the intensive daily treatment. Designed to be worn under, over,
or instead of your regular moisturizer, these super-charged
formulas contain high percentages of active ingredients *to*
target specific problems.

> **DEFINITION**
>
> *An active ingredient is*
> *the ingredient (or ingredients)*
> *in a formula that helps*
> *the product achieve its*
> *stated purpose*
> *effectively.*

Understanding antioxidants

If you're at all health conscious, you probably know a bit about antioxidants. These
naturally occurring substances include certain vitamins and plant extracts that fight
off free radicals. Free radicals damage skin by penetrating cells and damaging the cells'
ability to renew themselves, and by degrading the skin's collagen and elastin. When
applied to your skin, antioxidants help neutralize free radicals before they can do any
damage – some experts also believe antioxidants may be able to help repair past free
radical damage. Among the more popular antioxidants used in skin care are:

1. **Vitamin A:** There are over-the-counter products that contain one of two vitamin
A derivatives – retinol and retinyl palmitate. For a product to be effective, look
for a formula that contains at least 3 percent retinol or retinyl palmitate.

2. **Vitamin C:** Over-the-counter serums and moisturizers containing vitamin C are
among today's hottest-selling skin-care items. That's because they are especially
effective at treating the signs of sun damage. Get the most effective vitamin C
product by choosing a formula with a 10 percent or higher concentration of
ascorbic acid, which is thought to be the most effective of the vitamin C
derivatives. Other derivatives include magnesium ascorbate and sodium
ascorbate. Because vitamin C breaks down quickly in light, keep the product
in a dark place, such as a medicine cabinet.

3. **Vitamin E:** Often found combined with vitamin C, vitamin E is a perennial
skin-care favorite. Its chemical name is tocopherol, and it is known not only
as a particularly strong antioxidant, but as a natural preservative.

4. **Grape-seed extract:** If you're a label reader, chances are you've seen grape-seed
extract listed on quite a few skin-care ingredient lists. Literally the extract of
grape seeds, this product contains a compound of ingredients known
collectively as procyanidolic oligomers.

These ingredients help grape-seed extract strengthen capillary walls, reduce inflammation, and act as antioxidants on your skin.

5 **Green tea extract:** According to some studies, green tea extract may shrink precancerous skin lesions, thanks to its active ingredient, catechins.

6 **Pycnogenol:** Derived from the bark of Landis pine trees, pycnogenol is another antioxidant that contains procyanidolic oligomers.

Alpha hydroxy acids

Alpha hydroxy acids are naturally occurring substances that break down the dead cells that sit on the skin's surface, dulling the complexion and clogging pores. Alpha hydroxy acids also stimulate new collagen growth, giving users a slightly tighter, more youthful complexion. And the acids' light bleaching effect helps treat discoloration, freckles, and acne scars. For an alpha hydroxy skin-care product to be effective, it should contain at least 5 percent of the ingredient, and preferably 10 percent or more; stronger products are available through dermatologists and plastic surgeons. Here are the acids and where they occur:

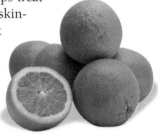

- Citric acid: derived from citrus products
- Glycolic acid: derived from sugar cane
- Lactic acid: derived from milk products
- Malic acid: derived from grapes
- Tartaric acid: derived from apples

■ **Oranges** *are a good source of citric acid, which promotes a clear and healthy complexion.*

If you are trying to improve skin and pigmentary imbalances, take fastidious care to use a sunblock, even on cloudy days. This will help prevent the return of any pigment that has been successfully bleached out by a treatment.

All about trentinoin

Retin-A® and *Renova®* are two examples of products that contain trentinoin. This vitamin A derivative is one of the few skin-care ingredients proven in medical studies to reverse some signs of sun damage and aging, such as fine lines, discoloration, and rough texture. Trentinoin is a powerful exfoliant that not only sloughs off dead skin cells but stimulates faster, more efficient cell renewal. It has also been shown to stimulate new collagen growth and destroy precancerous lesions. Results are visible after 2 to 8 weeks.

Trivia...

Cleopatra's famous milk baths were an effective way to harness the benefits of lactic acid. This alpha hydroxy acid works on skin's topmost layers to exfoliate and brighten the skin.

Trentinoin products are available only by prescription. You should be aware that because the ingredient can be irritating, you may experience redness, stinging, or itchiness that may or may not disappear with time. Some dermatologists believe trentinoin causes sun sensitivity, making it imperative that you wear sunscreens any time you are exposed to sunlight – something you should be doing anyway, whether or not you're using a trentinoin product.

Using Kinerase®

Kinerase rhymes with "line erase," which happens to be one of the product's functions. The chemical name for *Kinerase®* is furfuryl adenine, a natural plant-derived ingredient that has been shown in clinical studies to retard the aging process of skin by reducing discoloration, fine lines, and rough texture. Unlike trentinoin and alpha hydroxy products, *Kinerase®* is not an acid, does not irritate skin, and can be used safely with other age-fighting products, such as glycolic acid, *Retin-A®*, and antioxidant serums. While *Kinerase®* is not a prescription product, it is generally available only in dermatologists' and plastic surgeons' offices.

To see if you are sensitive to any particular treatment product, apply a small amount to the inner elbow. If you have any redness or itchiness 12 to 24 hours later, your skin may not be able to tolerate the product.

Skin bleaches

If you suffer from melasma, sun-induced blotchiness, or acne scars, you probably know a little something about skin bleaches. These products work on the skin's surface to lighten pigmented areas. The two most common bleaching ingredients are hydroquinone and kojic acid. Most cosmetic companies make hydroquinone-based skin lighteners, which contain 2 percent or less of the chemical; stronger 4 percent formulas are available through your dermatologist.

Not only can hydroquinone be irritating, it can actually cause an increase in darkness on black, olive, and easily scarred skins. For this reason, kojic acid may be a better choice for some of you. This naturally occurring substance is a derivative of a plant fungus. It has been used for centuries in Japan as a skin lightener and today is popular in over-the-counter skin lighteners. Whichever type of skin lightener you choose, be aware that progress can be slow: Most people don't see results for 2 to 6 months. Also, while some people experience dramatic lightening, most individuals see only a slight fading of blotchiness.

INTERNET

www.derm-info.net
www.dermatology channel.net

These informative sites contain information on a range of skin-care diseases and ailments and how they can be treated.

Sunscreens for the face

ACCORDING TO DERMATOLOGISTS, *the sun's ultraviolet light is your skin's biggest enemy – which means sunscreen may just be your skin's biggest friend. All sunscreen products today block out burn-causing UVB rays; very few adequately block UVA rays. Yet, it is these long, glass-penetrating UVA rays that are responsible for the wrinkles, collagen and elastin breakdown, brown spots, and broken capillaries associated with sun damage. To help your skin, you need a product that is labeled "broad-spectrum," which means it blocks both types of rays. You also need a formula that boasts an SPF of at least 15; with the thinning ozone layer, cautious dermatologists suggest an SPF that is no lower than 30.*

> **DEFINITION**
>
> *SPF is a somewhat confusing American term that stands for Sun Protection Factor; it refers to the amount of UVB rays a sunscreen protects you from. The higher the SPF number, the longer you can remain in the sun without getting burned. For instance, an SPF of 15 would allow you to stay in the sun 15 times longer than you could if you were unprotected.*

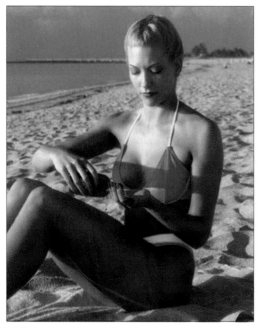

■ **If you're on vacation** *and spending a lot of time outdoors, use a sunscreen that offers adequate protection against both UVA and UVB rays.*

Chemical sunscreens

Chemical sunscreens use chemicals that absorb UVA and UVB light, preventing it from damaging surrounding skin cells. There are a lot of chemical ingredients currently used in sunscreen, but only Parsol 1789 blocks out both UVA and UVB effectively. Remember, it's important to block out both skin-ruining UVA and burn-causing UVB rays!

Don't use old sunscreen because these products lose their effectiveness after 1 to 2 years. If you can't find an expiration date and can't remember when you purchased your sunscreen, buy yourself a fresh bottle.

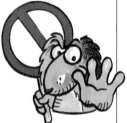

Physical sunscreens

Physical sunscreens are sometimes called sun-blocks because they form a barrier to block the entry of UVA and UVB light. Titanium dioxide, which protects against both UVA and UVB rays, is one of the most popular physical sunscreens – and it is an ingredient in most physical sunscreens. Because it leaves a white, flaky finish, it is best combined with zinc oxide, which is one of the most powerful UVA protectants around. Unlike the thick, white stuff that surfers and lifeguards once wore, today's zinc – which also goes by the names micronized zinc oxide and Z-Cote® – is transparent.

How to use sunscreen

When it comes to sunscreen, how you use it is as important as what kind you use. Make sure you use enough sunscreen for the protection you need. Don't rely on moisturizers or makeup that contain sunscreen. These can be additions to your sun-protection routine, but it is chemically difficult to blend a strong, broad-spectrum sunscreen into a moisturizer or foundation. You're safer using actual sunscreen as your primary defense against ultraviolet rays. Sunscreen needs a few minutes to meld with your skin before it can do its job. That's why many sunscreen labels suggest applying at least 20 minutes before sun exposure. Reapply even if a product says "waterproof," "rub-proof," or "all-day formula." Why? According to some dermatologists, most sunscreening agents have a 2-hour span when they're most effective.

Many sunscreens are heavy and greasy, which makes the acne-prone among us tempted to forego sun protection altogether. Experiment with light, oil-free gel formulas instead.

A simple summary

✔ Knowing your skin type is the first step in good skin care.

✔ You don't need to buy an expensive cleanser.

✔ Toning is a personal choice.

✔ You may not need a moisturizer.

✔ Masks are a fast way to make skin look great.

✔ If you have a skin glitch, you may need an intensive treatment to reduce its appearance.

✔ Make sure your sunscreen has an SPF of at least 15.

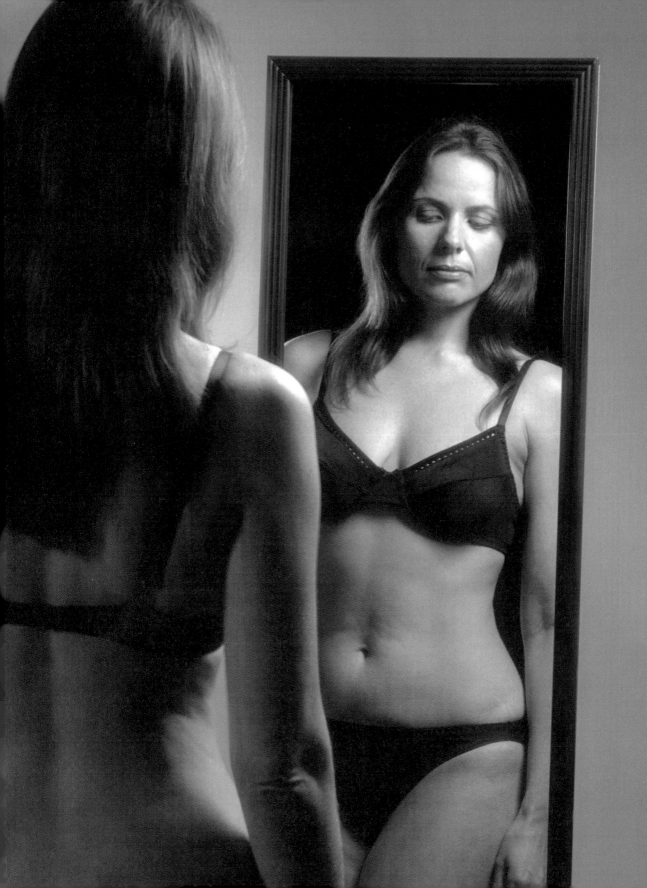

Chapter 4

What's Your Problem?

IF YOU'RE LIKE MOST PEOPLE, you were born with perfect skin – smooth, firm, seemingly poreless, lineless, and without a spot of discoloration. And, if you're like most people, you no longer have that skin. At some point in your life, you may have developed acne or the pores around your nose grew large and oh so visible. Perhaps a summer pregnancy left you with impossible-to-get-rid-of dark patches, or somehow you acquired two new moles on your face. While you may never regain the complexion of your childhood, I've got good news: there are products, people, and procedures to help bring your skin closer to the ideal.

In this chapter...

✔ Common skin conditions

✔ Go it alone or bring in help?

INSPECT YOUR SKIN REGULARLY TO CHECK ITS CONDITION AND LOOK FOR ANY CHANGES

Common skin conditions

FRECKLES, SCARS, SPOTS, *strange moles,*
skin cancer – unfortunately, unexpected things happen.
And yes, they can happen right on your face, and
when they do, they may make you feel embarrassed,
unattractive, or self-conscious. Often what plagues
you is painfully obvious. Yet sometimes, you may
not recognize what's developing there at the
bottom of your right cheek or above your left
nostril. Where did it come from? Why did it
target you? What can you do about it?

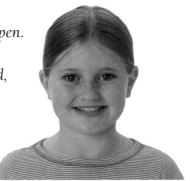

■ **Freckles** *that develop when you are a*
child usually remain throughout your life.

Discoloration

Discoloration is a kind of catchall word referring to any kind of dark
spots, splotches, or patches on your skin. Hyperpigmentation is
another term and is used interchangeably. Freckles qualify as
discoloration, as do melasma and *age spots*.

Discoloration is caused by an excess of melanin, the pigment that gives
skin its color. In some people, ultraviolet light, female hormones, and
even age can trigger cells to overproduce melanin in odd spots. To
avoid creating more discoloration, discontinue birth control pills or
estrogen-replacement pills (if you're on them) and begin using
sunscreens. Bleaching products, alpha hydroxy products, retinoids,
microbrasion, chemical peels, and laser therapy can also lighten marks.

Cystic acne

The word "acne" is often used as a general term to describe
any group of recurring blemishes. Yet a few whiteheads on
the chin around your period is a very different thing from
a scattering of scarlet nodular blemishes on your face,
neck, shoulders, or back. Dermatologists call this cystic,
severe, or nodular acne, and if you suffer from it, you
know it is not only painful, but deeply embarrassing.

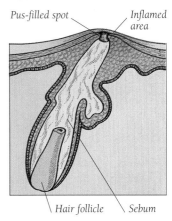

Pus-filled spot   *Inflamed area*

Hair follicle   *Sebum*

■ **An inflamed, pus-filled pimple** *can form when a hair follicle*
becomes blocked with excess sebum, allowing bacteria to collect.

Stress appears to play a significant role in the development of cystic acne. Deep breathing, meditation, and other tension-busting activities can help prevent it.

An acne cyst begins as a pimple deep in the sebaceous gland, where excess sebum and bacteria combine to create an infected nodule. Because this disease (yes, it's considered a disease) is disfiguring and difficult to treat with over-the-counter products, it is important to see a dermatologist, who may suggest a combination of oral and topical antibiotics, or even *Accutane®*. This is an oral drug that suppresses sebum production. Because *Accutane®* causes severe facial and ear deformities in fetuses, your dermatologist will require you to sign a document stating you will not get pregnant while undergoing treatment with this drug.

Large pores

Large pores are created in two ways. The first is through aggressive squeezing of blackheads and whiteheads, which stretches the pore. The second is heavy sebum production. When the sebaceous gland produces large volumes of sebum, the pore is forced to expand to release the oil and is therefore enlarged.

Unlike normal pores, large pores are visible to people around us. They are also easily clogged with sebum and dead skin cells. At the moment, there is no product or treatment available that can close these pores up to normal size. The best you can do is keep pores debris-free with thorough cleansing, exfoliation, masks, and professional facials – all will help make pores appear slightly smaller.

THE OTHER ACNE

Rosacea, or rosacea acne, is an ongoing inflammation of the cheeks, nose, mid-forehead, and chin. While it's not known what causes this mysterious disease, it is believed to be a disorder of the blood vessels, which are sensitive to emotional and physical stimulation. Treatment includes practicing stress management techniques; taking oral and topical antibiotics; and avoiding alcohol and hot and spicy foods.

■ **In some people,** *the inflammation caused by rosacea causes permanent and acne-like blemishes to appear on the reddened skin.*

Skin cancer

Skin cancer is more common than all other types of cancer combined. More than 90 percent of skin cancers are the cumulative result of a lifetime's exposure to ultraviolet light. In other words, even if you've been using sunscreens and protecting your skin from the sun for decades, the unsafe sun you got as a child and the tanning lamps you used as an adolescent count as ultraviolet exposure.

What does skin cancer have to do with beauty? Well, actually, quite a bit. Visit sunbelt cities like Las Vegas, Phoenix, or Dallas, and you'll find old-timers missing bits of nose, ear, eyelid, and lip where dermatologists have had to remove cancerous lesions. If left undetected, skin cancer can spread into cartilage and bone; it is common for people to lose an entire nose as a result of skin cancers on the face.

The sooner a scar is treated after forming, the more successful the results. If you suffer from acne, had a mole excised, or had past skin cancer removed, ask your dermatologist about treatments to soften a scar's appearance.

Trivia...

Some moles become raised with age, some stay the same, some become as wrinkled as surrounding skin, and some fall off.

ALL ABOUT MOLES

Nearly everyone has at least one mole. These marks on your skin are actually formed by nests of pigment cells. They can be tan, brown, black, bluish, or flesh-colored. When they appear on the face, they are known as beauty marks. A healthy mole will usually be flat, or slightly raised, and be even in color and texture. Not all moles are, or become, cancerous. In fact, they are usually harmless. However, if you hate your mole, or if you find that you keep catching it in clothing, ask your dermatologist if it can be surgically removed.

■ **Monitor changes** *in color, size, and texture of existing moles; and check to see if you have developed any new ones.*

Identifying skin cancers

Skin cancer occurs when skin cells divide rapidly and grow without any order. Some of these deviant skin cancer cells spread to other parts of the body to form new tumors. Call your dermatologist immediately if you spot any of the following signs:

- A crusty, red bump or sore that intermittently or continuously bleeds
- A flat, reddish spot that is rough, dry, or scaly
- A smooth, shiny, waxy, or pale bump that is ¼ inch (6 mm) or less in diameter
- A mole that is asymmetrical, has a jagged border, changes size or color, or is greater than ¼ inch (6 mm) wide

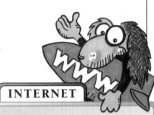

INTERNET

www.oneskin.com

Anything you could possibly want to know about skin and skin conditions, plus plenty of message boards devoted to particular skin ailments.

Go it alone or bring in help?

YOU'VE GOT A SKIN GLITCH *you want gone – or at least diminished. Where do you go for help? Well, it depends on the severity of the problem. Obviously, if you suspect skin cancer, you need to take yourself straight to a dermatologist. But for something that is more looks-threatening than life-threatening, you've got choices. You can opt for over-the-counter treatments, help from a professional skin-care therapist, or a visit to your dermatologist.*

Over-the-counter care

Pharmacies, chain drug stores, beauty emporiums, and department store cosmetic counters are great for the do-it-yourselfer. These places offer a range of treatment products (at a range of prices) that allow you to address your problem privately, conveniently, and relatively inexpensively. The downside to this? It's easy to either get swayed by the grand claims you read on a box of skin-care cream or get confused by a product's ingredient list. To avoid getting taken – and to ensure you find a product that works – you must do a bit of research not only on your condition, but also on product ingredients. You need to know what ingredients your skin finds irritating and avoid purchasing a product that contains these.

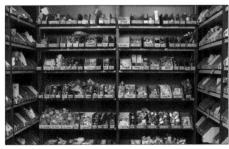

■ **There is a range of products** *available at drug stores to suit all types of skin problems – do some research before you purchase.*

Be aware that these "mass-market" items are designed to be used without professional supervision by an enormous cross-section of people. To avoid causing reactions in some of these people, manufacturers formulate their products with low concentrations of active ingredients.

You spent a good deal of cash on a cream that said it could banish freckles, and after using the whole jar, your freckles haven't lightened a bit. What to do? Contact the company that made the product and complain. In the US, you can also call the Food and Drug Agency and lodge a complaint: 800-532-4440; in Canada, contact The Cosmetics Program: 613-957-7926.

What is an aesthetician?

Aestheticians are most often found at skin-care salons, day spas, and even in dermatologists' offices. They give a wide range of facial treatments for a wide range of problems, from mild to moderate acne, to light wrinkling, to melasma; what they cannot do is perform surgery, work with lasers, prescribe medication, or diagnose dangerous skin ailments, such as cancer. A good aesthetician will tell you to visit your dermatologist if he or she spots something suspicious on your face. Think of an aesthetician as a skin-care partner. Most likely you will be visiting your aesthetician weekly, twice-monthly, or monthly until your problem is controlled. After that, you will go less frequently for follow-up and maintenance visits.

Many aestheticians and dermatologists use a Wood's lamp to view a patient's sun damage. The lamp projects a long wavelength of blue light deeper into the skin than visible light; sun damage shows up as dark, mottled areas.

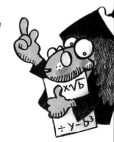

Visiting an aesthetician

If you decide to work with an aesthetician, a plan of specific cleansers, creams, sunscreens, and other regimens designed to treat your skin may be recommended. Aestheticians rely on professional treatment lines that are available for use only under an aesthetician's supervision. These professional products generally contain moderate levels of active ingredients; you may experience better or faster results from them than from over-the-counter products. The downside to aestheticians? The visits and products can get expensive.

Don't be shy when visiting an aesthetician or dermatologist. To help him or her choose the safest, most effective treatment plan for you,

INTERNET

www.skinema.com

This amusing web site was created by a dermatologist to expose the skin conditions of the stars.

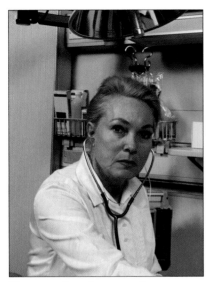

■ **Remember that** *everything you tell your doctor or dermatologist will be treated in confidence.*

you must speak up about your lifestyle and your health. Don't forget to mention allergies, reproductive plans, current medication, and even how many glasses of alcohol you drink in a week.

Get thee to a doctor!

A dermatologist is your only option if you suspect something serious, such as skin cancer, something appears abruptly, such as a rash, or you suffer from a particularly stubborn or severe case of something, such as cystic acne. But your visits don't have to be limited to these reasons – dermatologists treat minor skin-care gripes as well. In fact, because dermatologists are doctors, they can prescribe strong prescription medication that contains high levels of active ingredients. This means fast results and the benefit of someone monitoring you against any allergies or reactions.

Dermatologists can also perform cutting-edge procedures, such as laser, botox, and collagen, that you can't get anywhere else. Before choosing this option, however, you should consider that while some insurance plans do cover dermatology visits and prescription costs for "cosmetic issues" such as melasma, freckles, sun damage, and wrinkles, most do not.

A simple summary

✔ Relax, you're not the only one with skin glitches.

✔ For severe acne, prescription medication may be the best way to go.

✔ The sun is responsible for skin cancer and most skin discolorations.

✔ Consult a dermatologist if you are worried about a skin glitch.

✔ For most skin conditions, you've got options from simple creams to a dermatologist's care.

✔ For severe or life-threatening conditions, a dermatologist is essential.

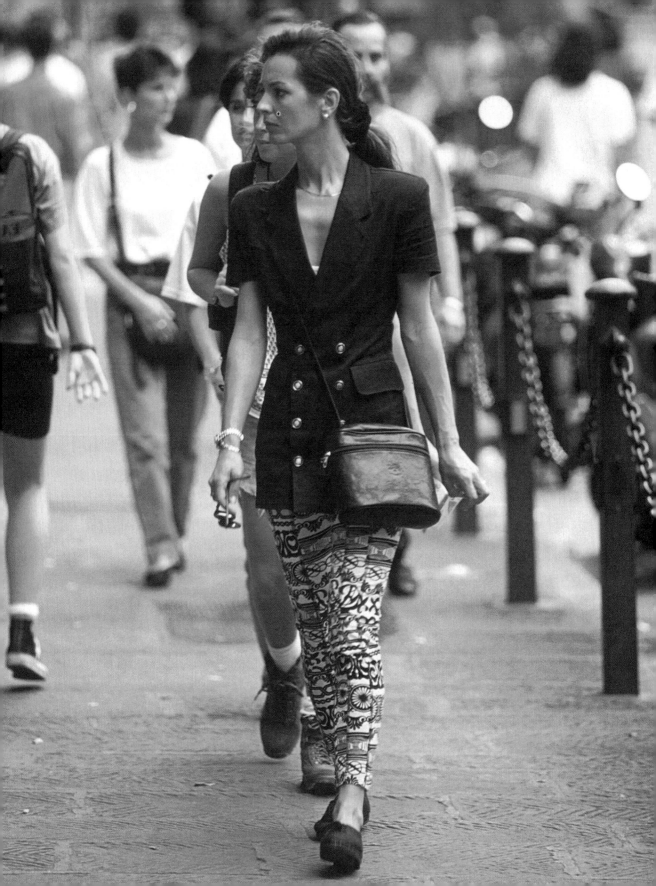

Chapter 5

Beyond the Basics

I F YOU SUFFER FROM ACNE SCARS, broken blood vessels, or some other complexion glitch, it's probably been a while since you felt comfortable letting people see you without makeup. In fact, you've probably been slapping on thick coats of coverup in an attempt to camouflage that brown patch on your forehead or that tangle of broken veins on your nose. You may be able to ease up. Almost yearly a new treatment comes along that is designed to soften the appearance of, or rub out, skin glitches that were previously unerasable. With the right procedure, you just may be able to leave your house without coverup at all!

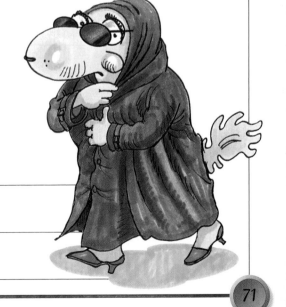

In this chapter...

✓ Quick treatments

✓ Doctors' fast fixes

✓ Big-deal treatments

SOME DERMATOLOGICAL TREATMENTS CAN BE CARRIED OUT DURING A LUNCH BREAK

Quick treatments

AT NO TIME IN BEAUTY HISTORY have there been a greater number of quick, "in-and-out" procedures than today. Dubbed "lunchtime" treatments, these procedures can generally be performed in under an hour and cause no disfiguring side effects – you can schedule one for your lunch break and then return straight back to work. In fact, some of these treatments are so gentle that even aestheticians offer them.

Be aware, however, that while these treatments may be straightforward, they are not for everyone. If you have sensitive skin, a medical condition, any type of allergy, are pregnant or lactating, or take prescription or over-the-counter medication, your skin may not react well to a certain procedure, or it could even be harmful to you. Before undergoing any of the following, please talk to your dermatologist or aesthetician about whether the treatment is appropriate for you.

Alpha and beta peels

Alternately called "acid facials," "exfoliating treatments," and "peels," treatments using alpha hydroxy (such as glycolic) or beta hydroxy (such as salicylic) acids are offered in stronger strengths by dermatologists and in more moderate strengths by aestheticians.

Avoid beta hydroxy peels and beta hydroxy products if you're pregnant, because most contain salicylic acid. This is chemically related to aspirin, which has been linked to fetal deformities and complications during delivery.

Here's how they work. Your face is thoroughly cleansed and a thin layer of acid applied. After 2 to 15 minutes – depending on your skin and the acid's strength – the acid is rinsed off. The results

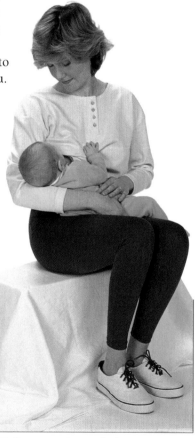

■ **If you are** *breast feeding, some skin treatments may have an adverse effect on you or your baby. Always talk to your doctor before going ahead with any procedure.*

are a softening of fine lines, lightening of skin discoloration, a brighter complexion color, and fewer pimples, thanks to the acid's pore-clearing action. Because their effects are cumulative, peels are usually performed in a series of six appointments; every week, or every other week, you return for a slightly stronger treatment.

PhotoFacials

The light-powered *PhotoFacial* addresses pigmentation problems, broken and enlarged capillaries, fine lines, scarring, and the flushing associated with rosacea. Developed by the Californian dermatologist Patrick Bitter, Sr., this noninvasive treatment uses intense, non-laser light. The treatment usually lasts less than 30 minutes.

Here's what to expect in a PhotoFacial. After you don a pair of protective goggles, a dermatologist or aesthetician will pass a special wand over your face – this wand emits repetitive flashes of light. When the procedure is over, you can get up, put on sunscreen and whatever makeup you want, then continue with your day. Most people experience no redness or dryness, though these are possible side effects. Because their effects are cumulative, PhotoFacials are performed in a series of three to six appointments: every 3 to 4 weeks, you return for another treatment.

> **DEFINITION**
>
> *Though the* PhotoFacial *sounds a bit like a laser treatment, it isn't. Lasers emit light over a single wavelength, and they are limited in how far they can penetrate the skin without causing damage. The PhotoFacial uses light that spans several wavelengths and can penetrate deep into the dermis – where abnormal skin pigmentation and dilated vessels are located – without harming skin cells; so the results are quite far-reaching.*

Microbrasion facials

Take a sandblaster, follow it with a vacuum cleaner, and what do you get? The much-repeated description of a microbrasion facial, also known as power peel, diamond peel, Parisian peel, and microderm peel. No matter what it's called, this treatment features a small tube-like device that sprays aluminum crystals, diamond dust, or salt (depending on the machine) across the skin to lift off dead skin cells and the outermost layer of the epidermis. A suctioning action simultaneously sweeps away exfoliated skin cells and the used abrasive material.

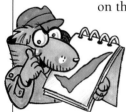

You may experience pinkness and chapping for a day or two after a microbrasion treatment, but nothing obvious.

If this sounds a bit unpleasant, it is. For many people, however, the treatment's slight discomfort is worth the payoff. This includes softening of acne pock-marks and other scars, lightening of dark patches and freckles, and removal of fine lines. Because their effects are cumulative, microbrasion facials are usually performed in a series of six to ten appointments; every week, or every other week, you return for a slightly stronger treatment.

Doctors' fast fixes

I CALL THE *following treatments "doctors' fast fixes" because they use lasers or needles, which push them into the realm of medical treatments. However, the procedures are every bit as fast as the lunchtime treatments mentioned earlier and, in some ways, they are faster. Unlike the lunchtime services, which offer cumulative results and should be repeated at regular, short intervals, the fix-ups outlined below generally offer instant rejuvenation in a single appointment.*

Collagen injections

In the late 1980s, collagen got a reputation as a lip-plumper thanks to Barbara Hershey's enhanced pout in the movie *Beaches*. Today, collagen is still popular, but it's more likely to fill indented scars and those deep lines that run between the nose and mouth, and the mouth and chin.

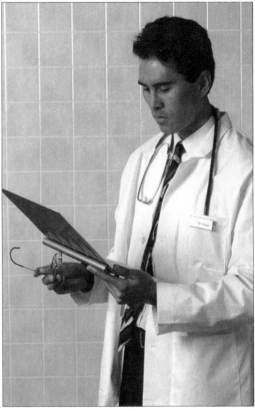

■ **If you have an unwanted scar** *or a skin glitch, talk to your doctor or dermatologist about the possible medical treatments open to you.*

Collagen lasts longer when injected into those areas of the face where there isn't a lot of muscle movement.

Vegetarians should keep in mind that collagen comes from cow cadavers, although there is a version called *Dermalogen®* that is extracted from human cadavers. If this gruesome information doesn't dim your desire to try collagen, visit your dermatologist. He or she will administer an allergy test; usually, this is a small injection of the material in the forearm. If after 2 weeks no redness or rash develops, you can return to have collagen injected into your face's dermis. While collagen is extremely natural-looking, its effects are short-lived, lasting anywhere from 2 to 6 months.

Laser vein removal

If you suffer from broken or dilated capillaries, you know how hard these scarlet squiggles are to hide with makeup. Fortunately, these unsightly marks are easily treated in a 15-minute appointment with a laser-wielding dermatologist.

When aimed at the offending capillaries, the laser emits a wavelength of light that heats the blood inside the small vein. When the heat reaches a certain level, the blood vessels' walls collapse and dissolve. You'll feel a small zap as the laser light does its work. If you are like most people, you'll need two to four treatments – spaced 1 or 2 months apart – to get the results you want.

Trivia...

To diminish visible facial veins, dermatologists generally use one of four lasers, depending on the results required: the Pulsed Dye, the Krypton, the VeraPulse, or the Argon. Each uses a slightly different type of beam to achieve its goals.

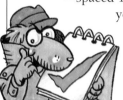

After laser vein treatment, you may notice redness around the affected area, but nothing severe.

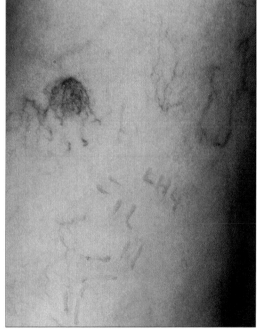

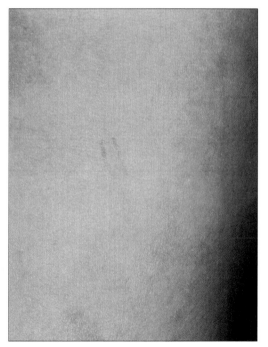

■ **Broken veins** *often appear on thighs. Before laser treatment, the dermatologist will mark your skin, as a guide to follow during the procedure.*

■ **After laser vein treatment** *on this thigh, the dilated capillaries are no longer visible, leaving the skin looking younger and virtually blemish free.*

Botox

If you read beauty magazines, you probably know about botox. This muscle-paralyzing substance is injected into muscles – usually in the upper third of the face – and it is particularly effective for eliminating or preventing crow's feet, between-brow furrows, and horizontal creases on the forehead. It smoothes the skin and prevents wrinkles by interrupting the nerve's signal to the injected muscle – when the brain sends a signal down along the nerve passageway, the message doesn't reach the muscle, the muscle doesn't move, and the area remains still and smooth.

INTERNET

www.asds-net.org

This is the site of the American Society of Dermatologic Surgery. Here, you can find professional advice on dermatologic surgery and information on particular procedures, as well as doctor referrals.

"Botox" stands for bacterium clostridium botulinum toxin, the same illness-producing toxin found in spoiled canned goods. Before you get alarmed, however, you should know that the form of botulism toxin used by dermatologists is not only purified and extremely diluted, but has been used safely for 20 years to treat medical conditions such as eye spasms, central nervous system disorders, facial paralysis, and excessive muscle contractions.

Always consider possible side effects before going ahead with a treatment.

While side effects are rare, botox can cause temporary eyelid droop in a small number of cases. This usually appears 1 to 2 weeks after the injection and can be countered with special eye drops. To reduce your risk of eyelid droop, go to a dermatologist or plastic surgeon who uses botox on a regular basis. Botox results last from 3 to 6 months.

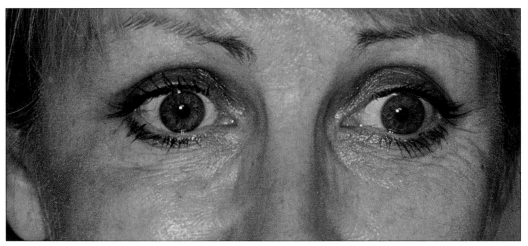

■ **This patient is undergoing** *botox treatments to help eliminate crow's feet around her eyes. The eye on the left has already been injected with botox, while the eye on the right is still to be treated.*

Big-deal treatments

WHEN IT COMES TO BEAUTY, a general rule of thumb is "the less the pain, the less dramatic the gain." Keep this in mind if you're looking for big results. For instance, if you'd like to create a satiny-smooth finish on pockmarked skin, eradicate moderate lines, or restore firmness to a slack area of the face, the quick "lunchtime" procedures we have just described probably won't give you what you want. However, there are more intensive procedures available.

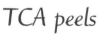

Not all big-deal treatments are performed in hospital. In fact, many are done in a dermatologist's in-office surgery suite.

TCA peels

With the advent of laser resurfacing, PhotoFacials, and microbrasion treatments, the TCA peel has waned in popularity. Named after its active ingredient, trichloroacetic acid, the TCA peel is a medium-deep treatment that "freshens" the skin, removes some sun damage and rough scaly patches, reduces freckles and irregular pigmentation, and softens fine wrinkles. There is some evidence that it may also reduce the risk of skin cancer by destroying precancerous cells. The treatment involves painting trichloroacetic acid onto clean skin until the skin whitens.

ABOUT PHENOL PEELS

Once upon a time, before skin lasers were invented, there were phenol peels – the deepest of all chemical peels. Little used today, phenol peels reach into the dermis, where they correct severe sun damage, acne scarring, and deep wrinkles. Unfortunately, the peels are so toxic that patients require a complete physical exam and an electrocardiogram prior to the peel, plus constant heart monitoring during the treatment.

Like glycolic, salicylic, TCA, and Jessner's peels, phenol peels involve a chemical solution painted onto clean skin. Healing time is relatively slow – approximately 2 weeks – during which the skin is red, swollen, and oozing until the tenth day, when scabs form. These scabs stick around for an additional 2 to 3 weeks.

During the 24 hours following the procedure, your skin will be slightly swollen and red. Over the next few days, the treated skin dries to a crispy brown; to keep things moist, your doctor may suggest coating your face with a thick layer of Vaseline®. Things get uglier: between days 5 and 7, the leathery skin begins peeling in large sheets.

As irresistible as picking at skin is after a skin treatment, let it peel at its own pace: pulling it can cause deep scars and infections. As soon as your face is done shedding, you can return to your regular skin-care routine.

Jessner's peel

The Jessner's peel resembles the TCA peel: a medium-deep treatment that is designed to remove the top layers of skin, thus evening pigmentation, improving the skin's texture, and minimizing fine lines. Instead of containing trichloroacetic acid, however, the Jessner's peel consists of a mixture of salicylic acid, lactic acid, and *resorcinol*.

> **DEFINITION**
>
> Resorcinol *is an intense, vitamin A-based exfoliating agent, often used as part of the ingredients for a Jessner's peel.*

The Jessner's peel solution is applied to clean skin. Immediately afterward, your skin will be red and slightly swollen, and after 3 or 4 days, it will become dry and tight. At this point it should begin to crack and peel; to keep things moist, your doctor may suggest coating your face with a thick layer of petroleum jelly. After 5 to 7 days, skin should be healed enough for you to return to your regular skin-care routine.

On dark skin, olive-toned skin, or skin that scars easily, chemical peels, laser treatments, and dermabrasion can cause scarring, light-colored patches, or dark patches. Do not consider any of these resurfacing treatments before getting a dermatologist's evaluation.

Laser resurfacing

Laser resurfacing was the "it" treatment of the 1990s – and with good reason. By removing skin's outer layer, the procedure can lighten or banish discoloration, scars, and fine and moderate wrinkles, as well as tighten slack skin, giving the face a firmer, younger appearance. The high-energy beam of light can selectively transfer its energy into tissue to treat the skin. A dermatologist will use one of two types of lasers for laser resurfacing treatments: the deeper-reaching carbon dioxide laser is usually used for deep scarring. The more surface-skimming Erbium Yag laser is generally used on areas of lighter scarring and has less of an effect. Prior to laser resurfacing, it may be necessary to take medication to prevent infection with herpes simplex virus.

If your dermatologist is using a carbon dioxide laser, intravenous sedation is generally used; local anesthesia is typically used for an Erbium laser treatment. After skin is cleansed, your dermatologist will pass the laser's light over your skin. The condition of your skin immediately following the procedure depends on the type of laser your dermatologist has used.

What if your face features both deeply scarred and lightly scarred areas? Your dermatologist may opt for a dual-Erbium Contour laser. Kind of a dual carbon dioxide-Erbium laser, the machine lets your doctor use the deep-tissue carbon dioxide beam on your severely scarred skin, and the Erbium beam on the more superficially flawed bits.

Laser effects

After a carbon dioxide laser procedure, skin is raw and oozy for the first 3 or 4 days. Next, skin crusts, peels, and is ready for makeup after 2 or 3 weeks. Skin can remain pink for up to 6 months after treatment. After an Erbium laser treatment, skin is slightly raw and feels sunburned for the first few days. Skin then peels and is ready for makeup after 5 to 7 days. Because both types of lasers stimulate new collagen growth, you may notice continued tightening and firming for up to 6 months after the procedure.

INTERNET

www.nih.gov/nia

Learn more about the aging process from this site, run by the US National Institute on Aging.

■ **Before laser treatment,** *your dermatologist will study your skin, looking for scarred areas, lines, slack spots, and discolored patches.*

LASER HAIR REMOVAL

Laser treatments are not only used to treat skin glitches, they are also used to remove unwanted facial hair. You may have been born with noticeable facial hair, or you may have developed it as you've got older. The point is that many women find facial hair embarrassing and laser treatment is an effective way of removing it. (In Chapter 16, we also look at laser treatment for body hair removal.)

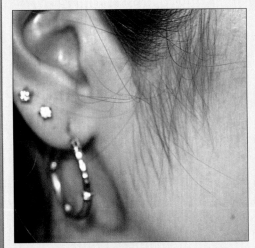

■ **Many women** *have fine hair that extends from the hairline and onto their upper cheek- and jawbones. They may be particularly self-conscious about it if they wear their hair up.*

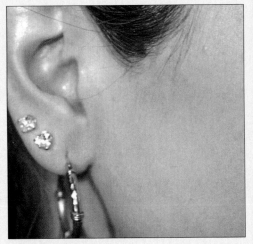

■ **Laser hair removal** *treatment can remove these fine hairs, creating a neater hairline. It can also help give a more flattering definition to the face by making the cheekbone appear longer.*

Dermabrasion

When it comes down to it, dermabrasion is a form of sandblasting for your face. The procedure uses a small rotating abrasive brush to sand away the top layers of skin. How many layers, exactly, is up to you and your dermatologist. The treatment has fallen out of favor since the advent of laser resurfacing, microbrasion, and PhotoFacials. However, dermabrasion is often more effective than any of these at evening scars out, and it is still used to improve the appearance of pockmarked skin.

The treatment itself is fairly quick, generally taking less than an hour. While the procedure is usually carried out under local anesthesia, you may be given a sedative that will relax you and make you drowsy. Immediately afterward, your skin will resemble raw steak; to keep it protected, your doctor will suggest thick coats of petroleum jelly or an antibiotic ointment. Scabs form (don't pick!) and fall off within 10 days to 2 weeks. After this point, skin will be pink for up to 3 months, but it will have healed to the extent that you can return to your regular skin-care routine.

Fat injections

Fat injections are ideal for plumping up those deep lines that run from nose to mouth and mouth to chin. They're also great for filling in indented scars or the depressed areas that show up on some of our lower cheeks as we age. One of the nice things about these injections is that the process uses a material that may already be hanging around your tummy, bottom, or thighs: fat. It doesn't require a lot of fat, usually just a few ounces. After choosing a donor site, your dermatologist will clean and anesthetize the area before making a small incision, from which fat is withdrawn. Before the fat can be reinjected, however, it must be purified of any blood or other material.

Dermatologists can also plump up old-looking hands with fat transplantation. After all, when it comes to broadcasting your age, your hands speak louder than your face.

Once the fat is cleansed, you can return to your dermatologist, who will numb the area to be treated before injecting it with fat cells. No bandages or other wrapping are required afterward. The entire procedure usually takes an hour. Results last about 3 to 6 months. With repeated treatments, however, the outcome can last longer. This is because some of the fat begins to incorporate into the surrounding tissue.

A simple summary

✔ Most skin glitches can be diminished or erased.

✔ Quick skin treatments should cause few visible side effects.

✔ Lunchtime treatments can usually be performed in an hour or less.

✔ Dramatic results usually require dramatic treatments.

✔ Talk to your doctor before you undergo any skin treatment, to make sure it is suitable for you.

✔ Laser treatments are available for skin and facial hair glitches.

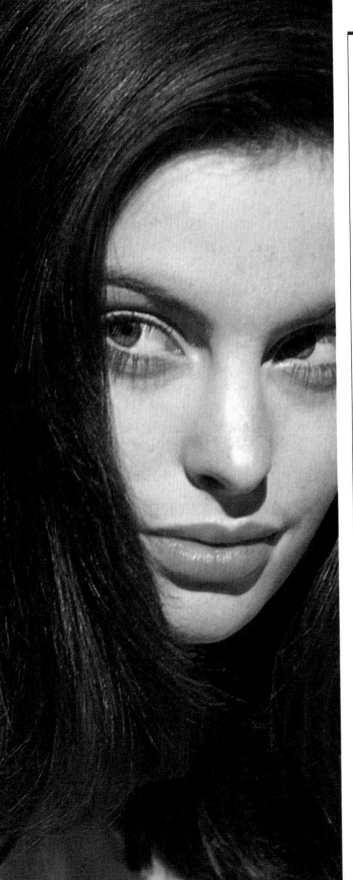

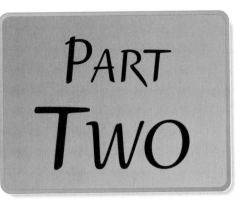

PART TWO

HEALTHY HAIR IS A BEAUTY ASSET

HAIR CARE

HAIR DRAWS PEOPLE'S ATTENTION. By studying a woman's *hairstyle*, we can gauge her personality, income level, intellectual prowess, health, line of work, place in society, and more. This is quite a feat when you

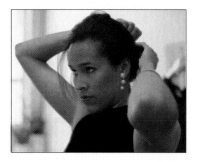

consider what hair is: stringy material comprised of dead protein cells whose purpose is to protect our scalps from environmental elements, such as the sun.

Beautiful hair is *healthy, strong, and luxurious*. This section takes a look at what hair is, how it grows, and the best way to care for it. From there, we move step by instructive step through choosing a hairstyle, the ins and outs of color, perm, and relaxing services, and tips for do-it-yourself styling. Keep reading and soon all your days will be *"good hair days."*

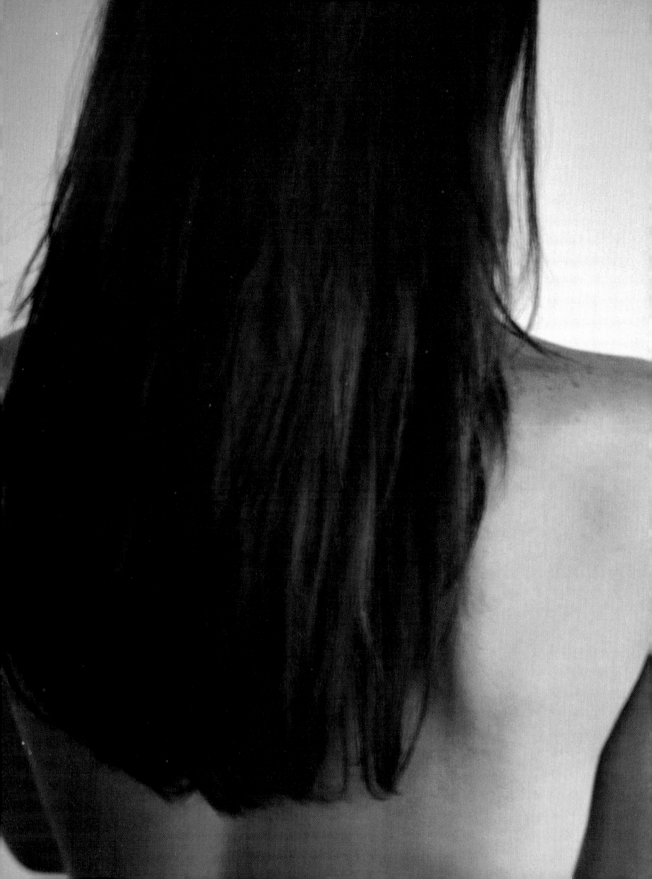

Chapter 6

All About Hair

HAIR – IT INCITES PASSION and pleasure, paintings, songs, and fashion, and is the basis of good (or bad) days. Pretty heady stuff when you consider what hair is: a vestige of our primitive past when humanlike creatures were covered with the stuff. Actually, if you count the downy fuzz on our face, arms, legs, and torsos, we're still covered with it, only most of the hair on our bodies is fine and hard to see. For our purposes here, however, I'll concentrate on the stuff coming out of our heads – the stuff that takes up so much time, thought, and worry.

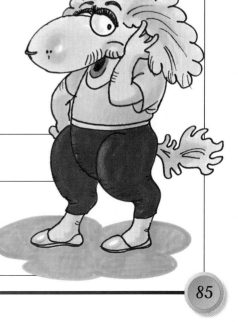

In this chapter...

✓ Hair: the whys and whats

✓ Enemies of healthy hair

✓ Hair loss

✓ How hair ages

EVERYBODY'S HAIR IS UNIQUE

Hair: the whys and whats

WHY DO WE HAVE HAIR? *The simple answer is protection. I've heard dermatologists argue about whether the scalp hair we modern humans have is enough to protect us from the elements. I have proof that it is: My bald grandfather's head gets cold when the temperature drops below 50° F (10° C), and his scalp and neck are covered with skin-cancer scars.*

Trivia...

Trimming your hair does not make it grow faster, but it removes splitting ends that can split up to 3 inches (7.5 cm) of your hair's length.

What hair's made of

You may have no interest whatsoever in knowing what the strands of your hair are made of, or how they grow. But the answers are interesting – and important, too. Once you understand how hair is built and how it functions, you'll find it easier to care for, be better able to pinpoint bogus hair-care claims, and know enough about how your locks behave to stop worrying about them and let them do what nature intended.

The only areas of the human body without hair follicles are the lips, the palms of the hands, and the soles of the feet.

Hair is an appendage of the skin. Each individual strand grows from a single live follicle that is anchored in the subcutaneous layer of your skin. A sebaceous gland that produces sebum is attached to each follicle. The oily sebum keeps the hair strand moisturized, shiny, and protected against toxic substances. Not everyone produces the same amount of sebum. The more sebum an individual produces, the oilier his or her hair is; the less sebum an individual produces, the drier his or her hair is.

Getting down to the roots

Before we go any further, let's return to the follicles, which contain the bulb-shaped roots of your hairs. These are nourished by tiny capillaries that carry minerals, proteins, vitamins, fats, and carbohydrates. It is here, at the root, that newly dividing cells force older cells upward, where they die and harden into the *hair shaft*.

DEFINITION

The hair shaft is the visible part of the hair. It is a synonym for hair strand, the individual hairs that grace most of our heads.

The hair shaft has three layers: the cuticle, the cortex, and the medulla. If you look closely at the cuticle under a microscope, you'll see that it is made up of layers of colorless, tightly overlapping tiles, much like a tile roof. The cuticle is the strongest part of the hair fiber and protects the fragile inner cortex. The cortex is comprised of a hard

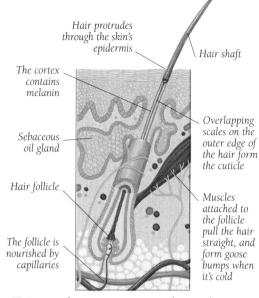

Hair protrudes through the skin's epidermis

Hair shaft

The cortex contains melanin

Overlapping scales on the outer edge of the hair form the cuticle

Sebaceous oil gland

Hair follicle

Muscles attached to the follicle pull the hair straight, and form goose bumps when it's cold

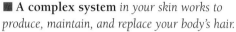

The follicle is nourished by capillaries

■ **A complex system** *in your skin works to produce, maintain, and replace your body's hair.*

protein called keratin. It is also the place where melanin – your hair's natural pigment – is located. The medulla – which for an unexplainable reason some people's hair happens not to have – does not extend all the way to the hair's tip. Though the medulla contains a small amount of pigment, it is essentially colorless; it does, however, help reflect the light that travels through the translucent cuticle and cortex.

Depending on your hair's natural color, it contains one or two different types of melanin: Eumalin is the most common and is responsible for darker hair shades, including chestnut, coffee, and black, while phaeomelanin contributes to light and reddish tones such as blonde, caramel, ginger, and auburn.

STRANGE BUT TRUE...

Those of you concerned with food safety may be interested to know that human hair is used as an additive in food – most notably in store-bought bread, pizza dough, and snack foods. The additive I'm referring to is L-cysteine (also known as L-cysteine Hydrochloride), an amino acid that can be made from petroleum, but is much more commonly made from human hair. Why? Because hair is cheaper than petroleum and it contains up to 8 percent of the natural amino acid cysteine, which is chemically converted to L-cysteine. Most of the hair comes from China's barber shops, where strands are collected, cleaned, and sent to processing plants to be chemically converted into L-cysteine – a powdery chemical. If you want to avoid this additive, check ingredient lists – however, it may be merely listed as "natural flavoring" or "dough enhancer."

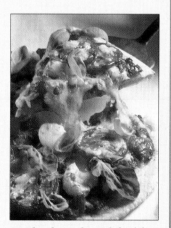

■ **Check packaged** *food for the additive L-cysteine – used as a preservative and flavor enhancer in bread and dough.*

How hair grows

As each strand of hair grows, it moves through three development stages: anagen, catagen, and telogen. The anagen stage is your hair's growth period, which typically lasts from 3 to 5 years. At the end of the growth period, the follicle prepares for a rest. The transition period – which typically lasts a month – is called the catagen stage. During this stage, the strand is still secure in the follicle but the lower portion of the follicle collapses. The telogen stage, the resting period, lasts for about 3 to 4 months. At the end of the resting stage, the hair falls from the follicle, a new hair begins to grow, and a new anagen phase begins.

Hair grows about one half-inch (1.2 cm) per month. A normal healthy hair is as strong as copper wire of the same diameter.

Straight or curly

I should also mention that your hair's curl pattern – or lack thereof – is formed deep in the follicle. Here, at the hair's roots, your strands are soft and pliable, adapting themselves to the shape of the surrounding hair follicles. If your follicles are genetically round, they'll create straight hairs; slightly oval follicles produce wavy hair; and flat-oval follicles produce curly hair. Study a cross-section of a straight strand, and you'll see the hair's round shape; study a cross-section of wavy hair, and you'll notice the oval shape; if you cut across a curly strand, you'll see the hair's ovoid shape.

What does all this have to do with curls? A circular cross-section of hair – or yarn, or string, or wire – boasts equal strength in all directions across the fiber. Because this shape features no weaker areas, hair hangs rigidly without coiling in on itself. As with all wirelike entities, an oval or flat-oval cross-section of hair is strongest across the wide part of the cross-section and weakest across the narrow cross-section. Weaker areas aren't rigid like strong areas. Instead, they are flexible and likely to twist around. This means wavy or curly hair boasts enough flexibility through its narrow cross-section to encourage strands to flex (wavy hair) or coil (curly hair).

As the wavy-haired daughter of a straight-haired mother, I feel obliged to offer this advice: Do not make your curly-haired child feel self-conscious about her hair! This can damage her confidence and lead to later abuse of blow-dryers and straighteners. Do not continually ask your child if she has brushed her hair – no amount of brushing is going to make curly hair smooth and it can make it even messier!

INTERNET

www.keratin.com

This comprehensive site features hair-related studies, hair biology lessons, hair news, hair links, and much more.

Enemies of healthy hair

HEALTHY STRANDS boast tightly closed cuticle layers. If hair is in good condition, it shines, swings, feels good when touched, and has no "cotton-candy" ends or split strands. The easiest route to healthy hair is to avoid as many of the following damaging things as possible.

Shampooing

Shampoo works by removing dirt and excess sebum from the hair's surface. Gentle shampoos remove just what they need to. Harsh shampoos, however, can take with them your hair's protective sebum, that necessary natural oil that keeps hair pliable, moisturized, and healthy. In some cases, harsh shampoos also disrupt your hair's cuticle layer, roughing up those tile-like portions and allowing damage to the interior cortex.

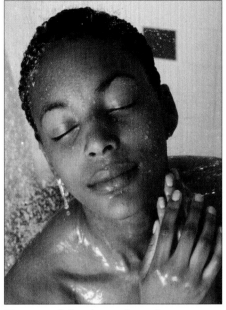

■ **Be careful** *with your hair when you are shampooing it, and when you rinse it out, don't use overly hot water.*

Wet hair is up to 30 percent weaker than dry hair, so handle damp strands carefully! Wait until your locks are dry before doing any heavy-duty brushing, combing, or styling.

Don't overdo it

In countries such as America, where people have a pathological obsession with squeaky-clean tresses, hair is often *overwashed*. (As an American, I am allowed to say all of this.) When strands are shampooed too frequently – this means washing hair when it doesn't need to be washed – there is no dirt for shampoo to remove, so it moves to whatever else happens to be clinging to your strands: This is usually your hair's protective sebum. Get into washing habits that suit your hair and you will benefit from healthy-looking, naturally shiny hair.

> **DEFINITION**
>
> Overwashing *is when you wash your hair more regularly than is necessary. This varies for different individuals. For some people, shampooing hair every day is overwashing, for other people shampooing twice a day, or even every other day, can have the same effect.*

Rough handling

Raking through damp strands with a fine-toothed comb, yanking at tangles, brushing hair 20 times a day, absent-mindedly tugging at locks, backcombing strands for a fuller finish – these all constitute rough handling, and they're all surefire ways to damage fragile tresses.

Every time you handle your hair, even if you just push your fingers through it, you put stress on its cuticle layer, causing the cuticle's tightly overlapping tiles to come unhinged; in hair-care circles, this is known as mechanical damage. Particularly aggressive treatment can even strip away a section of these tiles. When this protective armor is compromised or removed, hair splits, frays, or snaps off.

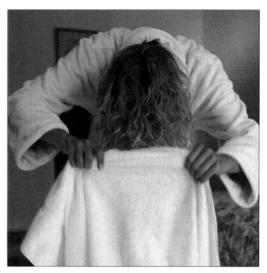

■ **When you dry your hair** *with a towel, gently pat it dry rather than rubbing it vigorously. This will help prevent split ends.*

Hair accessories

Ponytail holders, barrettes, combs, clips – most of us have been using these and other hairdo helpers since childhood. This is fine, as long as you don't use them more than one to three times a week. Wearing your hair day after day in the same style can wear away the hair's cuticle layer and cause breakage in those locks that are contained by the accessory. For instance, the hair directly under a barrette can be roughed up by the friction created between the hair and the ornament's metal clasp.

Similarly, if you're not gentle when removing them, hair accessories can damage locks in another way: Try not to yank free any tresses that become stuck in the hinge of a clip or a barrette or wound around a ponytail holder. Unfortunately, ripping strands out of a hair ornament's grasp can strip away a long swath of the cuticle layer.

■ **Choose hair clips** *with easy-to-remove clasps, and try to limit your use of hair accessories to social occasions, or for keeping it out of your face when you're playing sports.*

THE EVILS OF CHLORINE

Dull, dehydrated locks are a common complaint from those of you who swim often or live in areas with heavily chlorinated tap water. Chlorine is very drying and removes your hair's natural oils – those same oils that coat the hair and give it a shiny finish. Not only does chlorinated pool (and tap) water dry and weaken hair fibers, it can chemically react with hair to cause all kinds of hair glitches.

Crystallizing chlorine

Chlorine damages hair's structure, creating weak, brittle, easily broken strands. As you've read, your hair is protected by a scalelike layer called the cuticle. Chlorine is a type of chemical salt. When mixed with water, chlorine slips easily into individual hair fibers through small spaces between the cuticle scales. When you get out of the pool and your hair dries, the chlorine inside your hair's fibers crystallizes. During the crystallization process – which will take place inside your hair strands – the crystals grow bigger and literally push on the inside of each hair fiber. This pushing disrupts those bonds that give your hair its strength; when this happens, strands become very weak and can actually split apart. A long soak of around 20 minutes or more in pure water after a swim can help get rid of some of the chlorine crystals, but not all. This really is a case when prevention – a swimming cap, for instance – is the best treatment.

Turning a shade of green

Green hair is not news to people with blonde hair. Prolonged exposure to chlorinated water, which contains a high concentration of copper, can give you a slightly grassy-colored coif. The copper chemically reacts with chlorine to create a greenish chemical compound that binds to your hair's cuticle. Prevention is the best treatment: Wear a bathing cap or try swimmer's shampoos that contain edetic acid or D-penicillamine. These are designed to weaken the compound's hold on your hair, but be forewarned: these shampoos can also be drying.

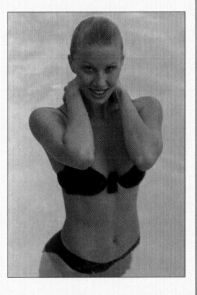

■ **Try combing olive oil,** *or vegetable oil, through damp hair before diving into chlorinated water.*

Heat styling

Ask any dermatologist or stylist what a surefire way to ruin your hair is and they will probably say heat-styling. Heat causes a number of problems: It lifts those tightly fitting tiles that create the cuticle layer, causing small spaces where water and other substances can enter and cause damage. Heat can also damage and remove small chips of the cuticle layer, causing a porous, hole-pocked surface that leaves hair weakened and prone to splitting, fraying, and breaking.

Research has found that blow-dryers operating at over 340° F (175° C) and curling irons, straightening irons, and hot rollers that reach over 250° F (125° C) cause splitting and fraying of the hair shaft.

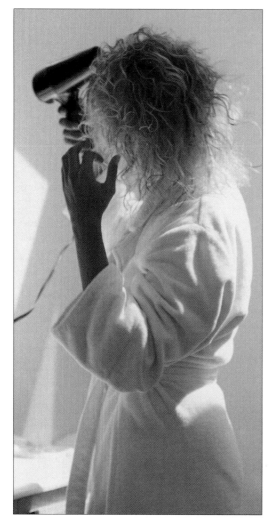

The best way to avoid heat damage is to air-dry hair and stay away from heated curling and straightening appliances. "But my hair looks terrible if I don't blow-dry," you say. First, try talking to your hairdresser about a style that looks fabulous when dried naturally. If you don't settle on an acceptable style, try and stick to the following rules: Blow-dry only when necessary (for example, when you're going out), prep hair with a leave-in conditioner for a bit of protection, and hold the blower at least 6 inches (15 cm) from the head.

As for the curling irons, straightening irons, and hot rollers, find a style that works with your natural texture and you won't need to fuss with these things again.

If you habitually twirl your hair, you're weakening your strands, and this could lead to splitting and breakage.

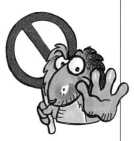

■ **If you blow-dry** *your hair, try to let your hair reach the damp-dry stage before you begin and use the lowest heat setting.*

THOSE ANNOYING FLAKES

An itchy scalp, a feeling of tightness, visible white flakes – if you've ever had dandruff, you've got plenty of company. It is a persistent skin disorder of the scalp caused by a tiny yeast fungus called *Pityrosporum ovale*, or *P. ovale*. This fungus lives on our bodies and scalp all the time, usually without incident. Yet stress, perspiration, hormonal fluctuations, a diet heavy in fat and sugar, or something else entirely can lead to a surge in the amount of *P. ovale* on your scalp. Although dandruff is associated with dryness, people with oily scalps are not immune – in fact, slick scalps are especially attractive breeding grounds for *P. ovale*.

There are numerous dandruff treatments available. Different individuals respond to different types of treatments, so you may want to experiment with the following:

1. **Ketoconazole** The active ingredient in many dermatological formulas and in the over-the-counter products, such as *Nizoral®*. These products are generally used one to three times per week, as long as needed.

2. **Salicylic acid** The beta hydroxy acid you may have read about in the skin-care chapters. When used to fight dandruff, it loosens the flaky scales stuck to your scalp and hair, so that these flakes can easily be washed away. Some dermatologists believe that removing a large portion of these scales makes it uncomfortable for fungus to continue breeding in large amounts.

3. **Selenium sulfide and zinc pyrithione** Two ingredients used in dandruff shampoos such as *Selsun Blue®* and *Head and Shoulders®*. Both ingredients decrease the number of pityrosporon cells on the scalp.

4. **Tar** Found in dandruff shampoos and topical scalp lotions such as *T-gel®*. It is thought that the ingredient is an anti-inflammatory that makes the scalp inhospitable to pityrosporon growth.

5. **Topical steroids** Anti-inflammatory and anti-itch ingredients that are available in shampoos and lotions prescribed by your dermatologist.

If your scalp is pink and you notice scales that are yellower and greasier than normal dandruff scales, you may have a severe form of dandruff known as seborrheic dermatitis and you should see a dermatologist immediately.

Over-processing with chemical treatments

Anything that temporarily or permanently changes the structure of your hair can damage strands. Hair colors, permanent waves, and chemical straightening treatments qualify as strand-wreckers. How much damage a chemical process causes depends on the process. For instance, semi-permanent hair color, which washes out in several shampoos, dries out hair, and lightly roughs up the cuticle. It isn't as injurious as hair bleach, which breaks open the cuticle and bleaches hair's natural pigment to create colorless strands. Similarly, a treatment designed to loosen a person's natural curls won't alter hair as much as a severe straightening service.

Trivia...

If you chew and swallow your hair, hairballs can develop in your stomach over several years. The strands become matted and trap undigested bits of food. They host colonies of bacteria. Surgery is the only way to remove them.

Hair loss

THERE'S A MISCONCEPTION OUT THERE *that hair loss is normal for a man and abnormal for a woman. True, hair loss is more common in men than in women – and society does make it easier for a bald man to feel attractive than it does for a bald woman. Still, women do suffer from hair loss.*

DEFINITION

Diffuse thinning *means steady, non-patchy thinning, either throughout the entire scalp or in a stretch of scalp.*

However, female hair loss is usually a bit different from male hair loss. Unlike men, most women don't get those shiny, bald patches that are completely devoid of hair. If we're going to lose hair, we're more likely to experience *diffuse thinning*. Like men, our hair loss can be the result of simple genetics, but it can also be triggered by a number of other things ranging from stress to illness.

According to conservative estimates, hair loss affects more than 60 million Americans – two-thirds of which are men. Genetic hair loss is the most common form of male and female hair loss. If you have genetic hair loss, you don't shed hair faster or more heavily than anyone else, but your new hairs simply do not grow at the same rate as your old hairs are being shed. The medical term for this inherited condition is androgenetic alopecia. There is no permanent cure for it, although many women find they can stop its progression – or even slightly reverse its progress – with hair loss medications.

In many cases of diffuse hair loss, more than 50 percent of the hair can be lost before the results are readily apparent.

Good health for healthy hair

Nutritional deficiencies can also cause temporary hair loss. The question constantly argued among hair loss experts is how many citizens of First World countries have diets poor enough to cause hair loss? While I can't answer that, I can tell you what deficiencies lead to thinning hair. Iron deficiency (known as anemia) contributes to hair loss. Anemia isn't uncommon in women, especially those of you who lose lots of iron-rich blood through heavy menstrual bleeding. Thinning hair is also a symptom of anorexia and bulimia – sufferers usually do not consume anywhere near the dietary requirements of fats, carbohydrates, and protein.

■ **Make sure you** *eat a well-balanced, nutritious diet if you want to enjoy healthy, shiny hair.*

Illness forces your body to conserve resources, prompting it to route nutrients away from "superfluous" appendages such as hair so that they can be used by vital internal organs. Depending on how long the illness – and how long strands have gone without nutrients – hair can fall out. Fortunately, this form of hair thinning is usually temporary and the hair will soon grow back.

Most people shed between 50 and 100 strands of hair each day; most also grow between 50 and 100 new strands each day.

The effects of stress and medications

Stress, regardless of its cause, changes the way your body works. When faced with an anxiety-provoking situation, your endocrine glands pump out adrenaline, cortisol, and other hormones. These substances have various effects on your body, including reducing blood flow to your hair follicles. The theory goes that a week or more of continual stress reduces nutrient flow to the hair for enough time to cause temporary hair loss. Get rid of the stress (or learn how to face it calmly) and give yourself a month: Your hair will return.

Medications have different effects on different people. For instance, birth-control pills may give you migraines but they may make your sister's skin break out. Aspirin may upset your mother's stomach but could be the only pain reliever that works for you. And so it is with hair loss: a drug that makes a friend feel slightly tired might leave you with temporary hair loss. While your body can react this way with any drug, some are notorious for causing hair loss, including chemotherapy drugs, antibiotics, and antidepressants. Also, if you have had, or are scheduled for, surgery of any kind, be aware that anesthesia can cause a week or two of temporary hair loss in some people.

A PREGNANT PAUSE

During pregnancy, your hair takes a break from shedding, which means that strands stick around for the entire 9 months without falling out. So yes, your skin might be doing unsightly things, you feel like a Buick, gross men can't keep their eyes off your ballooning breasts, and you've got undereye circles from lack of sleep … but gosh, your hair is full, lustrous, and downright gorgeous!

This is because, when you're pregnant, your body is awash in estrogen. This female hormone has an interesting effect on hair: it extends each strand's growth cycle, allowing individual hairs to grow longer than normal without falling out. Furthermore, during pregnancy there is a slight decrease in sebum. Sebum lubricates hair, thus weighing it down. A decrease in this oily material means hair appears less weighed down, which in turn makes your mane seem fuller and fluffier.

Once your pregnancy is over, however, estrogen levels return to normal and you must give up the extra hair. Within 2 or 3 months of giving birth, you'll notice your hair falling out at an alarming rate. Before you race to your dermatologist, remember: your body is making up for lost time. All those thousands of hairs that would have been shed each month during your pregnancy are now leaving en masse. Postpartum alopecia is the official name for this type of hair loss. Deal with it by getting a SMALL trim (post-birth is not the time to try a new coif) to make your hair look fuller, then ignore the defecting strands. This hair loss may go on for 3 to 6 months, until all those holdover strands leave. If your shedding has not slowed a year after the pregnancy, go ahead and consult your dermatologist: In rare instances and for unexplained reasons, some women never re-grow their prepregnancy hair.

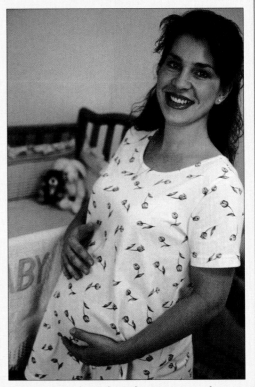

■ **Enjoy the benefits** *of pregnancy, such as having healthy, thicker-looking hair.*

Other reasons for hair loss

When worn daily for a month or more, tight hairstyles – such as cornrows, a severe ponytail, or braids – can damage the hair follicle, making it impossible for new hair to grow. This condition, called traction alopecia, is permanent. Damage to the scalp caused by chemicals used in hair color formulas, permanent waves or relaxer services, burns, or even a blow to the head, can damage hair follicles, causing permanent hair loss.

Sometimes hair loss just happens for no apparent reason. For example, a disease called alopecia areata strikes both men and women and causes diffuse thinning or even patchy baldness. In severe cases, it even causes sufferers to lose their eyelashes, eyebrows, and body hair. What is known about this disease is that it is an immune-system disorder that causes hair follicles to stop producing hair. In some people, alopecia areata is temporary, lasting from several months to several years. In other people, the condition remains, improving or worsening seemingly at whim.

In the United States, about 1 percent of the population have experienced alopecia areata, however about 90 percent of these people have had periodic episodes.

Dealing with thinning hair

One of the most common – and perhaps easiest – ways to deal with thin hair is to use hair-care products designed to add volume to skimpy strands. The thinking behind these products goes something like this: Even a small amount of hair looks like a lot when puffed up into frothy fullness. In addition to shampoos labeled "volumizing" or "thickening," there are also conditioning rinses, leave-in volumizing lotions, styling spritzes, and mousses. If you were born with lank hair and can't pin its causes on anything but heredity, this is a good route to try.

INTERNET

www.morehair.com

This site features everything you could ever want to know about hair growth and hair loss, including products, hairpieces, and medical options for thinning hair.

Stimulating hair growth

You've probably heard a lot about medications designed to stimulate hair growth. While most of the talk – and research – surrounding these drugs focuses on men, many can be used by women with similar effects.

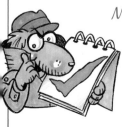

Many medical authorities view thinning hair as a cosmetic issue – which means that your treatment expenses may not be covered.

Minoxidil (or *Rogaine*®, as it is commercially known) began as a treatment for high blood pressure. It evolved into a popular scalp treatment when physicians noticed that it also promoted hair growth.

97

It isn't known exactly how minoxidil helps hair growth, but it seems to stop or slow hair loss and promote a little new growth. The product is massaged onto the scalp two times a day and has been proven to re-grow hair in up to 25 percent of users.

Minoxidil seems to be most effective at the crown and least effective around the face, while the hair it grows is fuzzy and probably finer than the stuff you lost. If you stop using the product, you lose whatever new hair appeared.

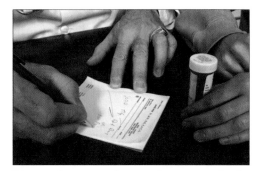

■ **Your doctor or dermatologist** *may decide to prescribe you a drug to help stimulate hair growth or prevent further loss.*

In a small number of people, cortisone shots can help slow or halt loss or stimulate the follicles to grow new hair. However, it has many side effects, including water retention, moodiness, and weight gain, and should be used with caution.

Propecia® is an oral prescription drug used as a treatment for male baldness. However, some maverick dermatologists are successfully using it on their female patients. The drug (also known as *Finestre®*) has been studied on men and has been shown to re-grow natural hair in two out of three men, while halting hair loss in five out of six men. The drug nudges affected hair follicles to re-grow hair that is nearly as thick as the original hair – it is most effective in the crown area. The bad news is that *Propecia®* takes up to 12 months to work, and any hair that re-grows can be lost if you stop taking the medication.

Androgenetic alopecia is the cause of more than 95 percent of both male and female hair loss.

Considering hair pieces

A visible scalp can be covered with wigs, partial hairpieces, and "hair integration units" – in which a web of fake strands is attached to your existing hair. The up side to these options is that none are medical. The down side is that they do not look like natural hair, can be expensive, and can come loose at inopportune times. With the hair integration unit, you must return to the physician or salon every 4 to 6 weeks to have the unit adjusted.

■ **Wigs are made** *from either natural or synthetic hair. You could choose one that matches your natural hair color, or opt for something completely different.*

Looking at the surgical options

While men who often suffer from bald spots are great candidates for hair-transplant surgery – a doctor can harvest a few follicles from a lushly forested area of a guy's head and "replant" the follicles in bald areas – women don't usually get totally bald patches. When we lose hair, we're more likely to suffer from all-over thinning, which makes hair transplants a less successful option for us. However, if you find that most of your thinning is in one place, for example, on your crown, a dermatologist or plastic surgeon may be able to "plant" a few hair-growing follicles through your sparse spots.

The hair follicle growth cycle is about 90 percent growth and about 10 percent rest. At any given time, about 10 percent of your hair follicles are resting and not growing new hairs. The resting follicles are randomly distributed over the scalp, so the resting follicles do not create bald spots.

How hair ages

THINK BACK TO YOUR CHILDHOOD. *Now focus on your pre-adolescent hair. It was probably more vibrant, shinier, fuller, and either lighter or brighter in color than your natural hair is now. There are a few reasons for this.*

During childhood, we have more hair in the growth stage than at any other time, giving us plenty of volume. At this time in your life, the sebaceous glands are working at the peak of their efficiency, which gives strands a high gloss. Hair pigment hasn't started to darken, so your hair color is vibrant, and you probably aren't yet messing around with hair-changing chemical processes, or using heat appliances – all of which can rough up strands' cuticles or strip them away entirely, leaving hair dull and brittle.

Teens and 20s

During your young adult years, hair slowly begins changing from its childhood state: Strands may become coarser, growth may slow just a bit, color grows progressively darker, and the sebaceous activity for most of us goes on overdrive, pumping out oil at a furious rate. (This is the same sebaceous activity that makes your complexion pimply.) The teens and early 20s are a time for experimentation – and rightly so: how else are you going to find out what works for you and what doesn't? Most of you have strong, slightly oily hair and can afford to rough it up a bit with the latest color or texture trends. Notice I said, "most of you." In beauty, as in life, there are no absolutes, and if you happen to be born with fragile hair or sensitive hair, take it easy.

Your 30s, 40s, and 50s

By the time you've reached your 30s, your hair has reached a plateau – the sebum is being produced at a more manageable pace and you have settled (I hope) into your looks and accepted your hair type. Your strands have reached their darkest shade and the biggest surprise awaiting you is probably the appearance of gray.

Blondes, redheads, and light brunettes are more likely to go gray, while deep brunettes have a better chance of going white.

Of course, when you go gray depends on your genetic makeup – if your father and mother didn't see gray until they were 95, then you probably can expect the same; if they both went gray in their 20s, you'll probably be gray by the time you hit 35. The 30s and 40s, however, are a kind of "human average age" for this rite of passage. And while we're on the subject of gray, keep in mind that gray hair does not mean your strands are no longer healthy. It simply means your cortex no longer

YOUR HAIR AND THE CHANGE

You probably know menopause is that time when your ovaries stop producing estrogen. Menopause can occur at any time during your adult years, but most commonly happens during your late 40s to mid-50s. Yet regardless of when it happens, menopause signals the end of your reproductive years, meaning no more pregnancies and no more periods. In my opinion, there are some fabulous benefits to this, including not having to worry about birth control and never suffering from menstrual cramps again. Menopause is not, however, so fabulous for your hair. That's because estrogen protects you against hair loss; without estrogen, your locks may grow noticeably thinner. For those of you who aren't near menopause, ask your mothers, aunts, grandmothers, or post-menopausal friends about how their mane altered after "the change"; most will admit their hair has not only grown a little (or a lot) thinner, but also finer in texture.

More bad news: For those of you genetically predisposed toward female-pattern hair loss, menopause is when you'll learn whether or not you're going to be affected – this also has to do with the sudden lack of hair-helping estrogen. Some women find hormone replacement therapy protects them near-totally or partially from all kinds of post-menopausal hair loss. However, hormone replacement therapy has been linked with breast, endometrial, and liver cancers; discuss the risks with your physician.

contains melanin. Another piece of information: Gray hair often has a wirier texture than pigmented hair, so don't be alarmed if these uncolored strands spring away from your head at strange angles. This is okay – even if you feel a like a Brillo pad.

Your 60s and beyond

By now you may be sporting quite a head of gray – or even white – hair. Sebum production has slowed considerably and your hair may grow drier and less in need of shampooing (and more in need of conditioning). Most humans experience thinning hair with age. By thinning, I don't mean obvious balding – although if you are prone to that, now's the time it will start happening. I simply mean that you will have less hair than you did in your youth. That's because as we age, our hair spends less time in the anagen, or growth, stage, and more time in the catagen (transition) and the telogen (resting) stages. At this point, there should be no great hair surprises for you. Instead, with each decade expect a gradual decrease in sebum production and a gradual increase in graying and thinning.

■ **As your hair thins,** *you may choose to have a permanent wave to help add volume to your hair.*

A simple summary

✔ Hair's primary purpose it to offer us warmth and protection.

✔ Hair is an appendage of the skin.

✔ The less you do to your locks, the healthier they will be.

✔ Hair naturally changes gradually as you age.

✔ The cuticle layer, which is hair's protective coating, is vulnerable to damage.

✔ Thinning is a common occurrence in women.

✔ If you're losing your hair, you have medical and non-medical options to choose between.

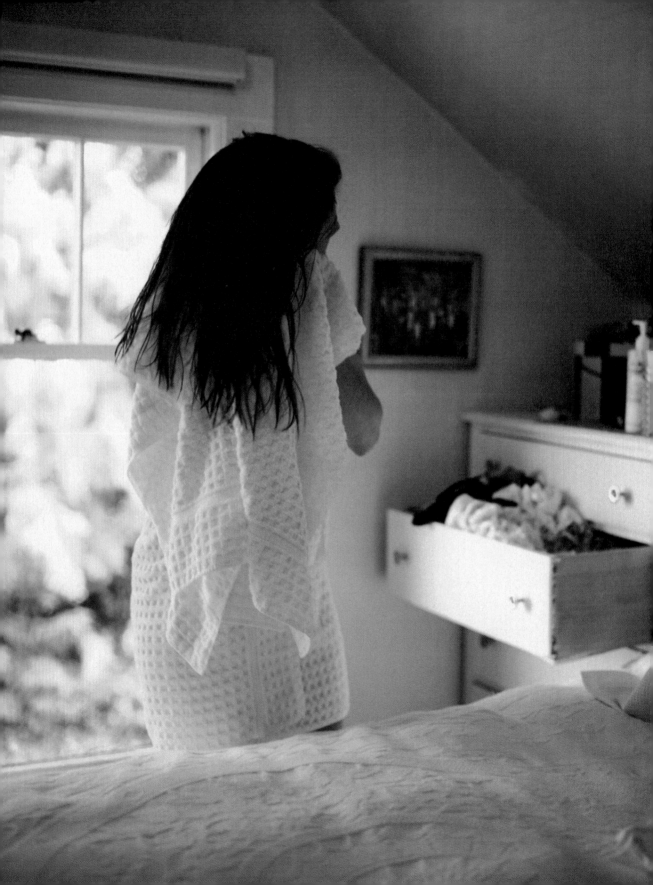

Chapter 7

Caring for Hair

MAGAZINE ARTICLES, OPINIONATED FRIENDS, stylists' advice – there is a lot of information out there aimed at telling you just how to care for your hair. Unfortunately, a lot of it seems contradictory. Should you brush hair 100 times a night, or should you avoid brushing altogether? Must you wash your hair every day or is it important to skip days? And what about conditioner – do you need it, or can you get away without using it? One reason for all the free-floating information: different people have different needs. Keep reading and you'll come away with a few of your own ideas about caring for your hair.

In this chapter...

✓ Brushing the right way

✓ Easy does it

✓ Pre-shampoo treatments

✓ Shampoo basics

✓ Conditioner basics

FIND A HAIRCARE ROUTINE THAT SUITS YOUR HAIR AND YOUR LIFESTYLE

Brushing the right way

I GREW UP SURROUNDED by hair-brushing lore: Brushing hair at midnight on the eve of a full moon was supposed to make strands grow faster and longer, brushing with someone else's brush gave you dandruff, and brushing your hair 100 times could make your hair oily or keep your scalp clean, depending on who you asked. On the other hand, brushing not at all – an idea that sounded pretty good to me as a child – proved you had been brought up badly.

Trivia...

The 100-strokes rule of hair-brushing has its roots in necessity: Before hair conditioners were invented, women relied on hair's sebum to moisturize strands. Getting the sebum from hair's roots to hair's tips required vigorous brushing.

INTERNET

www.helenecurtis.com

This trendy site features everything from information on hair health to picking a perfect hairstyle.

Despite all this advice, however, no one discussed what kind of brush I should use, or even how to use it. For answers to these questions I paid special attention to my friends' mothers as they cared for my playmates' hair. Every mom had a different method: One saturated her daughter's head with a spray-on detangler and reached for a wide-tooth comb. Another would fumble in her handbag for a small nylon-bristled brush, which she violently raked through her stoic child's tresses. Yet another mom would section her girl's locks into four parts and pull a wooden natural-bristled brush from root to tip, root to tip, until all strands had been groomed. I no longer have friends who live with their mothers, so for hair-care advice I turn to hairdressers, who have shown me exactly what kind of brush to use and how to use it – information I will happily pass on to you.

The right brush and comb

When was the last time you actually went shopping for a hairbrush? If you're like me, you have a drawer full of brushes that your hairstylist gave you, that came packaged with a bottle of shampoo as a promotional item, or that found themselves into your hair-care collection some other way. Still, you've never gone out and actually shopped for a hairbrush – nor a comb, for that matter. Well, perhaps it's time you did.

In high-quality brushes you might notice the bristles are set at uneven lengths. This prevents the bristles from snagging and pulling hair and it also makes the brush more effective at gentle detangling.

A high-quality brush is solidly built, with bristles that are strong enough to stand up to the toughest strands yet sensitive enough to move natural oils from your scalp down the length of the strands without scratching the scalp or causing splits, breaks, or other types of damage. Of course, your hair type is an important thing to consider when choosing a brush that works for you. Here's a rundown of various types of brushes:

Boar-bristle brushes

Natural boar-bristle hairbrushes have bristles made from the hair of the adult boar. If you look at these bristles with a magnifying glass, you can see that each bristle is scaly rather than smooth in texture; this helps remove dirt from the hair shaft and distribute the follicles' moisturizing sebum from the scalp to the hairs' ends. Thin hair, medium hair, straight hair, and wavy hair are all well suited to natural boar-bristle brushes.

Boar bristle brushes come in the traditional paddle, rounded, and half-rounded styles. Take care of them and they'll last decades.

■ **If you opt for a bristle brush,** *it is important to choose one with bristles that are long enough to contact the scalp in order to distribute the sebum.*

BRUSH CARE

A good-quality brush can be an expensive investment – but one that can last for many years if cared for correctly. Store your brush in a place where it won't get knocked around or banged against other objects. Make sure you gently remove hairs from bristles after using.

Wash your brush

Wash bristles weekly: add one or two tablespoons of mild shampoo to your bathroom sink and fill with warm water. Holding the brush by its handle, carefully dip the bristles into the sudsy water and swish around. Rinse the bristles in warm water. Take care not to get the base of the brush wet (or at least don't get it too wet) or you risk loosening the bristles from the brush's head.

Synthetic brushes

Nylon bristles do a good job of massaging the scalp. However, because the individual bristles are smoother than natural boar bristles, they do a poor job of cleaning the hair shaft and distributing moisturizing sebum along the hair shaft. Still, people with very thick or very curly hair may find a pure boar-bristle brush to be too soft to penetrate their hair, making nylon bristles a good choice. Choose a brush with rounded ends that won't scratch the scalp. Some nylon brushes feature a metal base that retains heat during blow-drying; this helps the brush act as a freestyle hot roller.

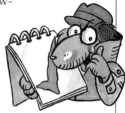

Like natural boar-bristle brushes, nylon bristle brushes come in the traditional paddle, rounded, and half-rounded styles.

Boar-synthetic bristle combination brushes feature a mix of natural boar bristles and nylon bristles. The combination of bristles makes these brushes ideal for anyone with thick or curly hair who needs the stiffness of a nylon bristle, but who wants the shaft-cleaning and moisture-distributing ability of boar bristles. Combination brushes are most popular in paddle styles, but can be found in round and half-round shapes.

The vent brush features inflexible plastic or rubber bristles imbedded in a vented base. It does not massage the scalp, help remove dirt, or distribute sebum; this type of brush is for styling only, and is often used during blow-drying. Because vent brushes can snag and pull hair, I don't recommend them.

■ **This synthetic vent** *styling brush is best for shaping hair while you are blow-drying.*

Using combs and picks

Combs and picks aren't necessary for everyone: some people use them, others simply rake gently through hair with their fingers. If you are a comb or pick user, look for a model with rounded, widely spaced teeth – these are gentler on hair than pointy-tipped, fine-toothed combs. Furthermore, make sure each individual tooth is smooth, without cracks or burs that can catch hair and rip away strands' cuticle layer. Hard rubber, hard silicone, and polished wood are the most hair-friendly materials.

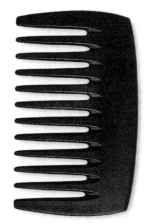

■ **Choose a comb** *with gently rounded ends to protect your hair.*

Brushing techniques

There are two reasons to brush your hair. The most obvious one is grooming – your coif looks messy, so you brush it into submission. For this type of brushing, work gently and do as little as possible: too much brushing can upset your style. The other reason for brushing is scalp and hair health. Now I realize that a bit of controversy surrounds this type of hair brushing. Some people believe the less you brush your hair, the healthier it will be; other folks claim that faithful brushing keeps the hair and scalp healthy by clearing away debris from the scalp and strands, massaging the scalp, and distributing moisturizing sebum through hair.

Regular brushing gives hair a natural shine and is said to create locks that are healthier, more manageable, and easier to style.

My own opinion is what I call "moderately pro-brushing." Through experience I've found a thorough brushing not only makes my hair look prettier, it dissuades oil from pooling around my roots and lifts dry flaky skin cells off my scalp. The best time to give your hair a thorough brushing is right before you hit the shower. I'll admit this is a bit arbitrary, so if you want to give yourself a thorough brushing in the middle of the day or before going out at night, go ahead. However, be aware that intense brushing loosens dead scalp flakes, which gives your hair a "dandruffy" look. Also, if you have wavy or curly hair, an in-depth brushing can create an electric, high-frizz finish. (Now you see why I like to hit the shower after brushing!)

■ **A good, thorough brushing** *helps keep your hair clean and your scalp healthy.*

Handy hints

You've been brushing your hair for years – do you really need someone to tell you how to do it? Maybe not, but I'm nonetheless going to tell you what I've picked up from several dozen hairdressers. Before you whip out the brush, take a wide-tooth comb or use your fingers and gently go through the ends of your hair to remove tangles, knots, snarls, and so on. Bend over at the waist. Start at one ear and, working around the neckline, brush in long strokes from scalp to tip.

I do not believe in giving tresses 100 strokes a day – after all, too much of any good thing can, with time, create damage. Each section needs only two or three "rake-throughs" before you move on.

INTERNET

www.hair-news.com

This site is dedicated to the "art and science of hair." Aimed at professionals, it still offers plenty of features for us regular folk, including "The Lab," which boasts dozens of hair, skin, and body recipes.

After you've finished working the neckline, remain bent over and separate your hair from nape to crown as if you were creating two ponytails. Starting at the nape and working toward the crown, brush strands on one side of the horizontal part. Repeat with the hair on the other side of the part.

Only dry hair should be brushed. Damp or wet hair is weak and vulnerable to breaking. If you must detangle wet hair, do it in the shower while you have conditioner in your hair. Work gently and use a wide-tooth comb or hair pick.

Stand up. Brush hair around the hairline by starting at one ear, moving toward the opposite ear, and directing hair back off the face. When you've finished, part hair in the center. Brush the hair on one side of the part. Repeat on the other side. Note: Those of you with curls or very thick hair may have to create a few more sections to ensure that every part of your scalp and hair gets brushed.

Those of us with longer hair, fragile hair, or hair that we're trying to grow must be more mindful of how we handle our strands.

DAMAGE CHECK

Wondering if your hair is in bad shape? Take one of the following tests and find out:

1. Pluck a strand, drop it in a bowl of tepid water, and give the strand a light nudge with your finger. If the strand floats, your hair is in fine shape. If the strand sinks, it's a sign your hair could use some tender loving care in the way of trims, gentle handling, pre-shampoo treatments, a gentler shampoo, deep-conditioning treatments and, yes, a moratorium on the heat-styling.

2. Yank out a strand and examine it under a magnifying glass. If you see signs of fraying or splitting, you need to take the action outlined above.

Easy does it

ROUGH TREATMENT of any kind – whether shampooing, brushing, or something else entirely – can damage individual hairs permanently. Unfortunately, once a strand is damaged, it can't be repaired. To keep the damage from moving up the strand and compromising more of the hair, a haircut is your only option. To keep hair shiny, and voluminous, you must be mindful of how you treat strands. Abuse them and you will be repaid in split ends, frayed shafts, and brittleness.

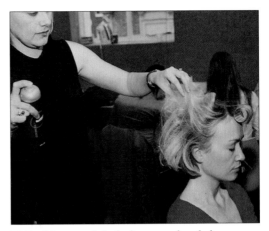

■ **Fashion models** *look groomed and glamorous but their hair is often subjected to extremely harsh treatments that can cause permanent damage.*

Styles to avoid

Each person's hair has a different personality. Except for the area around my face, where it's straight, my hair likes to wave in zigzags down my back. Perhaps your hair's natural inclination is to hang stick-straight or to leap away from your head in crazy curlicues. Fight your hair's disposition and you end up in a battle of wills for hairstyle dominance. Sure, you can make your ringlets straight, but you're going to have to beat them into submission with a relaxer service, or blow-dry them every morning, and perhaps you'll even need to use a straightening iron.

If you want to live peacefully with your hair, you've got to learn to accept it's natural tendencies, which brings me to this rule of thumb: The more a finished hairdo differs from your God-given hair, the rougher you'll need to be with your strands. For example, to look curly, straight hair must undergo permanent waves, curling irons, or being shaped by rollers. To look straight, curly locks must submit to relaxing services, the blow-dryer, or straightening irons. To look full, thin hair is often set on rollers and heavily *backcombed*. And so on. So when it comes to hairstyles, the least damaging looks (and the easiest to achieve) are those that go with your hair's natural flow.

DEFINITION

Backcombed is another word for teased. To backcomb, pull a small section of hair – about ½–2 inches (1–5 cm) wide – above the scalp. Insert a fine-tooth comb midway into the hair section and begin combing backward down toward the root. This lightly mats hair, which in turn forces strands to stand away from the scalp. While backcombing gives hair height and a look of fullness, it also has the effect of weakening strands and damaging the hair.

Using hair ornaments wisely

I grew up wearing barrettes. My sister always had ponytails. Every morning before school, I sat on my mother's bed. She would stand next to me and run a fine-tooth comb through my long, wavy, very tangled hair. After parting my hair, my mother gathered the tresses above each ear and forced the strands into metal drugstore barrettes. Then she would go to work on my sister's hair: pulling the strands tight for a neat, smooth finish, then winding the ponytail holder again and again and again around the blonde pigtails until my sister's coif was secure enough to withstand tag, monkey bars, kickball and grade school boys. When we finally stumbled from the house and onto the sidewalk, we were joined by neighborhood girls wearing beribboned hair clips, plastic headbands, red or yellow rubber bands, baubled ponytail holders, or small barrettes shaped like bows or puppies. As we walked toward the elementary school, one of us, then another, would move a hand toward our heads – but our strands were so tightly fixed in place that nothing ever moved.

■ **If you like to wear barrettes,** *avoid those with sharp edges that can catch and rip the hair, causing permanent damage.*

The average non-damaged strand is strong enough to suspend 3½ oz (100 grams) in weight.

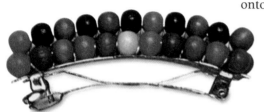

During our childhoods, it seemed essential that hair stayed put. Today we know better. When hair ornaments pull tresses tautly in place, or when they clamp down tightly around strands, they stress the hair shaft and weaken its cuticle layer. (I won't even go into the headaches that incorrectly worn hair ornaments can give.) When using hair ornaments, keep locks somewhat loose, do not overstuff the barrette, clip, or ponytail holder, and don't wear the same style day after day – another way to stress certain portions of the strand and cause breakage. Furthermore, when shopping for hair ornaments, look for barrettes, clips, and headbands with smooth finishes. Ponytail holders should be soft with no visible metal that can catch hair – and don't ever use rubber bands on hair. They are notorious cuticle-strippers.

■ **Use decorative ribbon** *to define a hairstyle, without pulling it in tight and damaging the hair.*

Pre-shampoo treatments

PRE-SHAMPOO TREATMENTS *are not necessary, so if you're the type who hates any kind of extras, head straight for the shampoo section. If, however, you love luxuries (even inexpensive ones), or have a special hair-care need you'd like to address, keep reading. As the name implies, pre-shampoo treatments are performed before shampooing. Some incorporate feel-good elements, such as massage, while others are strictly business.*

Scalp massage

There is a lot of controversy surrounding scalp massages. More specifically, there is a lot of controversy regarding whether or not scalp massage can help treat thinning hair. Proponents claim scalp massage stimulates blood flow to the scalp, which in turn helps nourish follicles, which in turn prevents hair loss and even prompts new growth. Massage has been proven to stimulate circulation, but whether or not it helps hair loss I don't know. But after having my first scalp massage, I no longer care. The treatment feels so good and leaves my hair looking so amazing that I am hooked.

The fanciest of scalp massages, often called scalp treatments, are given in salons or spas.

Specially prepared oils are massaged into your scalp, then brushed through the hair. These oils are specifically chosen to address your particular needs – perhaps oily scalp, sensitive scalp, dryness, or extreme hair damage. Next, your head is wrapped in a warm towel and you are encouraged to relax while the oil goes to work on your scalp and hair. If you're lucky, the treatment will also include a neck and even a shoulder massage. The service is then finished off with a shampoo and a deep-conditioning treatment for the hair.

■ **When having a scalp massage,** *oils are gently worked into the scalp and through the hair.*

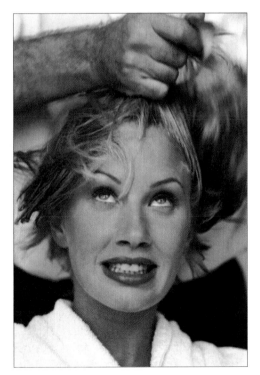

Try it yourself

To give yourself a home treatment, purchase a specially formulated scalp oil (Rene Furterer, Phytologie, and Philip B make them). A cheaper option for those of you with normal to dry scalp and hair is to use 2 to 4 tablespoons of almond or sesame oil (which are much easier to shampoo out than any of your everyday kitchen oils).

Start with dry hair and part hair into four or more sections. Drizzle a little oil onto the exposed areas of scalp and start massaging it in with the pads of your fingertips, working the oil gently and thoroughly over your entire scalp.

Use a natural boar-bristle brush to work the oil through your hair. Then, wrap your hair in a warm or room-temperature towel and relax for at least half an hour before washing your hair with your favorite shampoo, gently massaging your scalp as you go. Rinse, rinse, and rinse some more, to remove all traces of the shampoo and then apply your favorite conditioner. If your hair is very dry, you might want to use a deep conditioner, leaving it in for the full amount of time recommended on the product. Then, you must rinse your hair thoroughly again and leave your hair to air dry. You should feel relaxed, refreshed and pampered!

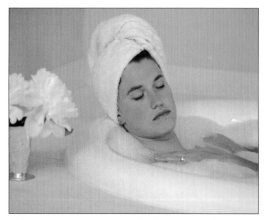

■ **Once you have** *applied oil to your scalp and brushed it through your hair, lie back in a fragrant tub and relax while the oil takes effect.*

Pre-shampoo conditioners

Conditioning your hair before shampooing helps give damaged hair protection against detergents, and it also gives dry, damaged, or chemically treated strands extra moisture. Available pre-shampoo treatments include moisturizing creams (I love J. F. Lazartigue's *Pre-Shampoo Cream with Shea Butter®*), hot-oil treatments (think *Alberto VO5®*), and homemade hot-oil treatments (heat 2 to 4 tablespoons of almond or sesame oil and apply to hair). These conditioners are usually applied to dry hair and left on for up to an hour. Hair is then shampooed and a regular rinse-out conditioner is used. Note: If hair is fine, thin, or oily, you may not need the after-shampoo conditioner.

Oily hair looks oily upon waking and generally must be washed every day or every other day. Normal hair can go for 2 or 3 days without shampooing, and dry hair looks fine for 3, 4, 5 days – even a week – without a shampoo.

Clarifying treatments

Most shampoos on the market are strong enough to clarify without help, but for people who frequently use styling products, *clarifying* treatments can help return locks to their original gloss and bounce. These treatments – which are available as pre-shampoo formulas or as actual clarifying shampoos – dissolve product remnants, allowing vestiges of hairspray, gel, mousse, and more to be rinsed from strands. Clarifying treatments are also helpful for people who live with deposit-causing, mineral-rich water. Overuse of clarifying products can strip necessary sebum from the hair, so limit treatments to once a month.

> **DEFINITION**
>
> *In hair-speak,* clarifying *means clearing hair of build-up – that shine-dulling stuff that remains on the hair after daily use of styling products.*

Shampoo basics

SHAMPOO IS LIKE SOAP FOR YOUR HAIR – in fact, until recently, soap was what most people used to clean their tresses. Its primary purpose is to clean dirt and excess oil from your strands. That's it.

Shampoo can contain any number of the following ingredients:

 Water is usually the first or second ingredient listed on a bottle of shampoo. It dilutes the detergent and gives shampoo bulk.

 Surfactants are detergents that cleanse and create lather. Because it is cheap to produce, sodium lauryl sulfate is the most popular detergent and is usually the only detergent used in supermarket and drugstore shampoos. Unfortunately, it is incredibly harsh – and, if you believe the rumors moving through the beauty industry – it may also pose a cancer risk. Other surfactants include sodium laureth sulfate, sodium cocoyl isetheoinate, methyl cocoyl taurate, cocamidopropyl betaine, cocamidopropylamine oxide, ammonium lauryl sulfate, ammonium laureth sulfate, and alpha olefin sulfonate.

c) Detanglers and anti-static agents are found in some shampoos. Quaternary ammonium compounds are common.

d) Humectants attract and retain water. Found most often in shampoos for dry, damaged, or chemically treated hair, the most common of these include glycerin, sorbitol, and hyaluronic acid.

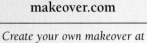

> **INTERNET**
>
> **www.visual-makeover.com**
>
> *Create your own makeover at this amusing site. Or just spend time reading about hair care and hair trends.*

Conditioning agents soften hair and retain moisture. Examples include amino acids, collagen, panthenol, proteins, and elastin.

 Thickening agents give shampoos viscosity and make them easy to handle. A commonly used thickening agent is hydroxyethyl cellulose.

 Preservatives prevent contamination from mold or bacteria. Search the label for methylparaben, quaternium-15, or propylparaben.

Cosmetic ingredients – and this includes hair-care products – are listed in descending order. This means a product contains most of whatever ingredient is listed first, and least of whatever ingredient is listed last.

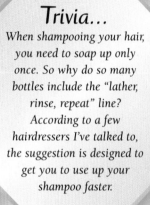

Trivia...

When shampooing your hair, you need to soap up only once. So why do so many bottles include the "lather, rinse, repeat" line? According to a few hairdressers I've talked to, the suggestion is designed to get you to use up your shampoo faster.

Choosing a shampoo

How a shampoo cleans your hair is what makes you fall in love with it or wish you'd never purchased it: Some shampoos are aggressive and not only sweep away dirt, but also your hair's protective sebum – in fact, some are so aggressive that they rough up your hair's cuticle layer. Others contain high doses of moisturizer – too much, perhaps, for your hair. To help you find a shampoo that works for your hair type, many manufacturers create formulas for specific hair types.

Daily or normal hair shampoos are middle-of-the-road shampoos with a balance of cleaning and moisturizing properties. Moisturizing shampoos contain less detergent than other shampoos. They also boast a generous dose of conditioners to attract and retain moisture, making them ideal for dry, damaged, permed, or color-treated hair.

Deep cleansing or oily hair shampoos contain a concentrated dose of detergents to remove impurities and oils. These often rough up the cuticle. For this reason, only the oiliest of the oily among you should use these – experiment first with normal hair shampoos. If they don't leave your hair as clean as you'd like it, then try an oily hair formula. Specialty formulas include shampoos to add body to limp hair, make gray hair sparkle, or coddle colored strands.

When washing hair, concentrate shampoo at hair's roots and allow shampoo to slide down the hair shaft as it is being rinsed out. Lathering the entire head creates tangles and dries out the hair's fragile ends.

DRUGSTORE VERSUS SALON SHAMPOOS

I have tried every salon shampoo around, as well as all of the drugstore and supermarket brands, and as much as I hate to admit this, the salon formulas are generally better than the mass-market versions. After doing some research, I think I know why this is: to keep prices down, mass-market shampoos use cheap ingredients, which are usually harsh and lack the finesse of high-quality ones. For example, I have yet to find a mass-market shampoo that doesn't use harsh surfactants – usually sodium lauryl sulfate, but sometimes sodium laureth sulfate or ammonium laurel sulfate. One of these detergents is usually the first or second ingredient listed, meaning there is a high concentration of the ingredient. Salon products, on the other hand, are more likely to use gentle, more expensive detergents, such as sodium cocoyl isetheoinate, methyl cocoyl taurate, cocamidopropyl betaine, or cocamidopropylamine oxide. Many salon products also bury detergent in the middle of the ingredient list, meaning the shampoo isn't as harsh and is less likely to strip hair of natural oils and cuticle bits.

Yet not everyone wants to spend $10 or more on something that will be on their hair only a few seconds. To "healthy up" a mass-market shampoo, dilute it (try 1 part water to 2 parts shampoo) or use the recipe below to make it a bit less harsh, and a bit more conditioning.

If you're on a limited budget, go ahead and buy a drugstore shampoo and reserve the rest of your hairdo dollars for a high-quality conditioner – a product that can make a huge difference to how your tresses behave.

Semi-homemade shampoo

- 2 teaspoons almond, sesame, avocado, or macadamia nut oil
- 1 tablespoon coconut milk or cow's milk
- ¼ cup shampoo of choice (you can also use an equal amount of liquid castile soap, such as *Dr. Bronner's®*)

Combine ingredients in a bowl and whisk for 2 or 3 minutes, or combine ingredients in a blender and mix on low for 25 seconds. To use, wet hair and massage appropriate amount of the mixture into your hair's roots. Rinse well. If desired, follow with your favorite conditioner. This makes enough for two shampoos. The remaining portion can be covered and refrigerated for up to 2 days.

Should I wash my hair every day?

Unless your hair is supremely oily, washing hair every day is not only unnecessary, it can be damaging. Taking every other day off from shampoo – or even 2 or more days off if your hair is dry or damaged – gives your hair a break from the detergents and the inevitable roughness that comes with shampooing, both of which can rough up hair's protective cuticle layer. A day away from shampoo also allows sebum – hair's natural conditioner – to get a foothold in individual strands. And for those who are trying to live life more simply (read: use less stuff), shampooing less frequently means using less shampoo.

Most of us like suds, which is why shampoo manufacturers often make high-foaming formulas. Yet suds have nothing to do with a shampoo's cleansing power. In fact, the lesser-foaming formulas are gentler on hair.

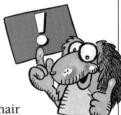

When I was a teenager, my friends and I never admitted to washing our hair any less than once a day – in fact, some of my friends used to brag about washing their hair twice a day. I told this story to a hairstylist once and he laughed. "For some strange reason, people get squeamish if you tell them to stop washing their hair every day. It's as if they think easing up on the shampoo is going to make them unclean," he said. After years of interviewing hairstylists and dermatologists, I've learned exactly what he is saying – and it has nothing to do with giving up bathing or showering.

Go ahead and get in the shower, go ahead and get your hair wet – just don't pull out the shampoo. I think you'll find that a good pre-shower brushing and a heavy dousing of old-fashioned plain water will do wonders for your hair. The brushing loosens up dirt, dead flaky skin, debris, and excess scalp oil, which the water then rinses away. If you're worried about tangles, go ahead and work a bit of detangler or a light conditioner through wet ends then rinse out – again, just no shampoo.

■ **Many shampoos** *create a lot of foam but this is not an indication of their cleansing ability. Try a low-foam product for a gentler wash.*

Conditioner basics

DO YOU NEED A CONDITIONER? Not every hair type requires it but most of us do. Conditioner adds moisture to the hair – some of the product may even sneak under the protective cuticle layers to infuse the inner strands with a temporary surge of moisture. It lubricates strands, helping to reduce static electricity, keeping hair from getting dry and brittle, and making locks easy to brush.

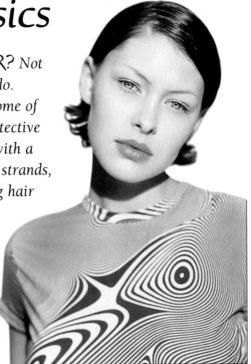

Conditioner acts as a temporary spackle that fills in chinks in the cuticle layer. This keeps strands from tangling around each other as you brush and style your hair. Conditioner also forms a protective seal around hair, which forces the cuticle to lie flat – this flat surface reflects light and makes hair shine.

■ **If your hair** *is short, oily, and in terrific condition you may not need conditioner.*

"LOOKALIKES"

Aveda, Matrix, Paul Mitchell, Nexxus – these brands are known as professional products because they are used by salon professionals. However, next time you visit a drugstore or supermarket, don't be surprised to find lookalike shampoos and conditioners that mimic salon products. Often the wannabe formulas will feature a tagline such as "Compare to Nexxus" or "If you like Aveda, you'll love this." What's the difference between the lookalikes and the real deals? Quality. Drugstore copycats generally contain the same fragrance and colors as the salon originals – some even contain minute concentrations of those pricey ingredients which salon brands use in high doses. Yet the mass-market formulas rely on harsh, inexpensive detergents and low-quality conditioners, both of which keep costs low enough for drugstore and supermarket shoppers to afford.

Lubricants and emollients are used in conditioners. They attract and lock in moisture. These can include vegetable oils, mineral oil, plant oil, and vitamin B derivatives. Proteins are popular conditioner ingredients and can include collagen, elastin, and amino acids, which are small, natural building blocks of hair that penetrate the cuticle to strengthen strands. Some conditioners contain shine enhancers such as dimethicone, which helps to smooth cuticles.

Choosing an after-shampoo conditioner

Because there is a wide variety of hair types and hair needs, there is also a wide variety of after-shampoo conditioner formulas. Sometimes called rinse-out, regular, everyday, or instant conditioners, these products are the ones you apply after every shampoo, leave on for 1 to 5 minutes, then rinse out.

Trivia...

When you are choosing a conditioner, you may sometimes see the term "hydrolyzed" in front of a protein ingredient. Most protein molecules are too large to penetrate a hair's cuticle layer. Hydrolyzed means that water has been used to break the proteins down to a smaller size so that they can better penetrate the hair's cuticle.

DEFINITION

A thermal formula conditioner contains ingredients that remain on the hair after rinsing. When exposed to heat – say, a blow-dryer – these ingredients penetrate the cuticle slightly to help insulate strands from high temperatures.

Detanglers are very light conditioners. Their main purpose is to smooth strands and keep hair from tangling. Because they are not moisture-rich, detanglers are best for fine hair, oily hair, or for use whenever you don't need a lot of moisturizing but still want hair to behave.

Body-building conditioners are great for fine, lank hair. Because they are so light, they don't add a lot of moisture. Instead they detangle hair and leave strands looking firmer, thicker, and fuller. Balancing or normal hair conditioners are middle-of-the-road conditioners that are not too light, not too heavy. This makes them ideal for normal hair. For those of you who can't give up your blow-dryers, look for *thermal formulas.*

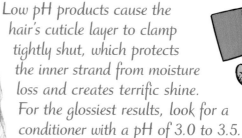

Low pH products cause the hair's cuticle layer to clamp tightly shut, which protects the inner strand from moisture loss and creates terrific shine. For the glossiest results, look for a conditioner with a pH of 3.0 to 3.5.

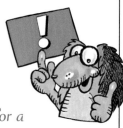

■ **The right conditioner** *can keep hair moisturized and tangle-free. Choose one that suits your hair type.*

MAKE YOUR OWN

If you like do-it-yourself projects, here are two conditioners for you to try:

Semi-homemade spray-on conditioner

- 1 tablespoon of your favorite conditioner
- 8-ounce (227-gram) spray bottle
- Water

Place a tablespoon of your favorite conditioner in the spray bottle, then fill it up with water. Shake well before using to control frizzies, condition dry ends, or to treat dehydrated hair. Note: For less conditioning, use less conditioner; for more conditioning, add more conditioner.

Homemade deep conditioner

- 4 teaspoons almond, sesame, or avocado oil
- 2 teaspoons coconut oil (available in health food stores and at West Indian grocers)
- 3 teaspoons honey
- 1 teaspoon cider vinegar

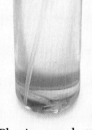

■ **Plastic spray bottles** *are readily available from most drugstores.*

In a saucepan, slowly heat all the ingredients except for the honey and vinegar. Remove from the heat, allow to cool, then stir in the honey and vinegar. After shampooing, massage the mixture into the hair, comb through the strands, and leave on for 15 minutes. Rinse well with warm water.

■ **Keep any suitable reusable bottles** *for storing your own homemade beauty products. Make sure that mixtures created from perishable products or foodstuffs are always stored in the refrigerator and used up within a few weeks, since they can deteriorate over time.*

Conditioners for dry or damaged hair

Conditioners for dry or chemically treated hair are heavier than those for normal hair and take into account the special needs of moisture-starved dry or chemically treated hair. These conditioners leave a bit of residue to lubricate and protect strands.

Conditioners for damaged hair use high concentrations of lubricants and proteins to nurture hair that is fragile, frayed, ultra-dry, or injured by color, permanent waves, or relaxing services. Damaged hair formulas leave some protective residue on strands to keep locks moisturized and insulated from further damage.

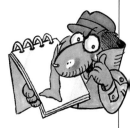

Spray-on conditioners are great for those of you with dry, damaged, wavy, curly, or frizz-prone hair. Just mist on craggy-looking spots whenever needed.

What are leave-in conditioners?

Leave-in conditioners are light moisturizers that are not rinsed out. They come in two forms: Cream is applied to damp hair, and liquid is misted on damp or dry hair. Because leave-in conditioners are so light, many hairdressers recommend them for people with fine hair. However, they can be used by anyone. I adore leave-in conditioners for the extra level of protection and frizz-control they offer my dry hair. I use a leave-in conditioner in addition to using a regular rinse-out conditioner for dry hair, but the fine-haired or oily-haired among you will do best with one or the other. For a really super shine, treat your hair to a cold water final rinse. Cold water forces your hair's cuticle tiles to lie tightly shut, creating a smooth surface from which light can bounce.

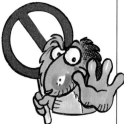

Do not use overly hot water to rinse conditioner from your hair, because it will damage your strands.

■ **After rinsing,** *wrap your hair tightly in a towel to remove as much excess moisture as possible before applying a leave-in conditioner.*

About deep conditioners

If your hair is oily, you don't need a deep conditioner. If your hair is fine in texture or normal in temperament, you probably don't need a deep conditioner. But if you are sporting dry, damaged, wavy, curly, or chemically treated tresses, a deep conditioner is a must. These intensive conditioners – sometimes called hair-repair treatments, moisturizing packs, or hair masks – boast super-concentrated levels of high-powered moisturizers. They are designed to penetrate the cuticle and condition hair, fill in gaps in the cuticle layer, add a degree of strength to fragile strands, and blanket hair in protective lubricants, as well as prevent tangles.

INTERNET

www.supercuts.com

At the official site for Supercuts salons, you can find such treasures as a glossary of hair products, ingredient lists for shampoo, conditioner, and styling products, plus a feature to choose the best hair-care products for your needs.

Most deep conditioners are used immediately after shampooing and allowed to sit for 10 minutes to 2 hours. Some require that you wrap your head in a towel, others suggest you apply heat to help the product better penetrate the cuticle layer, and others need nothing more than for you to sit around for a little while. If your mane is merely dry, a treatment every 1 or 2 weeks should be enough; if your tresses are fried you might benefit from a treatment after every shampoo – in fact, you might try replacing your regular everyday conditioner with a deep conditioner until your hair improves.

A simple summary

✔ Take your time when brushing your hair.

✔ Choose a brush that helps, not harms, your hair.

✔ An easy touch keeps tresses beautiful.

✔ Be careful when using hair ornaments.

✔ You probably don't need to shampoo every day.

✔ Most of us need a conditioner to maintain our hair's health.

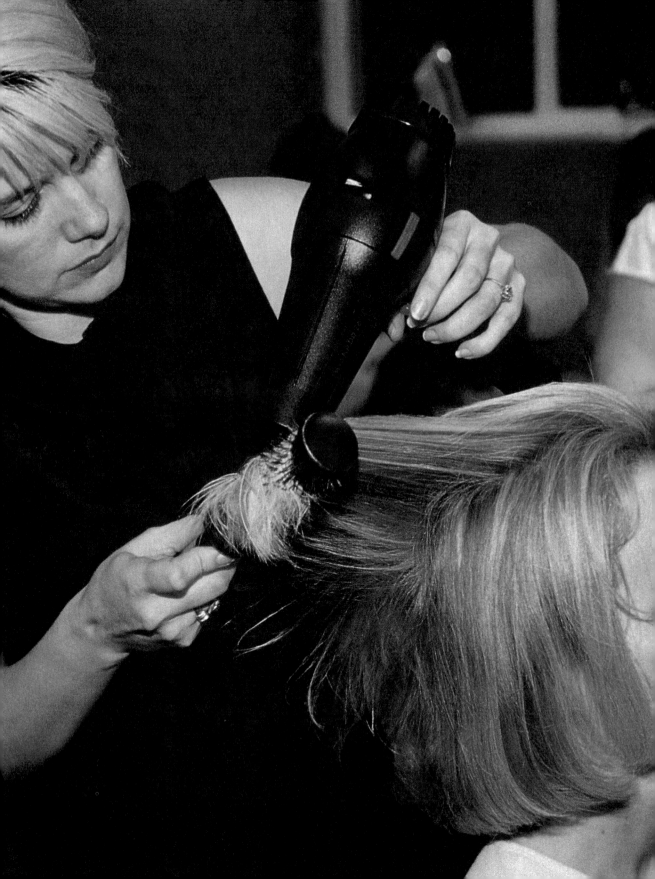

Chapter 8

Hairstyle Essentials

T HE PERFECT HAIRSTYLE — WHO ISN'T SEARCHING FOR IT? Most of us spend hundreds of dollars each year (and almost as many hours) in salons and drugstore hair-care aisles trying to create it. But what, exactly, is a perfect haircut? Something that can be styled with a flick of a brush? Something that plays up your eyes and makes your wide jaw seem slimmer? Something that makes you look 10 years younger? Yes, yes, and yes. Furthermore, the ideal hairdo suits your tastes, age, and schedule and is easily adaptable to a wide range of quick-change styling options. Do your homework and you can get just such a look.

In this chapter...

✓ What makes a good hairstyle?

✓ Creating a signature style

✓ Small changes: Updating your look

✓ A good hairdresser

CHOOSE A HAIRDRESSER YOU CAN TRUST BECAUSE YOU PUT YOUR HAIR IN THEIR HANDS!

What makes a good hairstyle?

THERE WAS A TIME when I had just one criterion for a hairstyle: sex appeal. It didn't matter that my thick, wavy hair would never sit still in a 1920s Louise Brooks bob, that I would need a blow-dryer and a straightening iron to create a long, waiflike finish, or that a pixie cut made my nose look big. If the look was hot, I wanted it.

Trivia...

Male hair is typically more dense than female hair. This holds true only if the male in question isn't balding.

During this period, I encountered a few hairstylists who refused to give me the exact look I wanted. "But your hair doesn't want to go forward," one would say. "With your busy schedule when are you going to find time to blow-dry your hair straight?" another asked. "This look doesn't work with your face; why don't we alter it a bit to suit your features?" asked another. But I was persistent; if one stylist wouldn't give me the precise look I wanted, I searched until I found one who would.

Living with your style

After living with the cut a while, I would grow frustrated. With the above-mentioned bob, for example, I woke up at 5 a.m. each morning to wash and condition my hair, blow-style, and say a prayer asking the weather gods for a perfectly arid day because even a touch of humidity would encourage my strands to return to their wavy ways. By the end of the day, my hair had begun creeping back to its natural position. If I had a dinner date, I needed to run home and either wet my hair down and re-blow-dry, or plug in a straightening iron and spend a half-hour removing kinks. My straight-haired friends literally woke up and ran a brush through their hair. That's it. Their strands fell effortlessly into place, which meant they could go from school to a night out without going home first. Yet even this wasn't enough to tell me I had chosen the wrong style.

At the time, I was a theater student: It took a comment from the drama department's costume and makeup director to make me rethink my coif. "Your hairstyle makes your chin look weak," she said. "You might want to try something softer." But the cut was such a sexy, late 80s, New Wave look! I loved it! "You like the haircut better than you like your face?" she asked. She had a point. I stopped blow-drying my strands straight and had a few softening layers added. The moral of this long-winded tale? A hairstyle should accentuate your total look – not be your look.

Tweak your look to keep it modern and to ward off boredom, but don't have a radical change simply for the sake of change. If you're happy with a cut and it works for you, why give it up?

Creating a signature style

A SIGNATURE HAIRSTYLE *is something that is "so you" that it becomes part of your overall look. Meg Ryan's short shag, Katie Couric's rounded crop, Goldie Hawn's banged pageboy, and singer Chrissie Hynde's choppy overgrown bowl cut are all signature 'do's. Though the wearer may regularly update her look by altering length, reigning in or adding fullness, changing a line, or playing with color, she's found a basic style that she likes, which works with her face shape and hair type, suits her personality, and fits her lifestyle.*

Working with your hair

You probably have an idea of what styles your hair can and can't pull off. For instance, if your hair is stringy-soft, there's no way it will look kittenish worn halfway down your back. Likewise, if your hair is incredibly thick it won't be sleek and swingy in a short, one-length bob; instead, you'll look like someone set a mushroom on your head.

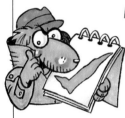

Icy blonde, Scandinavian hair is usually fine in texture, most Central European hair is medium, and Asian and Latin American hair is often strong and coarse.

You can attempt to overlook your hair type completely – if you can find a hairstylist who will let you. Most stylists, however, know that your hair type plays an integral role in determining which styles will and won't work for you. When a stylist talks about hair type, he or she is referring to a few different elements: how fine or fat in diameter your individual strands are, how many of these hairs you have on your head, and whether the strands are straight, wavy, or curly.

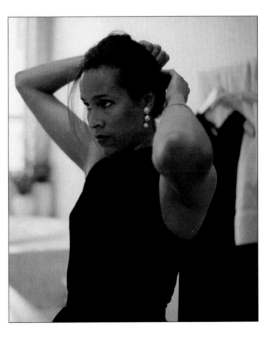

■ **It is most likely** *that you already have an idea of what your hair can and can't do, as well as what types of styles suit you best.*

Examining hair types

Hair with strands that are skinny in diameter is called fine hair and has a silky, baby-like feel. Although most people with fine hair have little of it, there are many fine-haired people who are blessed with an abundance of strands. Because it is so light in weight, fine hair is often flyaway and generally works best with unlayered or minimally layered cuts that don't remove too much weight.

Trivia...
"No other charm can quite compare with the allure of lustrous hair!" Advertising slogan for Drene *Shampoo, circa 1945.*

Medium, or normal, hair strands are those of middling width. These strands form the most common type of hair texture. Medium-textured hair is neither flyaway nor wiry; instead, it hangs where it's cut to hang – this makes it well-adapted to all kinds of haircuts.

HAIRDO DON'TS

I generally dislike categorizing hairstyles as "do's" or "don'ts." However, here are two looks that I cannot keep quiet about:

1 Mall hair is big. It is generally collarbone length or longer and might have a tight or loose perm. Mall hair's hallmark is a set of long, heavy bangs that are teased and gelled at the roots to fall like a giant wave onto or away from the forehead. Though the style went out of fashion in the mid-1980s, mall hair is still worn by rural and suburban teenagers and 20-somethings in English-speaking countries.

2 The mullet is another look from the 80s. During punk days, the style was worn by both females and males. Today, however, it is the male counterpoint to mall hair. From the front, the coif appears to be a typical men's short cut. It's not until you get past the ears that it becomes obvious a man is wearing a mullet; there, hair suddenly drops into a longer 'do. Interestingly, some men sport mullets that are very short up front and very long at the back. Other names for the mullet include the ape drape, the bi-level, hockey hair, the dual-cut, and the country & western. In addition to rural and suburban men in English-speaking countries, the mullet is popular among ice-hockey players, country singers, and in Central and South America.

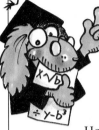

Hair that is fat is referred to as coarse. This type of hair is usually strong, easy to style, and may have a wiry look. While many people with coarse hair have a lot of individual strands, it isn't uncommon to find coarse-haired individuals who have so few strands that their scalp shows. Because coarse hair can have a bristle-like finish when cut too short, avoid styles that feature ultra-brief layers.

The circumference of a hair's individual strands indicates its fineness. The diameter of a medium strand of hair is 0.004 inches (0.1 mm).

Hair volume

How many strands you have per square inch (cm²) indicates your hair's thickness, which some hairdressers refer to as volume. To determine the quantity of hair you have, pull your hair back into a ponytail. If the diameter is approximately ⅜ inch (10 mm), you have thin hair; ⅝ inch (15 mm), you have normal hair; and ¾ inch (20 mm), you have thick hair.

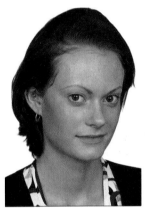

Another way of determining volume is to check whether you can see a lot of scalp when your hair is wet. If you can, your hair is probably thin. Because there aren't a lot of strands to give it a full, fluffy look, thin hair has a tendency to hang close against the head, making the scalp visible. If you can see some areas of scalp, your hair's thickness is medium, which just happens to be the universal norm. If there is little or no scalp peeking through, you've probably got thick hair.

■ **Worn against** *the head, thin hair can look lank.*

Hair of medium thickness works in many styles. Of course, hair's volume isn't the only thing to keep in mind when choosing a cut, but if yours is medium-thick, volume will be one less thing to consider. Because there is so much of it, thick hair often looks full – even puffy – in the way it blankets the head. Adding layers thins strands out, giving a sleeker finish and helping locks lie better. When short, thick hair needs some layering; if worn all-one-length, tresses look mushroomy.

■ **Thin hair** *works best in styles that are between shoulder- and ear-length. Any shorter and there is a danger that the scalp will become too visible through the hair.*

Hair waves

Your hair's curl pattern – or lack of curl pattern – is referred to as its wave pattern or its form. Confusingly, some hairdressers use the term "texture" – the same term used to describe hair's fineness – when talking about wave pattern. You can tell what kind of hair you have by allowing hair to dry naturally.

Many people have two or even three different wave patterns interspersed through their locks. This is normal! I, for instance, have straight hair through the top and crown; everywhere else, strands are tightly waved.

INTERNET

www.naturallycurly.com

Great for those blessed (or cursed, depending on your point of view) with waves, curls, kinks, or ringlets, this site provides support, suggestions, and styles.

Straight hair can have a slight bend to it or be completely without curviness. It hangs like a curtain, making it swingy, glossy, and great in barely layered or one-length styles, such as wedges, bowl cuts, bobs, and pageboys. Wavy hair features an S-pattern curve that travels the length of the strand. The wave can be tight or loose. Because wavy hair is loaded with body and movement, it looks great with longer layers and splicing, a technique used to add a slightly choppy finish to hair's ends. Shags of all lengths work especially well with curvy locks, as do short-layered cuts.

I love ringlets so much that at the age of 17 (right before school pictures) I begged my sister to give me a home perm. The results were disastrous enough that I vowed from then on that I'd get my curl fix by looking at other people's heads. With that in mind, I offer the secret to beautiful curls: moderation. Go too short and your hair looks severe, grow hair too long and strands look fuzzy and unkempt. Your best bet is a medium-short to medium-long 'do with a rounded shape and enough strategic layering to remove weight and keep ringlets springy.

DEFINITION

Low-maintenance cuts are those that are built upon your hair's texture, thickness, and wave. When these elements are incorporated into your hairstyle, hair falls naturally in place with little work. Low-maintenance cuts generally take 15 minutes or less to style.

Considering your lifestyle

I realize this is strange advice coming from a beauty writer, but the more we listen to these "authorities," the less time we'll have for life. This is my preachy way of saying your lifestyle – not a magazine, not a celebrity – should be among the first things you consider when choosing a hairstyle. If there are no friends, lovers, pets, or children in your life and if you have absolutely no hobbies and no interest in meditating or exercise, go ahead and get a high-maintenance coif. If your life is full-up, ask your hairdresser for a *low-maintenance* style. By the way, low maintenance doesn't mean frumpy – the best low-maintenance cuts are flattering and yes, even sexy.

Knowing your face shape

Have you ever spent weeks combing magazines for a new hairstyle, searching for looks that would work with your hair type? Upon finding one, you take the picture to your stylist who duplicates it down to the last layer. You stare at your new self – the style is gorgeous and works so well with your hair type. So why does it look so bad? You probably didn't take your face shape into consideration. A hairstyle chosen without your face shape in mind can distort your features by changing the balance of your face. A simple rule is that hair should be wide where your face is narrow and vice versa, and hair should have length where your face is square and vice versa.

There are several methods you can use to determine your face shape. The easiest is to ask your stylist. The next easiest is to pull your hair off your face and simply look. Often, your face is noticeably square, or oblong, or oval. If it's not, grab a bar of soap, a tube of lipstick, or an eyeliner and stand at least 6 inches (15 cm) from a mirror. Using whatever you've got in your hand, trace the shape of your face in the mirror. Match the shape you scrawled to one of the following descriptions:

1 Oval is considered the perfectly balanced face, making it a beauty ideal. Featuring a softly rounded hairline and a jaw line that is a smidge narrower than the temples, it can handle any hairstyle that works with your hair type. If you'd like to show off your lucky shape, avoid on-the-face looks that hide your features.

If you've got a round or square face, avoid center parts, which can emphasize the face's fullness. Instead, try parting your hair deep on the side to slim the face.

2 Round faces are, well, round. If creating a slimmer look is important to you, try to keep fullness away from the sides (no Farrah feathers or curly bobs) and create length at the top or bottom (or both) of the style.

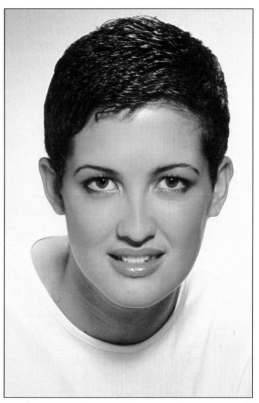

■ **Choosing a hair style** *to complement an oval face is relatively easy. Even really short styles work well as they accentuate the features.*

Styles to make a round face look longer include short or long cuts with ultra-short bangs, French twists, long-layered cuts with sleek sides, and side-swept bangs.

3 Square faces are generally full and feature equal or near-equal width at both the jaw line and hairline. The jaw line and hairline also have a squared line. The objective with a square face is to thin it a bit and soften the shape's blunt lines – easy to do with face-framing layers, soft waves, or large curls. Most hairdressers will advise you to keep locks well below the jaw to create the illusion of length. Stay away from blunt cuts, geometric lines, linear bangs, or anything severe.

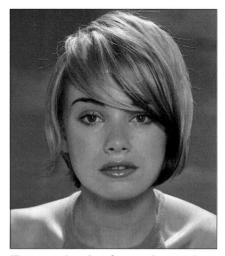

■ **Hairstyles that feature long,** *side-swept bangs flatter a round face.*

4 The oblong, or rectangular, face is long and slender. To flatter an oblong face, a hairstyle must do two things: de-emphasize length and create width. Therefore, long, straight hair is a no-no, while short and medium-length cuts with curls or plenty of fullness are ideal. Layered bobs are good and shags can work if the hair is directed off the face – if it falls on the face it will only make the face appear slimmer.

NECKLINES

As well as adding width, length, or slenderness to a face, the suggestions below show how a well-designed cut can also make your neck and jaw line appear more graceful:

1 **Receding chin** Keep hair collarbone length or longer to draw attention away from a weak chin. Add height at the crown to offer further subterfuge.

2 **Double chin** Keep the hair either below or above the jaw line – by 2 inches (5 cm) at least. A cut that is clipped to fall at the jaw or chin will draw attention to any extra flesh you have.

3 **Short neck** Opt for jaw-length or shorter, or collar-length or longer. Hair that stops anywhere along the neck only emphasizes your neck's stubbiness.

5. A diamond-shaped face features a narrow forehead, a narrow chin, and width through the cheeks. To normalize this shape, you should choose a hairstyle with width at the top and bottom and sleekness where the face is wide. A good option is a chin-length style that features wispy, temple-to-temple bangs. You can experiment with looks that are cut to fall onto the cheeks or try styles that are created to move off the face – I have heard various hairdressers claim one or the other is the best option for diamond-shaped faces.

6. Heart-shaped faces are characterized by wide foreheads and small, delicate chins. The right hairstyle can create a feeling of balance by making the forehead appear narrower and the chin seem wider. Looks with width at the jaw – such as chin-length bobs – are perfect for this. When swept to the side, longer bangs break up a wide forehead without adding too much width to the top portion of the face.

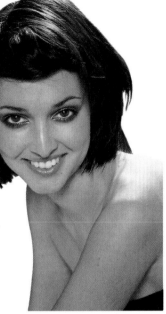

■ **This choppy,** *chin-length style adds width to a heart-shaped face.*

Is your face heart-shaped? Looking for something a bit different to give your hairstyle some oomph? Try sweeping hair to one side. It's an ideal way to de-emphasize the chin and make the forehead look narrower.

7. The triangular face is most narrow at the temples, slightly wider at the cheeks, and widest at the jaw line. Create balance with plenty of fullness in the bang area and at the temples, moderate width at the cheeks, and sleekness at the jaw. Does such a cut sound impossible? It isn't actually. Simply ask your stylist for a layered look with volume up top and tapering through the bottom. Plenty of short and medium-length cuts fit the bill, as do some shags.

8. The pear-shaped face is narrow at the forehead and flares out to great width at the cheeks and jaw line. Think symmetry by creating plenty of fullness at the temples and in the bang area, and sleekness at the cheeks and jaw. Full, layered looks that feature height at the crown are good, as are any kind of shag. Many hairdressers prescribe looks that fall well past the jaw.

Use your hairstyle to make close-set eyes look farther apart: add width at and below the temples and keep the top flat.

ANOTHER WAY OF DETERMINING FACE SHAPE

You can also find your face shape with a tape measure. First, measure the length of your face from the tip of your hairline to the bottom of your chin. Then, measure across the top of your cheekbones. Next, measure the widest portion of your jaw. Lastly, measure the widest point of your forehead. Review your measurements:

- An oval face's length equals one-and-a-half times its width.
- Your face is probably round if it is as wide (or nearly as wide) as it is long.
- A heart-shaped face is narrow at the jaw, wide at the cheekbones and forehead.
- A square face has nearly equal widths for forehead, jaw line, and cheekbones.
- An oblong face is longer than it is wide.
- Your face is diamond shaped if your cheeks are wider than both your forehead and your jaw line.
- Your face is triangular if your jaw is its widest feature, your forehead is the narrowest element, and your cheekbones are somewhere in between.
- You've got a pear-shaped face if your forehead is narrow and your cheeks and jaw line are wide.

Body shape

When it comes to finding a hairstyle to complement your body, balance is the word. The smaller your body – this refers to girth as well as height – the smaller the hairstyle should be. The bigger the body – again, this means girth as well as height – the bigger the hairstyle. A big coif emphasizes a small lady's stature by making her head seem enormous and her body even smaller. Similarly, a small coif on a big individual draws attention to her body by shrinking the appearance of her head.

Age

As we age, gravity takes hold, softening our features and silhouettes. A severe hairstyle often emphasizes these things. However, I don't believe length or lack of length influences a style's severity. True, a buzz cut is short and austere, but a tousled pixie is short and extremely soft. Yes, poker straight, waist-length hair with a center part is harsh, but long, curvy hair with plenty of body is gentle. The adage to keep in mind is that as you age, go softer.

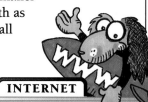

INTERNET

www.hairboutique.com

This charming site features a hairstyle gallery, plenty of hair gossip, regular columns, and loads of articles on everything from hairstyles for aging women to dealing with fine hair.

Small changes: Updating your look

ONCE UPON A TIME, *hair fashion moved slowly. A look that was popular in one century might still be just as current in the next. And when looks did change, they did so subtly – maybe the shape of a curl became more pronounced, or the curl disappeared entirely, or an up-do became a bit flatter and migrated from the crown to the back of the head. Today, however, fashion moves at lightning speed. Looks no longer survive a full year; most die after a season. To make matters worse, the changes are drastic. In 3 months, pixies can give way to long shags, only to move in another 3 months to sleek near-the-waist manes. No one I know has hair that grows that fast! So the best advice I can give you, and which has been given to me by countless stylists, is to disregard most of what's happening in fashion.*

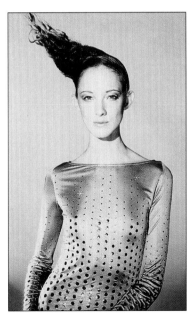

■ **Fashion is fun:** *It creates whimsy and keeps us from getting bored. But don't follow it slavishly.*

Staying in style

You probably don't want to ignore fashion totally – nor do most hairdressers want you to. After all, you want to look contemporary. Instead of changing your entire look to mimic what's going on in *Vogue*, however, try changing an element. Let's say you notice banged bobs in all the magazines – and indeed, you even read several articles on "banged bobs for spring." Perhaps you hate bobs, but wouldn't mind updating your look. The easy solution? After studying trends, choose an element that you happen to like. In this instance, get bangs.

Before you incorporate current trends into your 'do, talk to your hairdresser. For instance, if wispy looks make an appearance and your hair is too thin to carry off the layering needed for such styles, your stylist can create a slight touch of wispiness in your bang area.

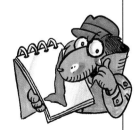

TRIMMING YOUR OWN BANGS

To trim your own bangs or not to trim your own bangs, that is the question. Unfortunately, I don't have a good answer. The hairdressers I know would suggest never cutting your own bangs. And I understand their position: Everyday they are faced with fringes that are crazily listing, oddly snipped, or downright butchered – all created by clients who were attempting to save themselves a salon visit. But I'm a realist. If your bangs are in your eyes, you have no time to see a stylist, and you've got an interview tomorrow which you need to neaten up for, I know you're going to prune your own bangs. I've trimmed my own bangs and nothing bad happened to me or my hair, so here's my official stance: Leave bang thinning, thickening, layering, or shape-changing to the professionals, but if you need a small trim to hold you over until your next salon appointment, then follow the directions below very carefully. And remember, you're trimming your bangs, not altering their shape or thickness.

1 Pull your hair off your face in a ponytail or headband. Comb only the hair you are trimming – your bangs – onto the forehead.

2 Search around for a pair of sharp scissors. A smallish pair with a sharp blade are best; new cuticle scissors are ideal. You don't want to use a pair of utility shears that cut paper, cloth, and cardboard – these will be too dull to clip hair well.

3 Hair should be dry; dry hair is easier to work with and also makes it easier to gauge results. Starting at the center, take a small section of hair – maybe ¼ inch (6 mm) wide – and hold loosely between your left thumb and forefinger (left-handed folks should reverse these directions). If you pull too hard you can remove too much length.

4 Snip away no more than ⅛ inch (3 mm), then continue, moving to the left. When you've reached the outer corner, return to the center and move to the right.

■ **For cutting hair,** *small, sharp scissors are essential. They give hair a clean, even cut, whereas blunt scissors tend to snag hair ends.*

5 Resist the urge to cut more.

A good hairdresser

MOST OF US HAVE A FIRM IDEA of what makes a good hairdresser: skill, experience, a pleasing personality, enthusiasm, the ability to listen, knowledge of the latest trends, and a way with our own particular hair type. Yes, such stylists exist – probably in your own town. You've simply got to know how to find and communicate with them.

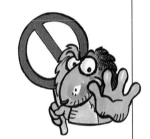

Trivia...
Though she may try dozens of stylists before deciding upon one, the average woman will have three to six long-term stylists in her lifetime.

Locating a good hairdresser

A good hairstylist is not impossible to find. You may have to search a bit, but locating a hair professional you trust and admire is very possible if you follow these suggestions:

1. Ask friends what salons they go to and if there are any stylists there who they think you would like. The salon your friend frequents may have the perfect hairdresser for you.

Don't overlook personality when deciding on a hairdresser. We're all different – a person I feel comfortable with may scare the pants off my mother!

2. If you see a woman whose hair you like, ask who her stylist is.

3. If you hear good things about a stylist, book a special occasion 'do. This provides a chance to try the hairdresser without pressure to get your hair cut.

4. Pick a salon with a good reputation. Usually, a salon gets a good reputation for a reason: professional, talented, caring stylists. Negative reports – slow service, indifferent stylists, gossipy assistants – can mean a negative salon experience.

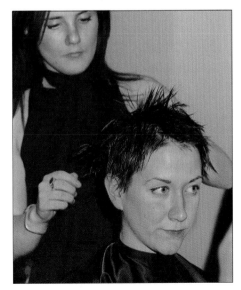

■ **Finding a stylist** *with whom you feel comfortable and can build up a rapport is worth all the research.*

5 Schedule a consultation. When you call, remember to tell the receptionist about your hair type and what kind of looks you like. Most salons don't charge for a consultation and it is a great way to get to know a stylist before committing to an appointment.

How to communicate

The most important element in the relationship with your hairdresser is communication. True, most of us struggle to communicate with our loved ones, coworkers, and even ourselves – how can we express ourselves to someone we see just every 2 months? When it comes down to it, you don't have to do anything. Keep in mind, however, that unlike those other people in your life, your hairdresser stands over your head holding a pair of scissors. That alone is enough to get me talking.

Make life easy on yourself – ask your stylist to show you exactly how to style your hair, what products are best to use, how to hold a blow-dryer, and so on. Stylists are professionals – don't be afraid to learn from them.

HAIR CONSULTATIONS

One of the things you should do when you have a hair consultation is watch how the stylist looks at you. Is the stylist studying your body type, your clothing, your movements? Is it almost as if he or she is looking for clues to your personality? Don't get unnerved. How else can the stylist suggest a look that works with your "total package"?

During a consultation, notice what kind of questions you are asked. Is the stylist interested in finding out your hair history? Does he or she want to know how much time you're willing to spend on home styling and salon appointments? Does the stylist ask about your feelings on trends, lengths, perms, layers, and so on? Now is not the time to be shy. You must tell this stranger every boring detail about your hair – and your hopes for your hair.

■ **Don't get dressed up to visit the salon:** *wear your regular clothing, shoes, and accessories. In order for your stylist to suggest looks that will work with your lifestyle, you must reveal what your lifestyle looks like.*

Start each visit by telling the stylist how the cut worked for you, how your hair is behaving, what is driving you crazy about your hair, what you might want to keep the same, and what you might want to change. If you've read anything about a new hair service or hairstyle, ask about it. If you've been seeing your hairdresser for a while, he or she probably knows what you mean by "take just a little off." If your relationship is a young one, however, you may need to physically show him or her how much you want off.

If you think the stylist is taking off too much or cutting an angle too steeply, speak up immediately. Don't remain quiet and then complain when the cut is over and the hair un-fixable.

Saying good-bye

You may reach a point where the relationship with your stylist isn't working. Maybe your hairdresser is burned out and it shows in wandering attention. More commonly, however, it's you who have changed. You want to grow your hair long, but your stylist works best with short hair. Or you have decided to go back to school and can't afford your stylist's recently raised rates. Or you are simply curious and wonder what "a fresh eye" would envision on you. If you find someone new to visit, are you under any moral obligation to call your previous stylist to say you won't be coming back? I asked a few hairdressers their thoughts. The surprising answer? No. Just quietly move on. To do any more can create awkwardness. If you run into your former stylist, be pleasant, but don't dwell on why you stopped seeing her. There's no need.

A simple summary

✔ To get a good hairstyle, you've got to know your hair type.

✔ If a hairstyle looks wrong on you, there's a good chance you didn't take face shape and body size into account.

✔ Choose a look that works with your lifestyle.

✔ Age should not keep you from wearing the looks you love and that work well for you.

✔ To find a good hairstylist, be willing to do some homework.

✔ Get the coif you want by communicating effectively with your stylist.

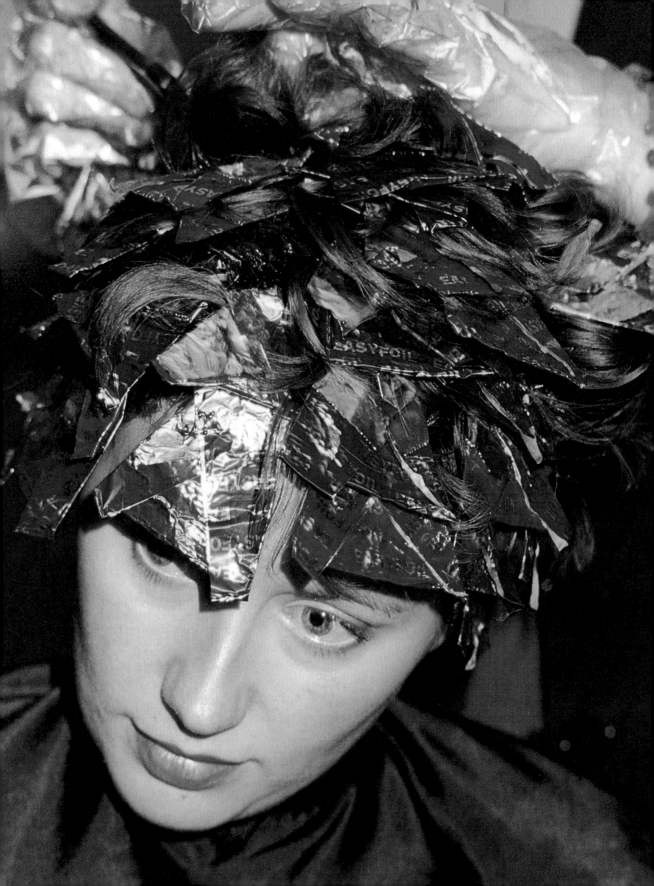

Chapter 9

Color you Beautiful

HAIR COLOR IS THE ULTIMATE HAIR COSMETIC. What else can make your eyes look brighter, your skin seem rosier, your cheekbones appear higher, or your gray hair disappear? Like makeup colors, shoe styles, and hem length, hair color can reveal what segment of society someone belongs to, what age a person wants to stay, and who a woman wants to be – and doesn't want to be. But what I love best about hair color is that it is democratic: it allows everyone to enhance what they were born with. We all want to look great. And if that means trying a shade we think is brighter, or sexier, or more mysterious than our own, so be it.

In this chapter...

✓ Is hair color for me?

✓ Types of hair color

✓ Home color versus salon color

✓ Maintaining your shade

A HEAD OF FOIL WILL SOON TRANSFORM INTO LOCKS OF YOUR CHOSEN COLOR

Is hair color for me?

IF YOU DON'T ALREADY COLOR YOUR HAIR, you may be ready to take the plunge if you find yourself utterly bored with your locks – so bored that not even a new haircut makes you feel perkier. At this point, you begin noticing hair color on other women, you study celebrities' locks, you see a magazine article on highlights and you can't help wondering: Should I try color?

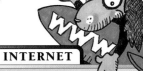

Whether or not you decide to color your hair is ultimately up to you. I will tell you this, however: There is no one who cannot wear hair color. Okay, maybe there are people who are allergic to some hair coloring ingredients – those folks should avoid color – but the rest of us live in a world filled with hair-color choices. So many choices, in fact, that it's easy to find a product to enhance your beauty gently or to downright alter the way you come across. You can try a no-pain, wash-out color, then slowly move on to more permanent choices such as highlights or double-process color . . . or you can keep experimenting with different temporary shades. That way, if you get tired of coloring your hair, you can simply stop.

Covering gray

I am just now beginning to see my first gray – a tuft at each temple. This confuses me: Both my parents were a full 15 years older than I now am when they started to gray. While there's nothing I can do to stop my premature gray, I can cover it. Apparently, I'm not the only woman who sees hair color as a way to cover silver. According to my hairdresser, half of his clients (both women and men) get their gray covered. This doesn't surprise me – after all, we live in a youth-oriented society, where even the smallest sign of age erodes a woman's sex appeal (or so we've all come to think). For those brave souls who want to keep their gray, a silver-enhancing shampoo can keep hair from looking dull or yellow.

■ **Graying hair** *affects people of all ages. How soon gray hairs appear is largely governed by genes.*

Gray strands are incredibly resistant to hair color: Depending on your hair, you may find that certain home hair-color formulas – especially the less permanent versions – simply can't cope with your silver strands. If you're having difficulty at home, why not go to a salon? Chances are, a color technician can hide every last trace of gray.

Adding excitement

Excitement is a subjective term – especially when it comes to hair color. To me, exciting hair color is color that is better (I know, another subjective word) than nature. On my own head that translates to "brighter than the *mousy*, light brown buried under my gold highlights." For someone else, exciting means brash, such as bombshell blonde or high-intensity auburn. Another person might see exciting as sensuous, embodied by a glossy espresso or cool aubergine. Blue streaks, green tips, pink ends – these can also be exciting, as can rushing to try every hair-color trend before it hits the streets. In short, the excitement of hair color is part fun, part self-expression, and part self-improvement. And yes, all of this is subjective.

Drawing attention to facial features

My eyes are my best feature. To play them up, my hair colorist has found just the shade of gold to make them look their greenest – a shade that he paints onto the strands that fall over my brows, my eyes, my cheeks. Can I scientifically prove these highlights make my eyes stand out? No, but immediately after getting my hair colored, cheeky men stop me on the street to say kind words about my eyes.

According to my colorist, this color trick is more visual manipulation than sleight of hand. This is how it works: Let's say you have gorgeous cheekbones. If your colorist applies a slightly brighter, lighter, or darker shade to the hair around your mid-face, your cheekbones will appear more prominent. Why? Simply because people's gazes are now drawn to that area. More proof of this technique's powers: The gorgeous brows of a friend became mesmerizing when she had her bangs tipped with a deeper color to draw people's attention; the lovely jaw line of another friend became a cocktail party topic after she had a lighter shade painted onto her hair's jaw-skimming strands.

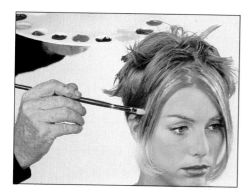

■ **Sections of hair** *can literally be painted with brighter or deeper colors.*

Types of hair color

WHEN IT COMES TO HAIR COLOR,
we live in exciting times. We can darken
hair for a day or a month, brighten strands
permanently, even make raven-colored tresses
as pale as sunlight. We can add lighter,
brighter, or darker stripes, as well as cloak
gray hair in the color it once was or paint
strands in a kaleidoscope of candy-inspired
shades. We can opt for hair color that
gradually fades with time (and leaves no telltale roots) or color that stays with the hair
strand as it grows out.

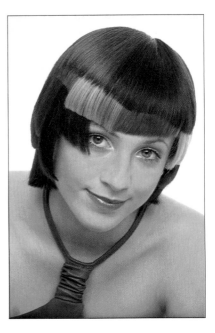

■ **Blocks of permanent hair color** *can be used to create
spectacular effects intended to make an impact. While striking,
this look is probably too extreme for most of us.*

*In the beauty world, enlivening or darkening your natural shade is not
a big deal. Making a dramatic change, such as lightening hair, is a
big deal. An easy-to-remember rule: the bigger the change, the more
chemicals needed, and the more chemicals needed, the harsher the process.*

How color works

Generally speaking, the more temporary a color formula is, the less damage it does to
hair; the more permanent a color, the more damage it does. Also, generally speaking,
the more temporary a color formula, the more subtle the
change it can create, while the more permanent a color is, the
more extreme the change it can produce. This has to do with
chemistry. Colors that wash out in less than 12 shampoos –
temporary and *semi-permanent* colors – simply coat the hair
shaft; because they aren't hanging around, they don't need
chemicals to push pigment molecules into the strand's cuticle
layer. Hair color formulas that last longer than 12 shampoos –
demi-permanent, permanent, and bleach – use one or two
chemical elements to open the cuticle layer and force pigment
molecules into the strand.

> **DEFINITION**
>
> *There is a difference
> between* semi-permanent
> *and* demi-permanent *hair
> color: Semi-permanent
> hair color lasts from 6 to 12
> shampoos; demi-permanent
> from 12 to 24.*

The basic chemicals

Peroxide is an ingredient in demi-permanent hair color, permanent hair color, and bleach and is used to help lift the cuticle layer so other ingredients can get into the strand and do their jobs. Peroxide also helps create longer-lasting color – in fact, the longer-lasting the color, the more peroxide a dye has.

Ammonia – or the ammonia substitute called monoethalonamine (MEA) – is found in many permanent hair colors and bleach. Ammonia dives into the strand and removes some or all of the hair's natural melanin. Why is all this necessary? Because the less natural melanin a strand has, the more readily it will accept new pigment from a hair-color formula.

Trivia...
"If champagne blondes turn his head . . . be one!" Clairol advertising slogan, circa 1957.

Temporary hair color

When I was in high school, I played on my school's volleyball and basketball teams. During my sophomore year, one of my teammates got the brilliant idea to paint patterns into the underlayers of our hair – nothing so overt that we'd be caught (there were strict rules against using makeup and hairstyles to distract players), but something subtle enough that it would take a few seconds for our opponents to figure out what the heck was going on with our hair. A few unguarded seconds were all we needed – so we thought – to get a ball safely over a net or through a hoop. When we got tired of using our school's colors (red, white, and black), we'd try our opponents' colors (purple and gold, green and black, burgundy and silver) or adopt a holiday theme (orange and black for Halloween, green for Saint Patrick's Day).

INTERNET
www.hairstylist.com

This site features a hairstyle search, hair color news, a Q&A section, hair-product finder, and much more.

The color we used for these experiments was temporary – shades that stayed in our hair only until the next shampoo. We preferred the foam (also called mousse and spray-on formula), but temporary color is also available as a rinse. Of course, not everyone wants to wear the fanciful shades my teammates and I favored; fortunately, temporary hair color comes in many natural hues. One more thing to keep in mind is that temporary color contains no ingredient to alter hair's structure and because of this, it cannot lighten hair. Instead, use temporary hair color to darken or slightly brighten strands.

If you have damaged, chemically straightened, or permed hair, temporary and semi-permanent colors are the safest choices.

Semi-permanent hair color

Semi-permanent color is terrific for hair-color newbies. It washes out in 6 to 12 shampoos, contains no potentially damaging peroxide or ammonia, and, once it's gone, leaves your hair the same color as it was before being colored. This means you can experiment with shades until you find one you want to use consistently. Because of its gentle nature, however, semi-permanent color can't change things very dramatically. It has a slightly translucent quality that makes it better suited to enhancing rather than altering your natural color. What semi-permanent hair color can do is take hair one or two levels darker, or maybe even a shade brighter. Gray hair, which is notoriously resistant to hair color, is rarely well camouflaged by semi-permanent shades. Furthermore, these shades' lack of chemicals means they have no lightening power whatsoever.

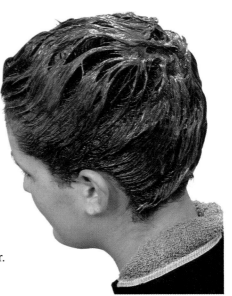

■ **Use semi-permanent** *color to give hair a change of tone rather than radically changing hair's color.*

If you're a brunette who dreams of being blonde, semi-permanent color is not for you.

Demi-permanent hair color

Demi-permanent hair color – which some people mistakenly call semi-permanent – lasts from 12 to 24 shampoos. It contains a small amount of peroxide – which means a small amount of hair damage – but no ammonia, making demi-permanent color a midway option between semi-permanent and permanent color. True to its middle-of-the-road position, demi-permanent color does a bit more than semi-permanent. First off, it stays in hair longer before fading away. In addition, demi-permanent color's slightly more opaque formula does a better job of darkening hair more than three levels (*see box opposite*), covers gray better, and boasts more power to brighten hair. That tiny amount of peroxide can lighten hair, but only slightly – usually less than half a level. Again, if you have dark hair and dream of light locks, demi-permanent color is not for you.

How do semi- and demi-permanent colors fade? Shampooing loosens their pigment molecules, causing color to progressively diminish until all the molecules are gone. Because of this, you'll never experience telltale roots with semi- or demi-permanent color.

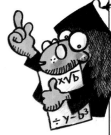

Permanent hair color

As its name implies, permanent color stays on your hair permanently. Its tenacity becomes especially apparent when the colored strands grow out: you'll see a line of demarcation between them and the new, untreated root growth. This, and the damage permanent color can cause (the formula contains both peroxide and ammonia), are its negative aspects.

On a more positive note, with permanent hair color you don't need to worry about losing the color you love after 6 or 24 shampoos, you get superior gray coverage, you can brighten or darken hair as dramatically as you like, and you can lighten hair up to four levels. Be aware, however, that if you'd like to lighten hair more drastically, you're better off with double-process color. Permanent color can lighten hair only so much – go beyond four levels and it won't be strong enough to remove all the natural melanin in your hair. The not-so-gorgeous result? Strands that are brassy, brassy, brassy.

ON THE LEVEL

When a stylist talks about "taking you three levels lighter or darker," he or she means trying a shade three levels lighter or darker than your own. To confuse matters, many drugstore hair colors use the word "shade" as a synonym for "level." In the salon world, however, "shade" refers to a color's brightness and whether it has a gold, red, blue, or neutral undertone. In other words, a medium brown and medium auburn are both level 4, but are different shades.

Color level categories

In the world of salon hair color, hair is categorized from 1 to 10 depending on how much pigment it has. Since black hair has the most pigment it is labeled as level 1, while the palest platinum blond is considered level 10.

- Level 1 – true black, blue-black, violet-black, espresso-black
- Level 2 – deep brown, aubergine
- Level 3 – dark brown, dark red-brown, dark auburn
- Level 4 – medium brown, medium auburn
- Level 5 – light brown, light auburn, true red
- Level 6 – dark blonde, dark strawberry-blonde, light auburn
- Level 7 – medium blonde, medium gold, medium strawberry-blonde
- Level 8 – light blonde, light gold, light strawberry-blonde
- Level 9 – pale blonde, pale gold, pale strawberry-blonde (pink-blonde)
- Level 10 – platinum blonde, platinum-gold

Highlights and lowlights

If you've ever sat in the sun and ended up with a head full of blonde, gold, or red streaks, you know what highlights are: stripes of color that are lighter or brighter than your own. Highlights can be as subtle or dramatic, as thick or thin, or as few or plentiful as you like. They grow out gracefully and, because they can go from 2 to 4 months without attention, are terrifically low-maintenance. Highlights are created with permanent hair color that is painted onto, or combed into, small sections of hair. To create dramatically lighter highlights, double-process color can be used. Lowlights are the near-opposite: a darker color is painted onto the hair to create contrast. Lowlights may be used to tone down hair that is overly light.

Do not use clarifying shampoos if you use any type of hair color. They can leach color pigment from treated strands. Dandruff shampoos and formulas for oily hair can also strip hair color from strands.

HIGHLIGHTS

The techniques used to create highlights may vary from salon to salon but the principles are the same: Hair is sectioned and then the strands are separated out according to whether a dramatic or subtle result is required.

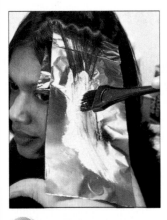 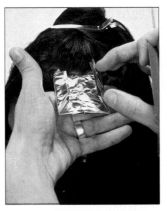 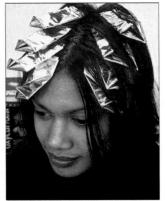

1 Applying the color

The hair is sectioned onto strips of aluminum foil. Color is applied from the roots down.

2 Folding the foils

The colored hair is folded up into the foil to keep the color away from the untreated hair.

3 Developing color

Once all the foil packages are in place, the hair is left for the required processing time.

Double-process color

Have you always dreamed of having pale blonde hair? If your locks are dark blonde, any level of red, or any level of brown, you'll need double-process color to get what you want. Double-process is so named because hair is first bleached of all (or nearly all) color. Some people choose to leave hair in this state, but a more polished option is to treat your decolorized tresses with a semi-permanent or permanent hair color in the blonde shade of your choice (champagne, wheat, ice, moonlight – there are quite a few options). I suggest going with the semi-permanent color. It's less damaging to hair and gives you room to experiment with various shades until you find the one you adore.

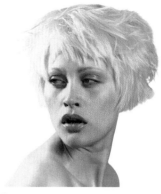

■ **Icy blonde** *may be the color you long for, but bleach can damage your hair.*

Henna

Henna is a natural vegetable tannin that stains the hair. I love the idea of using a nature-made color on my hair, but I must confess, henna scares me. That's because, while henna generally produces some shade of red, you won't know exactly what shade until after you've completed the treatment. If you don't like the results, you're stuck – you can't remove the color, nor can you use any of the more conventional hair color formulas to hide the color.

That said, I've seen some amazing hennaed hair. Henna seems to strengthen strands, making them shiny and healthy-looking. Furthermore, the people I know who use henna swear that, since their conversion, they've never had a split end. So it comes down to this: If you like red and you want to try henna, get help. If you can't find a henna expert in your area, get on the Internet and start surfing until you know everything possible about henna's behavior.

> *Trivia...*
> *Henna has been used for more than 6,000 years. In fact, the Muslim prophet Mohammed colored his beard with henna, as do many devout male Muslims today.*

Do not mix henna with conventional color. This creates a chemical reaction that turns hair green or a greenish black, or can make the hair break off.

■ **Using henna** *usually produces a reddish tone, but the actual shade will depend on your natural hair color and type.*

SEEING RED

I have a theory: Humans love what's rare. Red is the hair color least seen in nature, which (according to my theory) explains why it is one of the most popular salon and home hair-color shades. Help celebrate humankind's love of red with the following trivia:

 Only 2–3 percent of the entire human population has naturally red hair.

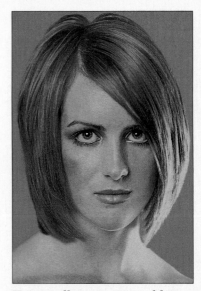

 In England and Scotland, redheads comprise up to 10 percent of the population.

c Because red hair is a recessive genetic trait, scientists believe that red hair might totally disappear in the future.

d Jesus is often depicted as having auburn hair and blue eyes.

e Judas (Jesus' betrayer) and Eve (of Tree of Knowledge fame) are often depicted as redheads.

f England's Queen Elizabeth I often wore a red wig.

■ **Naturally occurring red hair** *is much rarer than its blonde and brunette counterparts.*

g During the Middle Ages, female redheads were viewed as witches. In addition to being persecuted, red-haired women of the time were in danger of being executed for witchcraft. (Could today's lack of redheads have anything to do with these "witches," who may not have had a chance to pass on their red hair?)

h During the 16th and 17th centuries, red hair became fashionable among upper-class men and women.

i Within some Christian groups of the 18th and 19th centuries, red-haired children were "evidence" that their mothers had slept with Satan.

Home color versus salon color

SHOULD YOU COLOR *at home, or should you leave it to a salon professional? There's no one answer that fits all situations. I, for instance, have done both. When I was in high school, I enlivened my dark-blonde hair with a permanent medium-gold hair color, which I bought in a local drugstore and applied in my bathroom. Today, I prefer to go to the salon for highlights and lowlights. My experience of hair color has shaped my personal philosophy: The easier a technique is and the less harsh the formula, the more likely I'll try it at home. The more complicated a technique is and the harsher the formula, the more likely I'll go to my stylist.*

Choosing a shade

When you go to a salon for hair color, you have a color specialist – someone familiar with skin tones and what hair colors flatter them – at your disposal. This expertise is essential if you crave a big change, whether you're a dark brunette and want to be strawberry-blonde or have deep auburn hair and want to be platinum. A color technician can tell you whether you can carry off such a change; if you can't, she'll steer you toward a more realistic (but no less exciting) choice.

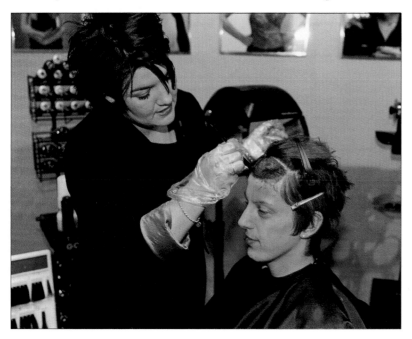

■ **If you're planning** *a drastic color change, a color specialist is the best person to advise you on what you can achieve and, most importantly, on what shades will best suit your skin tone.*

If you're coloring at home, however, you've got to choose a shade yourself. It's best to choose something that is no more than 1 to 3 levels different from your own – and try to stay in the same color family. Mother Nature provides us with natural hair colors that flatter our skin and eyes: make things easy on yourself and stay near what she's given you. For instance, if your hair is golden in tone, choose another golden shade. If your hair is red, look for something in the red family; if it is *ashy*, choose an ashy shade. If your hair has none of these tones, it is neutral – choose a shade in the neutral family. For example, if you have auburn hair and crave something lighter, go for a dark strawberry-blonde; if you have medium-brown hair and want something darker, go with an ashy deep brunette.

> **DEFINITION**
>
> *Ashy is another way to say cool. If your hair has cool, almost grayish tones, consider it ashy.*

If your hair is below shoulder length or very thick, you may need to use two boxes of coloring product to fully saturate your hair.

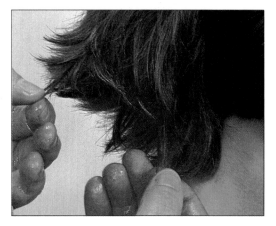

Preparing color

Whether you're going it alone or heading to a salon, there are a few things you can do beforehand to ensure gorgeous color:

1. Wash hair 24 to 48 hours before coloring. Shampooing the same day as your color service strips the natural oil that protects hair and scalp.

2. Deep condition hair's ends. The older a strand is, the more likely it is to have been damaged by sun, wind, or styling. These damaging elements make hair's ends more porous than the hair closer to the scalp. Porous areas suck up color, creating a result that is noticeably more intense through the ends. Deep conditioning the ends 24 to 48 hours before color is added can help temporarily close the cuticle so strands don't absorb as much color.

Coarse hair generally takes more time to absorb hair color, while fine hair absorbs color more quickly.

■ **Have a consultation** *with a colorist before your appointment to assess your hair's condition. Applying a leave-in conditioner to the ends is beneficial if the hair is especially damaged.*

When searching for a home hair-color shade, don't choose a color by the model on the box.

The result you achieve from a home hair color may not be exactly what you expect. A given hair-color shade actually produces a range of end results, depending on the hair-color shade you start with. That's why the back panels of most hair-color packages show you a range of color swatches so that you can determine your end result based on your starting color.

Here are a few additional steps for the home-colorists among you:

1. Do an allergy test, also known as a patch test, to determine whether you have any allergies to a given hair color. At least 2 days before you plan to color hair, mix a small amount of the color – you'll find instructions for patch-test mixing included with your box of hair color. Using a cotton swab, apply a ½-inch (1-cm) patch of color to the inside of your elbow. Leave the area uncovered, unwashed, and undisturbed for 48 hours. Save the remaining mixture for use in the strand test (*see below*). If no redness or irritation appears after 48 hours, the product is safe to use. If you do experience a reaction, you are allergic to the product so get rid of it.

Trivia...

Many women start with semi-permanent hair color and slowly work their way up to more permanent formulas.

2. Do a strand test with the color you mixed for your patch test. A strand test shows you exactly what color a home hair-color product will create on your hair. It will also give you an idea of how long a product takes to treat your hair type. Clip a few strands of hair – you want a sample that is ¼ inch (6 mm) in diameter and at least 1 inch (2.5 cm) long – preferably from the darkest area of your hair. Bind one end of the strands with tape to keep them together. If the instructions say to apply color to wet hair, dampen the strands. Otherwise, leave hair dry. Paint the strands with some of the mixed hair-color solution, then place strands in a plastic container. After about 10 minutes, rinse and dry the strands. If the color of the strand is not as rich as you would like, reapply the color solution and check every 5 minutes, up to 20 minutes for gray patches. When the strand is the color you want, note the amount of time the color has been on the strand. This indicates the amount of time you should leave the color on during the overall application.

3. Gather your supplies. Find some old towels, a second-hand shirt to wear, petroleum jelly or a heavy moisturizer to put around your hairline (this keeps color from seeping onto skin), and anything else you'll need – you don't want to be wandering through your house with hair color on your head. Remember, permanent dye really is permanent.

READY, GET SET, COLOR!

I'm going to assume your hair-color comfort is similar to mine and offer you directions applicable to semi-permanent, demi-permanent, or permanent hair color. If you want highlights, lowlights, or double-process color, I suggest visiting a salon.

1 Read the package directions. If the instructions say to apply color to wet hair, get in the shower and wet your hair. Otherwise, leave your hair dry.

2 Section your hair in four parts. Start by making a center part from your forehead to your nape – as if you were going to put your hair in two ponytails. Make a second part from behind one ear over the top of the head to behind the other ear. Clip each of the four sections of hair loosely against the head.

3 Most home hair-color kits come with plastic gloves. Put these on, or use an old rubber pair. Mix the hair color according to the package directions.

4 Touching the nozzle to your scalp, squeeze the color onto the roots between each section and down the center part. If you need to, unclip the hair and use your fingers to spread the color across the roots. Apply the color section by section until all of your roots have been colored.

5 If you haven't already done so, unclip the hair. Apply color to any gray hair.

6 Finish by applying remaining color to untreated strands. Remember the strand test you did? It gave you the ideal processing time for your hair type. Set your timer.

7 Time's up! Check the color by wiping off a small strand behind the ear. If the hair doesn't seem done, leave the color on for 2 to 5 more minutes.

8 Follow the directions for rinsing and conditioning. Generally, you will be asked to rinse your hair and follow up with a conditioner. While most hair-color products come with a single application of conditioner, feel free to use whatever deep conditioner you have on hand. Leave conditioner on for up to 5 minutes, then rinse hair in cool water.

Maintaining your shade

ONCE YOU'VE COLORED YOUR HAIR, *you must treat it gently if you want to maintain that gorgeous shade you (or your stylist) worked so hard to create. Fortunately, color care isn't difficult.*

Preventing color from fading

Always be aware of water temperature when you wash color-treated hair. Hot water is a no-no when it comes to color-treated hair because it causes the cuticle to swell allowing pigment molecules to escape. This leads to dull, faded color. Opt for lukewarm water.

You should also avoid strong sunlight. Think back to your childhood. Do you remember how brassy – or blonde – your hair used to get in the summer? You can blame that on the sun, which has a color-bleaching effect. The sun's ultraviolet rays are especially hard on chemically colored locks, turning treated strands brassy and causing color to fade.

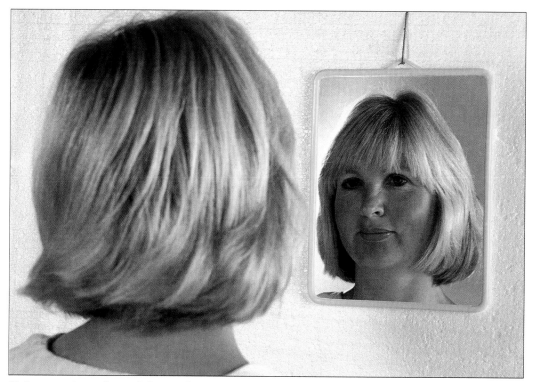

■ **Once you've achieved the perfect shade,** *take care to protect your new color from the color-altering effects of hot water, chlorinated swimming pools, saltwater, certain hair products, and environmental factors, such as the sun.*

Products for color-treated hair

There are products specifically designed for chemically treated hair and using these is a good way to coddle colored strands. Color-formula shampoos are less detergent-laden and more moisturizing than normal hair shampoos, while color-formula conditioners often contain more concentrated doses of emollients and may even include ingredients such as UV screens to protect against the color-fading effects of the sun.

Like color-formula products, color-enhancing shampoos and conditioners are gentle on color-treated strands. What makes them different, however, is that they contain small amounts of pigment to keep hair color looking just-from-the-salon fresh.

HAIR-COLOR HORRORS

Let's say you color your hair with permanent hair color: What if you hate the result? Is there anything that can take the color out? Go to a beauty supply store and purchase a color-remover kit, which will pull a portion of the hair color pigment from strands. You can also wash your hair three or four times with hot water (to force open the cuticles) and clarifying shampoo. (Dish soap also works well.) Don't forget to deep condition afterwards, or your hair will be more brittle than straw.

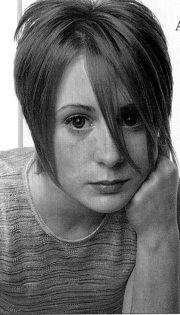

A better solution, in my opinion, is to visit a salon that specializes in corrective color and let them fix the mistake. Color chemicals are funny things; you never know how they are going to react. A professional who is trained in fixing color mistakes can not only extract the offending color, he or she can nudge your hair back to your natural shade – or another desired color – with as little damage to your hair as possible.

■ **If you change your mind** *about your new color, do not despair. A color specialist can help you return your hair to its previous shade – or even a new shade – with minimum damage.*

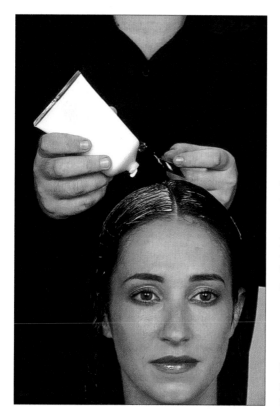

Color-enhancing shampoos and conditioners are available in a large range of shades. Rotate color-enhancing products with color-formula products.

Regular deep-conditioning treatments will also help to maintain your color. If you use demi-permanent, permanent, or double-process color, expect your hair's cuticle layer to get a bit roughed up. Consider a weekly, deep-conditioning treatment to add moisture and smooth bristly strands.

A leave-in conditioner not only blankets hair in all-day moisture, it protects locks against damage from sun, tangling, styling, and more.

■ **Salon conditioning treatments** *can be applied regularly between your color appointments to maximize the condition of your hair.*

A simple summary

✓ Reasons for coloring hair include covering gray, adding excitement, and drawing attention to features.

✓ Looking for a no-damage way to color your hair? Think temporary.

✓ The more permanent the hair color, the more effective it is at covering gray.

✓ Complicated hair coloring processes are best left to salon professionals.

✓ If you want your hair color to remain its lustrous best, treat colored hair gently.

✓ Hair-color mistakes can be rectified; seek advice.

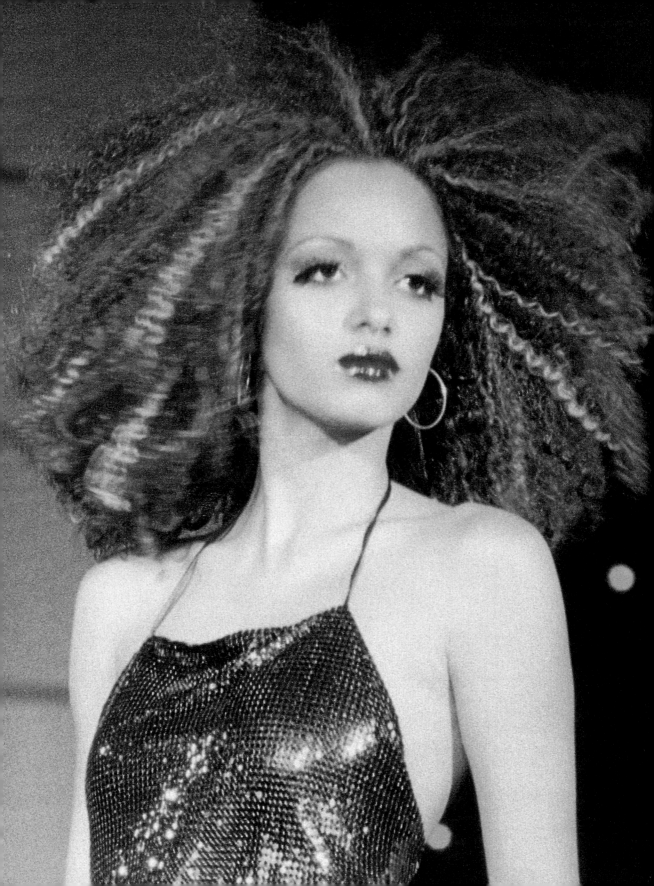

Chapter 10

A Change in Texture

HUMANS ARE FUNNY: Those of us with curly hair long for smooth tresses and those with straight hair often wish for curls. Of course, I am as guilty as everyone else. I've used roller sets to coax my waves into curls and I've spent mornings with blow-dryers and straightening irons. If you're certain you want to change your hair, it may be easier on you and your tresses to try something that's longer-lasting – I'm talking about a permanent wave or a chemical straightening service.

In this chapter...

✓ About permanent waves

✓ At-home versus in-salon waves

✓ Caring for your permed hair

✓ Give it to me straight

✓ At-home versus in-salon relaxers

✓ Caring for straightened hair

RUNWAY MODELS MAY SHOW OFF EXTREME WAVES, BUT YOU CAN OPT FOR SOMETHING MORE SUBTLE

About permanent waves

A PERMANENT WAVE IS A SERVICE that creates permanent curl, waves, or body. To achieve this, hair is wound around small plastic curlers, called rods. Once every strand is rolled, locks are saturated with waving lotion. This lifts the individual tiles that comprise your hair's cuticle layer, seeps into the hair strand, and breaks down the bonds that give your hair its individual shape. This lotion is sometimes called "reducing" lotion because it actually reduces the interlocking ability of hair's bonds.

> **Trivia...**
> In hairdressing, "alkaline" generally means any solution that has a pH of 7.9 or higher, "neutral" has a pH of 7.0 to 7.8, while "acid" means anything that has a pH lower than 6.9.

Following a perm, it takes up to 48 hours for your hair's keratin to completely re-bond and your cuticle layer to close. That's why you are not supposed to wash, wet style, or brush your hair during this period.

When the hair's bonds have been broken apart, the hair is then doused in neutralizer; this forces hair's bonds to re-form according to the configuration of the rods the hair is rolled on. This neutralizer is often called an oxidizing liquid because it contains either hydrogen peroxide or sodium bromate. These ingredients inject oxygen into the hair, which in turn combines with the hair's natural hydrogen molecules to form new hair bonds.

There are two types of permanent waves: alkaline and acid. Each type has its own pros and cons:

1. **Alkaline permanent waves** These are standard permanent waves. Their waving lotions use a strong, alkaline chemical called ammonium thioglycolate, hence their nickname "thio perms." They work quickly, give strong curl, and are great for hair that is resistant to permanent waves, such as coarse or Asian hair. The bad thing about alkaline perms is that they do not offer subtle, soft results, and can be very damaging. In addition, they are not recommended for those with artificial color in their hair or for people who have very dry or damaged locks.

2. **Acid waves** These are gentler than alkaline perms; their waving lotions use a kinder chemical called glyceryl monothyioglycylate. If you have fragile, colored, or damaged hair, acid waves are your perm. Unfortunately, acid perms are more likely to give subtle ripples, or lots of body, rather than firm, crisp curls. Note: Endothermic acid waves require an application of heat; exothermic acid waves don't.

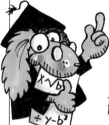

A combination of ammonia and ammonium thioglycolate is what gives a permanent wave its telltale odor.

Full perms

For a full perm, or standard perm, an alkaline or acid formula product can be used – it's the way hair is rolled that gives the service its name. The hair is sectioned in five forehead-to-neckline sections – the center section up top is rolled away from the face, while the rest of the hair is rolled under horizontally. Depending on the hair's length and the size of rods used, the resulting curls can be loose and jumbled, tight and kinky, or bigger up front and smaller toward the back.

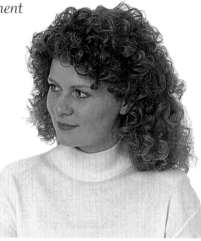

■ **A full perm** *is a traditional permanent wave that creates all-over curl.*

Partial perms

If you're like me, hair on different parts of your head does different things. Perhaps the hair at the back of your head is curly, while all other strands are stick-straight. If you'd like the straight locks to match the curls, ask your stylist for a partial perm, also called a spot perm. As the name implies, the perm is performed only on specific areas – the remaining hair is left untreated.

Got a cowlick? When perming your hair, roll affected strands in the direction you want them to fall.

Body waves

If you've got limp hair that would rather hang against your head than hold a style – even after you've tried all kinds of bodybuilding haircuts, experimented with styling products, and backcombed it repeatedly – a body wave might be for you. Think of a body wave as a kind of support measure that encourages hair to behave when you blow-dry it under, stays when you comb it back, or goes along with whatever you like doing to it. Because oversize rods are used for the service, you won't get curls with a body wave; you may or may not get large, very loose waves.

INTERNET

www.shampoo4me.com

Aimed at professional stylists, this site also has plenty for the general population. Content includes interesting information on perming, color, hair care, and salon products.

Root perm

For people with flat, stick-to-the-head hair, a root perm can add lift without curl. Large rods are placed at the hair's roots – and just the roots. This gives volume and height to perpetually lank locks. Think of it as a body wave for your hair's roots.

ROLL WITH IT

How your hair is rolled, and what kind of rods are used, are both essential to your permanent wave's finished look. Read the tips below to achieve the look you want.

1. Generally speaking, the tightness or looseness of a permed curl is determined by the size of the rods used. The smaller the rod, the tighter the curl; the larger the rod, the bigger the curl.

2. A basic perm set is the five-section set: it features five nape-to-forehead sections.

3. For the crispest curls, hair should be parted no wider than ¼ inch (6 mm) before being rolled onto rods.

4. To create a strong curl that is unmarred by rod marks or unevenness, strands are rolled "off-base." This means a section is combed and held at a 45° angle from the head.

5. End papers are small pieces of paper that are folded over the strands' ends before rolling. These help protect the ends from damage.

6. Hair that is longer than 5 inches (13 cm) does best when rolled in two rollers per parting – called piggyback rolling – or rolled onto tube rods that can be looped around strands; this looks a bit like a rag-roller set.

■ **To create a perm,** *sections of hair are wound around the rods starting from the top of the head and working down the length of the hair to the ends.*

If hair doesn't look curly after a perm service, it's said that the hair "didn't take." Culprits could include styling buildup on the hair, a medication you are taking, or imbalanced hormones, such as those caused by pregnancy. To prevent damage, don't re-perm hair immediately — wait 1 to 3 months. And if you're pregnant, wait until you've delivered the baby and are no longer nursing!

Spiral waves

You know those gorgeous, coiled ringlets you see on some naturally curly heads? That's what a spiral perm aims to duplicate. The curls are created by perm rods that are rolled vertically instead of horizontally. There is a downside to spiral perms: The vertical rod placement doesn't create the same firm, tight curls as the more traditional horizontal placement, which means your ringlets may be looser than you'd like.

Reverse perm

In a way, a reverse perm is a kind of curl-softening service. The treatment takes tightly or moderately curled locks and sets them on oversized rods. The result is softer, looser waves.

Touch-up perm

It's not healthy to re-perm strands that have been previously treated. The best way to keep damage at bay is to simply perm the new, untreated growth. This treatment is known as a touch-up perm, a re-touch perm, or sometimes a root perm.

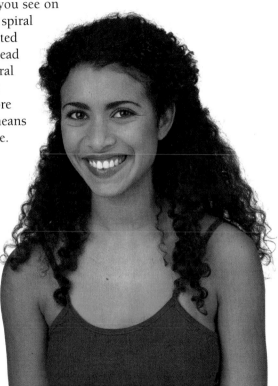

■ **If you were** *born with kinky-curly hair, a reverse perm can slightly soften your hair's curl pattern, creating a looser look.*

Heat styling is downright dangerous on degraded, fragile permed hair. If you can't live without your styling appliances, limit yourself to occasional heat styling and always protect strands with a leave-in conditioner before you begin.

At-home versus in-salon waves

WHEN MY SISTER AND I HIT OUR TEEN YEARS, *we became interested in permanent waves – she wanted something to create long-lasting curls in her straight hair and I wanted something to create long-lasting curls in my wavy hair. Yes, we'd heard awful tales of poodle-frizz home perms, but at that point we were already experimenting with home hair color, and because we cut each other's hair (and our friends' hair and boyfriends' hair), we figured home perming would be a cinch. So we sought out the best-stocked drugstore, and spent an hour reading perm boxes and studying bags of rollers. In the end, we concluded that we each had resistant hair, and purchased accordingly.*

When we returned home, I spent 45 minutes fumbling with those rods. After I'd finished my arms were aching. But the pain was worth it: My sister's hair looked great! There was some breakage, but the overall effect was a soft cascade of loose curls.

Encouraged, we decided that she'd do my hair the following week. The result was so frizzy, so unevenly curled – so ugly – that not a single picture of me exists from that time.

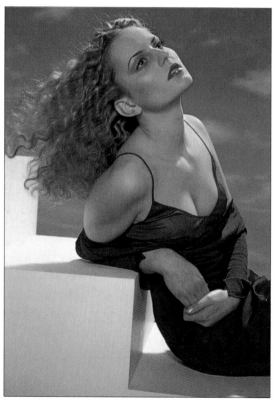

As you've probably guessed, I am not a proponent of home perming: Too much can go wrong. Changing your hair's wave pattern is one of the most complicated things you can do to your locks. The perm process is intricate enough in a salon, where there are professionals who will assess issues, such as your medical history and your hair's texture and condition. At home, there is no one but you and perhaps a well-meaning friend. Yes, salon perms can be expensive, but, in my opinion, you're worth every penny.

■ **For a beautiful result,** *a perm is best left to the professionals – they've been trained to consider all the variables and all the possible outcomes.*

Caring for your permed hair

WHEN YOU GET A PERM, *you put your locks through a complicated process designed to break down, then reconfigure strands' structure. All this quick-changing is hard on hair, leaving tresses fragile. Coddling is required to prevent treated locks from looking or being damaged.*

Careful handling

You used to rake through your hair with a vent brush, or tug at wet strands with a fine-toothed comb. Maybe you scraped locks back into a tight ponytail that you held in place with a rubber band you removed from a bundle of newspapers. Or perhaps you were constantly twirling your hair or nervously fiddling with it in some other way. All this has got to stop now that you have a perm. Think of your strands as something precious and very delicate, akin to the fibers that make up a silk blouse or angora sweater. Careful handling doesn't require any special instructions – simply use common sense: detangle hair gently before brushing, don't style or touch or play with strands more than necessary, pull hair back in windy weather so locks won't become knotted, and so on.

Trivia...

Before chemical waves were developed, permanent waves were given by a machine! The invention is credited to British hairdresser Charles Nestle, who created the machine in 1906. In America, Marjorie Stewart Joyner, who took out a US patent on her version of the permanent-wave machine in 1928, is often credited with its invention.

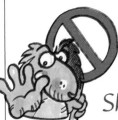

Don't get a permanent wave if your head has scratches, nicks, pimples, or if your skin is in any way broken – the chemicals can severely irritate your scalp.

Shampoos and conditioners for permed hair

If, before your perm, you were using shampoo and conditioners formulated for oily or normal hair, or if you were using bodybuilding or dandruff shampoos, post-perm is the time to switch. Harsh detergents rough up your permed hair's already manhandled cuticle, damaging strands, drying hair, and turning locks into a frizzy mess. You see, products for chemically treated hair not only have gentle detergents, they boast concentrated emollients, which do several things: they protect hair from moisture loss, condition and help repair perm-abused hair, and keep curls fit and bouncy. It's true – moisturized curls are springier than their dehydrated cousins.

The right styling products

To emphasize individual curls, some people use gel, sculpting lotion, and/or mousse on permed hair. I don't. Not only can these products dry already-dehydrated hair, they create a "crunchy" finish. Have you ever tried to run your hand or a brush through crunchy hair? Because these products behave like adhesive, hair loses its flexibility and you end up accidentally pulling strands of hair from the root or trying to bust apart glued-together ends. Instead, opt for conditioning creams and sprays.

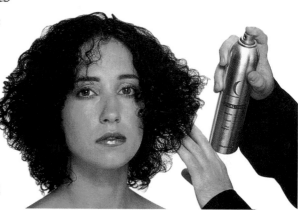

■ **Healthy styling options** *for permed hair include volumizing sprays, styling cream, and styling wax that can be applied just at hair's ends.*

Give it to me straight

RELAXERS STRAIGHTEN HAIR – NOT ALL THE WAY, but enough to make tightly wound coils of hair look like soft curls or even loose waves. Long used by people of Afro-Caribbean descent, relaxers are also popular with curly-haired women of European ancestry. Like permanent waves, relaxers work by breaking down hair's bonds, then restructuring them in a different configuration. Unlike permanent waves, rollers are not used, which makes the procedure a bit easier and faster – but no less harsh. In fact, relaxing services often begin with an application of petroleum jelly or cream to the scalp; this protects skin from the harsh chemicals that follow.

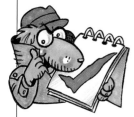

If your hair is damaged, but not extremely so, don't be surprised if your stylist asks you to undergo a series of deep-conditioning treatments before she will relax your hair. If the damage is slight, she may agree to relaxing your hair on the spot after applying a protective conditioner – called a filler – to the porous, damaged areas of your hair.

Next comes an application of the relaxing solution, which is painted on hair, then pulled through tresses to ensure all strands are coated. The longer the solution is left

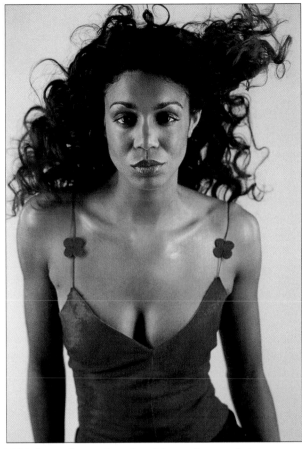

Tight curls can be *relaxed into soft, wavy hair or very straight hair depending on hair type and the chemicals used.*

on, the straighter the hair will be. However, because of its harshness, relaxing solution usually remains in place just 5 to 8 minutes to avoid harming hair. Note: Some chemical technicians actually comb relaxing solution through strands, although many experts feel this leads to severe breakage.

Fixing the relaxer

When the hair has finished processing, the relaxing chemicals are rinsed away with warm water. This is a long rinse – some stylists keep their clients under the faucet for 10 to 15 minutes. Afterward, hair is shampooed for up to 10 minutes. Next comes a neutralizer solution – often called a fixative or a stabilizer. Like the one used in a permanent-wave service, this neutralizer encourages the hair's bonds to stay put in their new configuration. Some stylists finish the service with a deep-conditioning treatment to re-moisturize strands.

Depending on the company that makes them, some relaxers use a neutralizing shampoo instead of separate applications of shampoo and neutralizer solution.

Among the several types of relaxers are:

a **Sodium hydroxide relaxers** These are also known as lye relaxers. As the strongest of the relaxer types, sodium hydroxide formulas provide the fastest results and the most dramatic straightening effects. While they are capable of making super-kinky hair super-straight, the chemicals are so damaging that it is not often recommended. A better option for most people with really curly hair is to go for a loose wave, which can be worn naturally, or, occasionally, blow-dried straighter for special occasions.

b **Calcium hydroxide relaxers** These are often referred to as "no-lye" relaxers and contain a mixture of calcium hydroxide and guanidine carbonate. While calcium hydroxide relaxers are slightly less damaging than sodium hydroxide relaxers, they tend to create frizzy, fuzzy, rough-looking results – the chemicals simply aren't strong enough to evenly break down the hair's bonds.

c **Ammonium thioglycolate relaxers** Often called thio relaxers or perm relaxers, they use the same ingredients as many permanent waves. The results, while thorough – none of that no-lye relaxer fuzziness here – are gentle. Thio relaxers are better at gently softening curls than aggressively turning kinks to waves. For this reason, they are popular with Caucasian curlytops and others whose original curls are on the moderate side.

> ### Trivia...
> In African-American hair salons, relaxers are often called perms, due to their permanent (or somewhat permanent) ability to loosen curls.

At-home versus in-salon relaxers

YOU PROBABLY ALREADY KNOW WHERE I STAND *on home relaxing: I think you should leave it to the professionals. As talented as you may be with hair – and I bet you are talented – you haven't gone to beauty school nor do you have the experience that comes from spending day after day facing all kinds of straightening situations.*

Making your choice

Here's another way to think of it: If you do your own hair, think how tired your arms are going to get from reaching behind your head to apply relaxer to your nape, your crown, and the spots behind your ears. How are you going to see what parts of the back are done, or even if you've applied the relaxer formula evenly? What are you going to do if the relaxer doesn't seem to be working – or if it seems to be working a bit too well? If you go to a respected stylist, you can sit back, relax, and let the professional do all the work. Your turn to work will come after the service.

I suggest choosing color OR a relaxer or permanent wave. Do both and you risk very damaged, very dull hair. If you positively cannot live without changing your hair's wave pattern and wearing hair color, wait 3 or 4 weeks after the relaxer or perm, then head to your salon for semi-permanent or demi-permanent hair color. Your strands can't take the ammonia and peroxide found in permanent color.

Caring for straightened hair

YOUR STRAIGHTENED HAIR IS MUCH MORE *delicate than your pretreated strands. To ensure your tresses remain healthy, you must do everything possible to shield them from harm. This means gentle treatment, vigilant conditioning, and perhaps giving up some of the things you used to do such as using straightening irons, backcombing, or regular use of curling irons.*

Careful handling

You probably already know that rough treatment damages your hair. You probably also know what rough treatment is: brushing wet hair, tight roller sets, overly vigorous shampooing, hair clips that snare strands, and many more methods of styling.

RANDOM THOUGHTS

When you use a thio-type relaxer on top of sodium hydroxide relaxer, hair is melted away. For this reason, it is important to always ask your hairdresser what type of relaxer he or she uses. Here are a few more relaxer facts:

- Relaxers shouldn't remove every iota of hair's wave. Taking hair from curly to stick-straight is extremely damaging to strands.
- To keep hair and scalp healthy, relaxers should be scheduled no more often than every 3 months.
- Excessive use of relaxers can permanently damage hair. For this reason, it's imperative that you avoid re-relaxing previously treated hair: Stick to touching up the re-growth.

DEFINITION

Mechanical refers to physical activity, such as brushing, twirling between your finger, or backcombing.

If you're new to this hair-coddling business, however, keep in mind that relaxed tresses are especially vulnerable to all kinds of stress, be it *mechanical* or thermal. A good rule of thumb: If you have to ask yourself whether an activity is hard on hair, it probably is. Avoid harsh styling and leave your hair as natural as possible whenever you can.

Shampoos and conditioners for relaxed hair

If your hair is relaxed, you probably know first-hand the changes that have occurred in its texture, the way it feels in your hand, how it responds to styling products and so on. It's probably drier, less vibrant, more brittle, and much more easily prone to damage. For this reason, choose products that are labeled "for chemically treated hair" – or go a step farther and find shampoos and conditioners formulated specifically for relaxed tresses. These low-detergent, high-emollient products won't rough up your delicate cuticle layer nor will they strip your hair of important natural oils. What they will do is infuse parched hair with moisture and create a protective barrier to help fragile strands withstand styling stress.

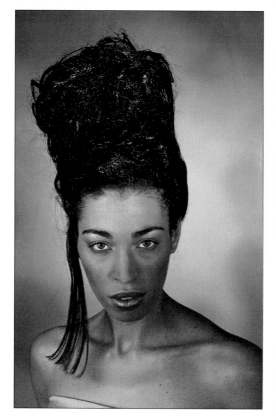

The right styling products

If you were using moisture-filled styling products before your relaxing treatment, keep on using them. In fact, you may even want to kick the conditioning up a notch and seek out products designed solely for chemically treated hair. Don't go overboard though: Use too much conditioning oil, pomade, or styling wax and your hair will get grimy, forcing you to the shower for more frequent shampoos. Styling products to avoid? Go easy on dehydrating products such as sculpting lotion, gel, or alcohol-based hairsprays.

■ **When styling hair** *for a night out, make sure you use products designed to protect relaxed hair. To further safeguard hair's health, limit the amount of heat styling you do.*

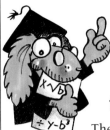

If your hair is in good shape prior to relaxing, but begins breaking heavily after the procedure, there's a good chance that your strands weren't properly neutralized.

Heat styling

The less you do to your relaxed hair, the healthier it will be. This means that if you opt for a wash-and-wear look, your hair will be stronger and suffer from less breakage than if you blow-dry or use a straightening iron, a curling iron, or hot rollers. Occasional thermal styling is fine, but if you have to use heat several times a week, ask yourself this: Could it be that you're not used to seeing yourself with relaxed waves? Or do you truly believe your hair looks unpresentable if it's not blow-dried to a stick-straight state? If it's the first, try wearing your hair in its post-relaxed waves and see if the look grows on you. If it doesn't, ask your stylist for a good cut that works so well with your relaxed waves that you no longer think about forcing it straight.

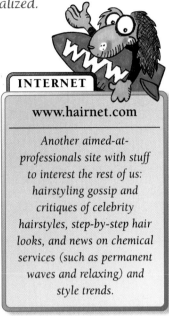

INTERNET

www.hairnet.com

Another aimed-at-professionals site with stuff to interest the rest of us: hairstyling gossip and critiques of celebrity hairstyles, step-by-step hair looks, and news on chemical services (such as permanent waves and relaxing) and style trends.

A simple summary

✓ Instead of fighting your hair's natural tendencies, a permanent wave or relaxing service can make your life easier.

✓ Permanents and relaxers use similar chemicals to break the hair's bonds apart.

✓ Chemically altered hair must be coddled to avoid breakage.

✓ Special shampoos, conditioners, and products are essential to maintain treated hair.

✓ Heat styling is hard on both permed and relaxed strands.

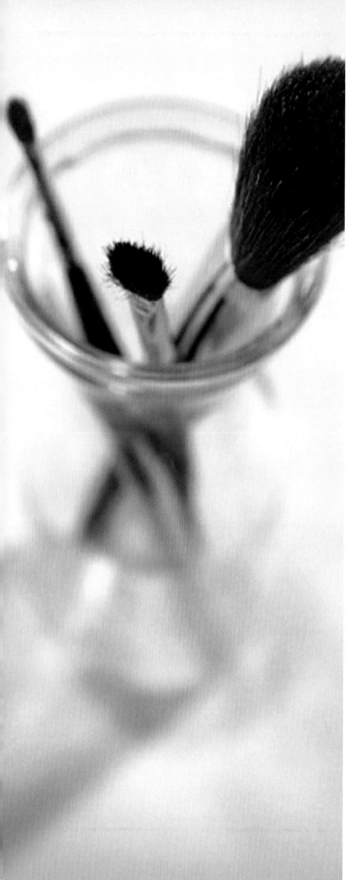

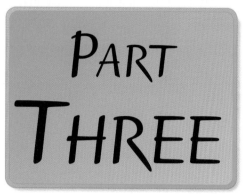

PART THREE

INVEST IN A FEW QUALITY MAKEUP BRUSHES

MAKEUP

D O YOU NEED TO WEAR MAKEUP? Do you want to wear it? If so, how do you decide what products are for you? After all, there are *thousands of cosmetics* out there – including foundations, lip pencils, brow products, and more. It's easy to get carried away and buy too many items, but think of it this way: Do you really want (or need) eight or ten products on your face? If you're like most of us, you can *dress up your looks* with a lot less paint if you choose products carefully and apply them well.

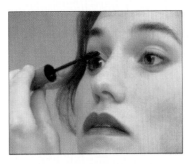

Yes, deciding what to wear is only the beginning. At some point you'll have to apply your makeup – with a light hand, please! – so it looks *natural and alluring*, like you, only better. The following chapters will help you do just that.

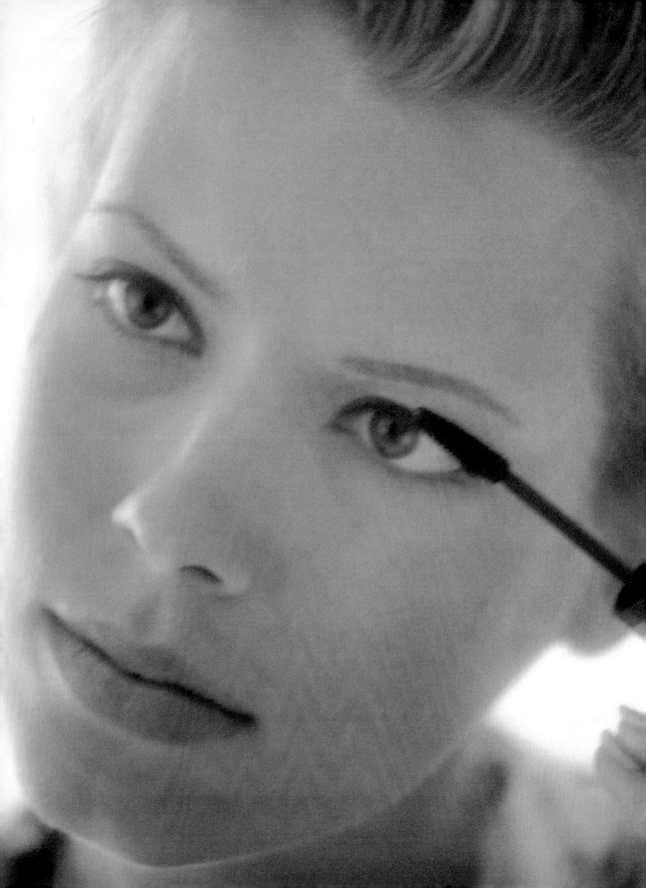

Chapter 11

Makeup Fundamentals

IT WAS THE ROMAN DRAMATIST PLAUTUS who wrote, "A woman without paint is like food without salt." I do understand what he's saying – makeup complements human beauty. Indeed, people have been wearing makeup throughout history. In 4000 BC Egyptians were painting their eyebrows with kohl and in 1100 BC Greeks were wearing rouge. Today, we have a larger variety of cosmetics at our disposal than at any point in time and the freedom to choose what's right for each of us.

In this chapter...

✓ Why wear makeup?

✓ Instant bone structure

✓ Lip service

✓ Making eyes

✓ Makeup tools

✓ Cruelty-free cosmetics

EYE MAKEUP CAN ACCENTUATE THE NATURAL BEAUTY OF YOUR EYES

Why wear makeup?

YOU DON'T NEED MAKEUP
to be beautiful. We all know gorgeous women who never touch the stuff, as well as less attractive women who are never seen without a full face of paint. Makeup helps those of us who wish our cheekbones were higher, our skin more evenly toned, or our jaws more prominent. Makeup is also a way to celebrate those features we love and want to draw attention to, such as almond-shaped eyes or a rosebud mouth. And lastly, makeup is fun – or should be. From an unusual shade of eyeliner and long, flirty eyelashes, to a brighter-than-usual lipstick and a bit of sparkle across the cheekbones – makeup is the grown-up equivalent of playing dress-up.

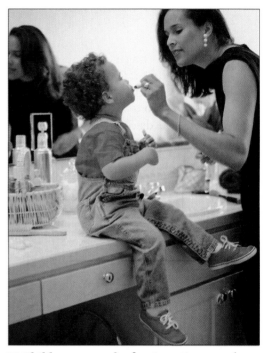

■ **Children sense the fun** *in putting on makeup – they love the colors, pots, and brushes, and often want to get involved too.*

Complexion perfecters

I have been on photo shoots where the makeup artist spent most of his or her time working on a model's skin. At first, this didn't make sense to me: Why not devote more energy to features like the eyes or mouth? Then a makeup artist explained to me that skin is the foundation of the complete look. If skin looks flawed, no one will look past it to see the eyes or mouth. That made sense. After that, I made more effort with foundation, coverup, and powder. I also started looking more closely at my skin-care regimen – after all, makeup can help hide skin glitches, but it can never be a substitute for good skin care.

■ **A powder compact** *is an invaluable accessory for a busy woman. You can quickly powder your face during a busy day and keep your skin looking even, free from oil, and blemish-free.*

Considering foundation

A lot of people are hesitant to wear foundation, or "base" as it's sometimes called, because they're afraid of an unnatural result. Yes, foundation can look like a mask, but only if you choose the wrong product or apply it incorrectly. Take the time to think through a foundation regimen so that you achieve results that suit your skin and your lifestyle.

First, decide how much coverage you need. Sheer foundations – also known as light or natural coverage – provide a see-through wash of color with only enough camouflaging power to hide minor imperfections. Moderate coverage is a good choice for those of us with some discoloration, a few acne scars, maybe some freckles, or broken blood vessels. Heavy coverage foundation offers the heaviest coverage. It is good for covering burns, birthmarks, bruising, melasma, and scars.

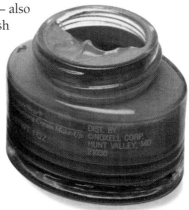

It is important to consider your skin type. If you have dry skin you should avoid oil-free and oil-absorbing makeup, which will give your skin a parched, flaky finish. Those of us with oily skin should eschew moisturizing makeups that will make skin look slick and greasy, and normal skin types should stick with a formula for normal skin. Most cosmetic companies make several types of foundations, each geared toward a different skin type. If you are having trouble deciphering foundation formulas, ask a salesperson – they're paid to help. If you're in a drugstore, look for clues on the product's label or packaging.

■ **Make sure you** *choose a foundation suitable for your skin type.*

Choosing a product

Don't be afraid to experiment with different products. Most foundations are liquid or cream, but some come in cake form and are applied with a sponge. Another type of foundation is wet-to-dry – you apply it with a damp sponge and it dries to a powdery finish.

Do not use foundation to change your skin color! These products are designed to enhance your complexion, not to alter it.

Be sure to choose the right shade. Avoid overtly pink, peach, orange, or russet shades, which rarely occur in nature. To create a flawless finish – and to prevent a masklike look – a foundation's color must be matched as closely as humanly possible to the color of your own facial skin.

If you're in a department store or makeup artist's shop, a salesperson can help you find your perfect match. If you're in a drugstore, search for testers and a mirror.

You will achieve a more even finish if you apply foundation correctly. Dot the makeup onto your forehead, nose, and chin, and then blend it down under the eyes, outward to the cheeks, and toward the jaw. This keeps makeup concentrated in the area of the face where most of us have the greatest number of imperfections, and also keeps makeup from building up at the jaw line, where it can look fake. You can use your fingers to do the blending, or you can use a makeup sponge. Just be aware that a sponge absorbs some of the makeup, which means less product on your skin and a sheerer finish than you'd get if you were using your fingers.

Trivia...

A tinted moisturizer isn't strictly a foundation. It's a moisturizer with a small amount of sheer pigment added. Similarly, a tinted sunscreen is a sunscreen with a small amount of sheer pigment added.

SHOPPING FOR MAKEUP

Does it matter where you buy your cosmetics? For the most part, no, but loose powder, foundation, and concealer are three products that are best bought from a department-store brand or makeup-artist line. There are three main reasons for this:

1. **Color:** The more expensive foundations and concealers generally have a natural-looking yellow cast, while cheaper products tend to have very pink, peachy, or orangey shades – tones that are unnatural even for Caucasian women and impossible for women of African, Indian, Pacific Island, or Asian descent. Furthermore, department-store brands and makeup-artist lines boast wider ranges of shades. Some lines even offer custom blending to ensure the shade is exact.

2. **Quality:** Cheaper brands may include inexpensive ingredients, such as talc, that sit atop the skin and create a chalky, unnatural finish.

3. **Your needs:** If you want a talc-free, finely milled loose powder that gives your skin a flawless finish without dryness, go with a loose powder from a department-store or makeup-artist line. If you're simply looking for something you can throw in your bag for midday touch-ups or to sop up extra oil, head to the drugstore for a compact of pressed powder.

■ **To help you find** *the right foundation tone for your skin, test a variety of different products – ideally, on your jaw – and ask the sales assistants for advice.*

Using concealer

I love concealer. Also called coverup, this highly concentrated product is like a super-coverage foundation. I use it on a bright, broken blood vessel on my nose and on the small dark patches I have on each cheek. Other people pat it under their eyes to lighten up dark circles, or dab it on pimples to mask them. When choosing coverup, look for a product that is a half shade to a shade lighter than your complexion. The most popular concealers come in swivel-up sticks that look like lipsticks, although they are also available in small tubes or pots, or containers with sponge-tip applicators. The thicker the formula, the more concentrated the product, and the better the product's ability to hide skin glitches. Thus, the stick usually has the greatest coverage, followed by the pot, tube, and sponge-tip container respectively.

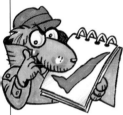

If you've ever wondered about those color-tinted coverups, here's the scoop: Yellow-tinted shades lighten brownish discoloration and purplish or grayish scars, while green-tinted shades help neutralize redness.

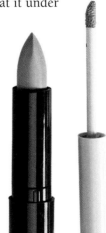

■ **Concealers** *come in a variety of forms and consistencies.*

If you've got particularly good skin, you can skip the foundation outright and simply pat a bit of concealer onto areas that you feel could use some help. Alternatively, you can use concealer in conjunction with foundation. Although some makeup artists apply concealer under foundation, I agree with those professionals who use concealer as a finishing touch to cover those things that foundation couldn't. Besides, if you apply concealer after the foundation, this helps prevent concealer from being accidentally wiped away. When applying coverup, use your third or fourth finger, and liberally pat the product onto the area to be covered. You can use a makeup sponge, but the sponge absorbs so much of the product that you're better off with your finger. Whatever you use, remember to pat, not rub, so that you don't accidentally wipe off any makeup.

Powder: pressed and loose

Powder is terrific for *setting* foundation, absorbing oil, and creating a flawless finish. I prefer loose powder because of its natural-looking, slightly see-through finish.

Unlike loose powder, pressed powder contains extra ingredients to bind powder particles together so that they stay pressed in a compact. Unfortunately, these binders can also clog pores and contribute to pressed powder's heavy look. Still, I do keep a compact of pressed powder in my bag for quick touch-ups when I'm out.

DEFINITION

In makeup-speak, setting *refers to fixing something in place so that it will last longer. Powder sets foundation by absorbing excess oil and moisture on the skin, both of which could cause foundation to melt.*

Translucent powder is a sheer shade that works well with most fair skins, especially those with a bit of pink. The rest of you, however, should look for a powder in a shade that is not only near your own skin tone, but that contains no unnatural looking pink, peach, orange, or russet tones. One last powder point: Many cosmetic companies make powders with additions, including UV protection, moisturizers, and zit-zapping ingredients – something to consider if your skin has special needs.

■ **Use loose face powder** *to fix freshly applied makeup; you may need to rely on a powder compact during the day.*

Instant bone structure

A STRONG bone structure gives a face a certain presence and definition. If you have prominent cheekbones and a confident jaw line, it doesn't matter how close-set your eyes, how bulbous your nose, or how lopsided your lips, you're still going to turn heads. Yes, I developed that theory myself, but only after looking at hundreds of strong-boned beauties (many of them models) whose other features were average, asymmetrical, or unusual. I, unfortunately, wasn't blessed with prominent bones. I rely on blush to draw attention to my cheeks. If you must do the same, keep reading.

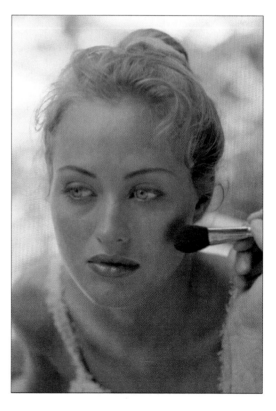

■ **Even a light tone** *of blusher can attractively accentuate the line of the cheek bone.*

Cheeky color

I have sallow skin, which is one reason I like cheek color: it makes my skin look vibrant. But perhaps what I like best about cheek color is how a hint of pink on my cheekbones, on my chin, and at the temples makes it appear as if I actually had some kind of bone structure!

Cheek color comes in several forms. The most common types are blush and rouge. Blush is a colored powder you brush on with a makeup brush, and rouge is a cream – usually packaged in a small pot – that is applied with your fingers or a makeup sponge. Other forms of cheek color are translucent gel (packaged in a tube); swivel-up cheek color sticks; and liquid cheek color, which looks like colored water and creates a budge-proof translucent stain on your skin.

■ **Brush on blush powder** *is convenient to carry in your purse. It's also easy to use, and it gives you subtle, effective results.*

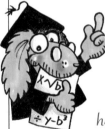

What type of cheek color should you use? The drier your skin, the creamier your makeup should be – rouge and swivel-up cheek color sticks are great for dry complexions. Gel and liquid cheek color are terrific for normal skin. Brush-on blush – which can be used successfully on all skin types – is a must for oily skin, and will help reduce shine on the complexion.

Achieving effects with highlighting cream

Highlighting cream – also called highlighter – is a makeup-bag extra, something that's nice to have but not necessary. This pale, slightly pearlescent cream catches the light, making a feature appear more prominent. When I use highlighting cream – usually for a night out – I pat a minute amount under my brow bone, on the tops of my cheekbones, and on my jawbone. The result is not at all obvious, but very, very pretty.

Highlighting cream is available in shades with a pink, peach, silver, pale yellow, gold, or copper undertone. It is most often packaged in a small pot, but you can find it in swivel-up sticks, as powder, with a wand applicator, or as a liquid. If you like, you can use a pure white coverup stick as a kind of makeshift highlighter – you won't get the light-catching gleam of a highlighter, but the pale color can make features look more prominent.

Trivia...
In the year 2000, the American cosmetics and beauty industry tallied more than $20 billion in sales.

Using bronzer

Bronzer is used to give skin a tanned look – and it is a much safer option than sunbathing. Its color is a close approximation to bronze, such as deep tan, red-brown, or golden tan. I am not a big bronzer user, but I have friends who love the sun-splashed glow it gives cheeks, temples, chins, and other areas. Bronzer looks like blush and is applied in exactly the same way. It is available in powder, cream, gel, and bead forms.

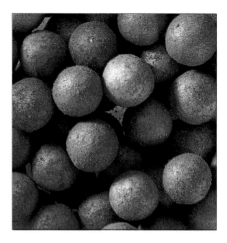

■ **Bronzing beads** *usually have two or three tones of color. Run your makeup brush over them and apply to your face.*

WHAT IT ALL MEANS

Ever wondered what terms like hypoallergenic or ophthalmologist-tested mean? Here are some of those confusing terms defined:

a **Fragrance-free:** This does not mean a product has no natural odor; it simply means a product has no separate fragrance added to it. In other words, a fragrance-free product may contain several ingredients – such as botanical extracts – that happen to have odors, but it cannot have fragrance added simply for the sake of fragrance.

b **Hypoallergenic products:** Many people with sensitive skin look for these thinking they won't cause an allergic reaction. While hypoallergenic products are free from the most common allergens – such as mica, glycol, lanolin, and SD alcohol – they can still cause allergies if you happen to be one of the individuals sensitive to one of their ingredients.

c **Non-comedogenic:** These products don't contain common pore-clogging ingredients such as mineral oil. However, if you are breakout prone, even non-comedogenic products can contribute to breakouts.

d **Ophthalmologist-tested:** This term simply means a product was tested by an eye doctor and found to be safe for use around the eye. If you have sensitivities, keep in mind that this term refers only to a product's safety, not its allergy-generating quotient.

Contouring secrets

During the 1970s, contouring was popular – at that time, nearly all powder blushes were accompanied by a deep shade that was meant to be applied to the hollow of the cheeks. While light colors bring features forward, dark colors make features recede, therefore a bit of contour could slim chubby cheeks, as well as soften the look of a double chin or make the sides of a person's nose look slimmer. Outside of a few swivel-up contour sticks, I haven't seen many contouring products on the market lately. That doesn't mean, however, that contouring doesn't exist. Many makeup artists simply use a darker-than-skin shade of foundation or coverup as a face contour. The secret to natural-looking contour is to use a product that is only one or two shades darker than the skin and to apply it with a light hand.

Glitter – either packaged loose in pots or suspended in transparent gel – is a trendy and fun way to draw attention to cheekbones, eyelids, browbones, or lips. Just be sure to use it very sparingly.

Lip service

OUR LIPS BECOME FLUSHED *and rosy when we're sexually aroused and we wear* lip color *to mimic this effect – or so say human sexuality experts. I, however, wear lip color not because it makes me look sexier, but it makes my face look prettier and more balanced. For many women, lipstick is an essential makeup item and they don't feel dressed without it. I favor lip pencils, although during my teen years, lip gloss was the only thing I'd wear. A rundown of each follows.*

> **DEFINITION**
>
> *When I say lip color, I mean any product that adds color to the lips – lip pencils, lipstick, and colored lip gloss are all examples.*

Lip pencils

Lip pencils are sometimes called lip liners because they are often used to outline the lips. This outline helps create more symmetrical-looking lips and prevents lipstick from migrating into the skin surrounding the mouth. Lip pencils can also be used to color the entire lips; they offer precision and are generally longer-lasting than lipstick.

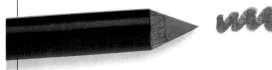

■ **Look after your lip pencils** – *make sure you keep the tip well sharpened so that you achieve maximum definition and accuracy.*

Lipstick allure

It wasn't until I was 20 and on vacation in Paris that I considered wearing lipstick myself. Like many American girls, I'd heard a lot about that elusive French allure. Hoping to capture some of that allure myself, I spent a good part of my stay staring at people. I noticed that French women didn't seem to wear much makeup, but they all wore lipstick – mostly red, but that year, tangerine was trendy and many of the younger women sported bright orange lips. Instead of looking ridiculous, it looked sexy and fun. When it was time for me to leave, I spent my last francs at the airport duty-free shop on a Christian Dior orange. Yes, I wore it in the States and yes, I actually liked the way a colored lip looked.

Thick lip pencils are sometimes referred to as lip crayons.

All about lipstick

Lipstick usually comes in stick form – hence its name. It also comes in pots and in compartmentalized compacts, both of which are applied with a small lipstick brush. You can find lipstick in sheer, almost gloss-like finishes; matte finishes, which are flat, opaque, and not a bit shiny; regular finishes that are somewhat moist and dewy; and shimmer or luster finishes, which are slightly pearlescent. There are long-wearing lipsticks available – these stay on for 4 hours or more, but they can be terribly drying.

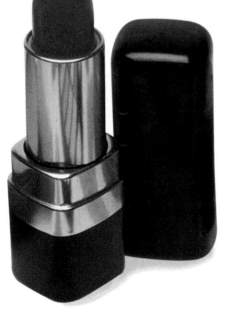

If you dislike the dry finish and unnatural peachy cast of long-wearing lipsticks, you may want to try makeup sealant. A kind of cosmetic shellac, sealants come packaged in tubes or small bottles and can be brushed over any type of lipstick to make it longer wearing.

■ **Lipsticks come** *in a wide variety of colors and finishes; some are also moisturizing and may even provide sun protection.*

Lip gloss

When I was a teenager, lipstick seemed so obvious, so fake, so old-fashioned – something my friends and I would never, ever wear. Looking back, it seems strange that we were worried about fake-looking lips considering all the eye makeup we wore! Instead, we opted for more natural-looking lip gloss.

Today, I wear gloss slicked over lip pencil or dotted on the center of a lipsticked lip to create a subtle shine. Lip gloss comes in pots, tubes, sticks, and wands with sponge-tip applicators. The colors are usually transparent and very subtle, but there are some highly pigmented versions available that give lips a wet, shiny finish.

Making eyes

A FEW MONTHS AGO I was getting my hair colored, when a discussion developed among the stylists and clients about what makes a person attractive. My hairdresser said, "It doesn't matter what the rest of a person looks like – if he or she has beautiful eyes, he or she is beautiful. End of discussion." And so the discussion ended, for who could argue with that? Eyes are the windows to the soul. They are also one of the first things we notice about each other, which helps explain the popularity of eye makeup. No other kind of makeup does so much to enhance – and change – our features as eye makeup.

Mascara

For many of us, mascara is the one thing we put on before answering the door or ducking outside to get the newspaper. Long, lush lashes are considered youthful and sexy, but I suspect the real reason we like mascara is the way it makes our eyes "pop" without making us look done up.

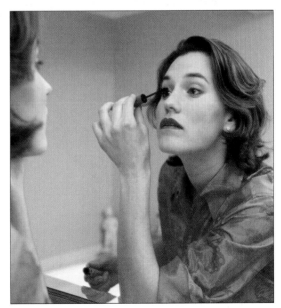

■ **Mascara defines** *the shape and length of your lashes and helps to add volume. It can also make the wearer appear naturally doe-eyed.*

Mascara comes in a wide range of formulas: waterproof, lash-thickening, lash-lengthening, lash-curling, conditioning, glossy-finish types, and even non-flaking versions for contact lens wearers. Although black, black-brown, and brown are the most popular shades, mascara also comes in russet brown (great for redheads), aubergine, purple, royal blue, navy blue, forest green, teal, and other fashion shades.

When I was a teenager (you may have gathered by now that I lived in a small country town with not a lot for us to do), my friends and I were addicted to colored mascaras. We spent hours trying on different colors, trying to decide which shades made green eyes brighter, brown eyes more gold, or blue eyes seem icier. We liked our mascaras as bright as possible, but today I prefer more natural tones.

■ **After applying** *a black or brown shade of mascara, try adding a blue or green tone on top, to give a subtle hint of color.*

Eyeliner

Eyeliner can be drawn above upper lashes or below lower lashes – or both. Its primary purpose is to make the lashes look lush, but it also draws attention to the eye and can enhance or even change the eye's shape. Eyeliner is available in a wide range of hues, from the common black, brown, and gray to more adventurous shades such as bright primary colors, pastels, frosty silvers and golds, white, and even glitter-flecked colors. The most common type of eyeliner is the pencil form, but liner also comes in a tube with a thin brush, in a felt-tip pen, and in cake form to be applied with an eyeliner brush. That said, there is no need to go out and purchase a special eyeliner – simply use a small brush dipped into the eye shadow of your choice.

Trivia...

Mascara used to be available in cake form only – you moistened it with water, passed a brush over the cake, and then applied it to your lashes. Cake mascara is now making a comeback, thanks to its natural finish and ability to build up even the puniest of lashes.

Eye shadow know-how

Eye shadow's primary purpose is to enhance the eye's shape. A dark tone makes an area recede, while a light or bright shade will bring an area forward. This is why eye shadow is often sold in kits of two shades – a dark and a light.

Eye shadow's other use is to draw attention to the eye, which accounts for the many shades of purples, blues, greens, yellows, and oranges that come in and out of fashion. Eye shadow is commonly found in powder form, but it is also available in cream, with a sponge-tip wand, and in crayons.

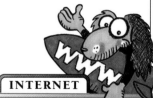

INTERNET

www.makupmania.com
www.ebeauty.com.

For more beauty and cosmetic hints and tips, check out these helpful web sites.

Makeup tools

DO YOU NEED SPECIAL *makeup applicators or can you simply use your fingers? Your fingers or even cotton swabs will work – but in most cases, makeup goes on more precisely, more smoothly, and blends better when you're using good makeup tools. Notice I said "good" makeup tools. Cheaply made, clumsily designed tools actually do more harm than good to your final look, so if you're going to buy makeup tools, be prepared to invest.*

Most makeup-artist lines feature makeup tools; My favorite brushes are from Tony & Tina and are made by master calligraphy brush craftsmen in Japan.

Trivia...

Can you make your lips plumper without a trip to the doctor? Yes, but only temporarily. Lip plumpers, made by companies such as BeneFit, Joey's New York, and English Ideas, fill in small grooves on the lips and coat lips so that they seem puffier. The results last 3 to 6 hours.

Makeup sponges

A makeup sponge is one makeup tool you can pick up for very little money. While sponges are available in flat disks and round shapes, my favorites are the triangular wedges that allow you to apply foundation to large areas or work it into the creases around the nose and eyes, as well as to pat the face clean of excess dirt or oil.

■ **Makeup sponges** *are available at drugstores and are very inexpensive.*

Makeup brushes

Name a type of cosmetic and there is probably a brush to help apply it. These brushes, depending on their intended use, are large, mid-size, small, or downright tiny and are usually used dry – although they can be dampened and used wet. When shopping for makeup brushes, look for sturdy handles and tightly anchored brush hairs. Here's a rundown of brush styles:

1. Powder brushes are big and fluffy with long hairs, all the better to dust on a light, even application of facial powder.

2. Blush brushes are slightly smaller than powder brushes, but have the same rounded shape.

3 Contour brushes aren't as popular as powder and blush brushes, probably because contour isn't as popular as facial powder and blush. If you do use contour, you may want to invest in one of these compact brushes, which look a bit like small blush brushes with shorter, stiffer bristles.

4 The small, rounded heads of eye-shadow brushes allow them to smooth eye shadow onto the lid.

5 To create those darker shades of shadow that are swept into the eye's crease, eye-contour brushes are slightly angled.

6 Eye-blending brushes are larger than eye-shadow brushes and are to be used to blend eye shadows so that one shade blends seamlessly into another.

7 The small, angled heads and stiff hair of eyebrow brushes allow them to work brow color into the brow area.

8 Eyeliner brushes have pencil-thin heads and can be used wet or dry to paint super-slim lines at the base of the lashes.

9 Lip brushes are small with compact, slightly flat heads. They are used to apply lipstick or lip gloss and are terrific for those mix-masters who like to combine colors to create new shades.

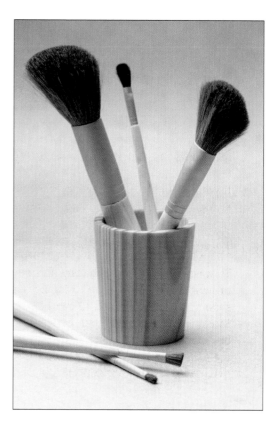

10 Concealer brushes feature stiff bristles and squared heads that allow you to work concealer into small or awkward areas.

Don't assume the best makeup brushes are made from camel or other animal hair; some of the best brushes are entirely synthetic.

■ **Invest in a quality** *set of makeup brushes so that you can achieve the best possible results when you apply your makeup.*

Pencil sharpener

If you use any kind of lip or eye pencils, you'll need a pencil sharpener. These look exactly like those small pencil sharpeners you kept in your school bag as a child – they work the same way, too. Look for a sharpener that has two openings, one for regular, slim pencils, and one for fatter "crayon-type" pencils.

Eyelash curlers

I know big-time makeup artists love eyelash curlers for the way they curl lashes and create a more "open-looking" eye. Still, I don't use an eyelash curler. Then again, my lashes are curly to start with. If yours aren't, you may want to give this contraption a go. Choose a lash curler that fits your eye comfortably – this means it must be wide enough to fit your entire row of lashes – without pinching or pulling any of your lashes.

Lash and brow combs

Lash and brow combs are two-sided tools featuring what looks like a mini-toothbrush on one side and a mini-comb on the other. The brush side is used to brush up brows and blend brow color, while the comb side is for separating lashes.

■ **Use a lash and brow comb** *to brush your eyebrows and lashes, so that they always look well groomed.*

BRUSH CARE

If you use makeup tools every day, it's important to wash them regularly – every 4 to 6 weeks is a good rule of thumb.

Cleaning brushes

To wash a makeup brush, first dampen the head, taking care not to get the base or handle wet (doing so can loosen hairs). Then gently work a tiny amount of shampoo or mild soap into the brush hairs, without splaying or crushing them. Rinse the brush heads under warm running water, again taking care not to get the brush base or handle wet. Gingerly squeeze out excess water with a towel, reshape the hairs, and lay brushes flat on the edge of a sink so that the heads can hang over the brim and drip into the basin. Drying generally takes 5 to 10 hours.

Cruelty-free cosmetics

THERE ARE SOME THINGS ABOUT MAKEUP *you probably don't want to know – such as the animal testing performed by some cosmetic companies. I don't blame you. It is heartbreaking to hear how animals suffer for something as trivial as a lipstick or blush ingredient. But to be an informed consumer, you need to be aware that animal testing exists. The "basic four" animal tests commonly performed by companies involve dripping caustic substances into restrained rabbits' eyes, smearing ingredients onto guinea pigs' raw skin, pushing substances down mice's throats, and forcing rats to inhale cosmetic ingredient fumes. Animals subjected to these tests commonly shake, vomit, bleed from the nose, mouth, or eyes, and can convulse before dying.*

The good news is such tests are not required by US, Canadian, or British law for cosmetic or household products, nor have animal tests been shown to guarantee a consumer's safety.

■ **Many beauty and cosmetic products** *are now manufactured without any animals having to suffer in the process.*

ANIMAL-FRIENDLY BEAUTY

In the market for cruelty-free makeup? Check out the offerings from some of the following compassionate cosmetic companies:

- Avon: www.avon.com
- Bonne Bell: www.bonnebell.com
- Chanel: www.chanel.com
- Christian Dior: www.dior.com
- Ecco Bella Botanicals: www.eccobella.com
- Estee Lauder (Aveda, Bobbi Brown, Clinique, Jane, Origins, Prescriptives, Stila): www.esteelauder.com
- Hard Candy: www.hardcandy.com
- Mary Kay Cosmetics: www.marykay.com
- Merle Norman: www.merlenorman.com
- Revlon (Almay): www.revlon.com
- Tony & Tina: www.tonytina.com
- Urban Decay: www.urbandecay.com

Fortunately, more than 550 companies have banned all animal tests and use modern testing methods, including cell cultures, chemical appraisals, or human volunteer testing. Many of these modern products carry claims such as "not tested on animals" or "cruelty-free." Because knowledge gives me the power I need to be a smart consumer, I research a company's animal-testing policies before I fall in love with its makeup.

There are a number of sources of information you can refer to for advice on products and to find out whether a company uses animal testing. The People for Ethical Treatment of Animals, for example, produce a list of international companies that do and don't test on animals, as well as providing information on ordering *The Shopping Guide for Caring Consumers* – a guide filled with cruelty-free items. You can find them on the internet on www.peta-online.org/liv/cc.html

INTERNET

www.aavs.org/DOC/
cruelty.htm
www.hsus.org/programs
/research/cc-brochure

The American Anti-Vivisection Society publishes a free guide to compassionate shopping and the Humane Society of the United States gives the low-down on cosmetic testing on animals.

A simple summary

✓ Spend time searching for the right foundation. This is one cosmetic you don't want to make a mistake with.

✓ If you have "flawless" skin, concealer is the best option.

✓ Wish you had high cheekbones? Don't despair. Try using a blush to accentuate your features.

✓ Yes, a drugstore lipstick can be as good as an expensive brand –

but be prepared to do some testing before you find one.

✓ Mascara does more than make lashes look long. It also enhances the eyes.

✓ No, you don't need makeup brushes, but they sure make making-up easier.

✓ There are still cosmetic companies that test on animals. Check before you buy.

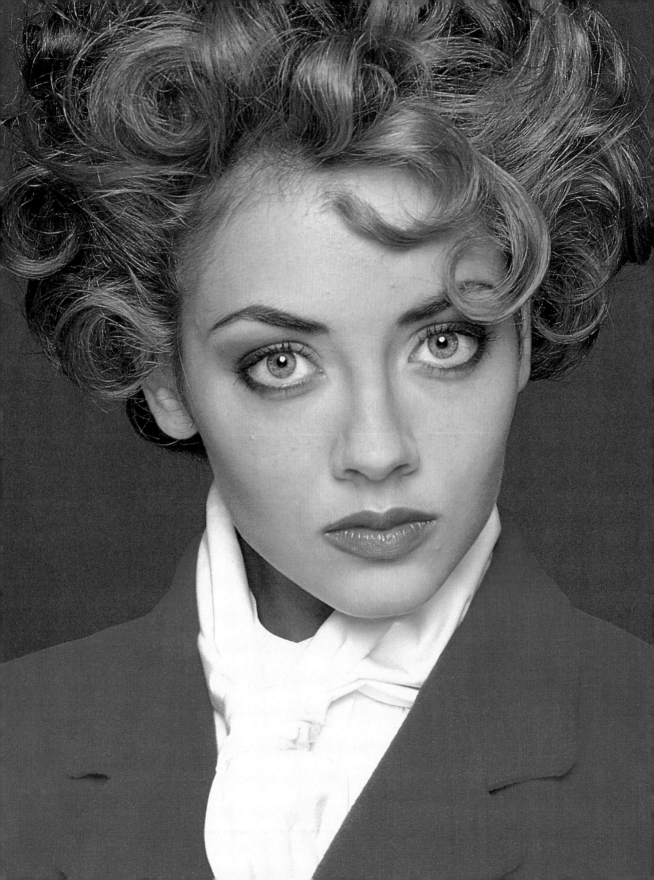

Chapter 12

Giving Good Face

I S THERE A SECRET BEHIND PUTTING ON MAKEUP? In a word, no. Applying makeup is about knowing how makeup works – how it makes one area stand out and another recede, why it glides over dry skin or stays put on oily skin. The best way to learn about makeup is to experiment. Use this chapter as a guide, but remember, all advice is simply advice. Have fun! That's what makeup is for.

In this chapter...

✓ Getting to know you

✓ Just the basics: creating an everyday look

✓ Face shape

✓ Evening glamour

✓ Makeup for special situations

✓ Makeup looks by age

YOU CAN USE MAKEUP TO CREATE A STUNNING LOOK

Getting to know you

*MY BLUE-EYED, SCANDINAVIAN-BLONDE SISTER looks gorgeous
in icy shades; every time we go to a makeup counter together I reach for softly-
colored lipsticks, blushes, and eye shadows to swipe on the back of her hand.
After 15 minutes, her skin is covered with rose, carnation, lilac, lavender,
mauve, and silver streaks. "I am not buying anything pastel!" she says, trying
to move out of my reach. No matter how pretty she looks in these shades, she
will never wear them; she says she hates pastels because they are "too girly,
too prissy." Still, I press these colors on her, although I always promise to stop
because I know how she feels.*

When makeup artists see my yellowy
skin, dark blonde hair, and green
eyes, they immediately move toward
me with terracotta and apricot eye
shadows, bronze blush, and bright,
brick-red lipstick. While these shades
do complement my eyes beautifully,
they make my teeth and the whites
of my eyes appear yellow, in turn
making me feel even more yellow
than I already am. For this reason,
I will never buy orangey-earth shades
no matter how many compliments
I get while wearing them. Why am
I telling you all this? To point out
the importance of personal tastes.

Establishing what you like

Maybe several cosmetic salespeople
have suggested that cream foundation
would work well with your dry skin,
but you detest the product's rich
texture. Perhaps you adore loden
eyeliner even though everyone tells
you navy blue would better suit your
complexion. People may recommend
some contouring in the hollow of your

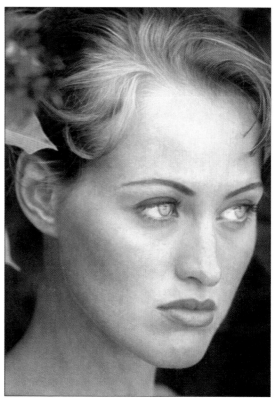

■ **Lovely eyes** *can be created by using makeup you
like and feel comfortable with. Don't be persuaded into
wearing colors you don't like, even if they are supposed
to suit your skin tone and coloring.*

cheeks to accentuate your bone structure, despite the fact you hate contour. What to do? I am all for ignoring other people's advice and following your own tastes – after all, makeup is not only for helping us look and feel better, but also for expressing ourselves, and our likes and dislikes come into that category.

Interested in trying out a certain type of blush, color of eye shadow, or new type of mascara? Head to the cosmetic counter at a nearby department store or makeup artist boutique, where you can test makeup for free. If you like the item after wearing it for 3 or 4 hours, you can return and purchase it.

That said, don't dismiss a cosmetic until you've tried it – which means wearing it in public for a day. This is important because you can't always immediately tell what you will love or hate. For instance, one of my favorite cosmetics is a highlighting cream from *Face Stockholm®*. I had never considered wearing highlighter – for some reason, I always associated it with disco. But one day, I was in New York City's *Face Stockholm®* store with my sister (yes, I was painting pastel stripes on her hands) when I saw a display of several highlighting creams. A month earlier, someone had told me that Caroline Bessette Kennedy used to wear this particular highlighter. Being envious of Bessette Kennedy's naturally glowing skin, I decided to dab some highlighter on my cheekbones and temples. It looked great and not at all disco-like. After wearing the highlighter around Manhattan for a few hours – and still loving the way it looked – I returned to the store and bought it.

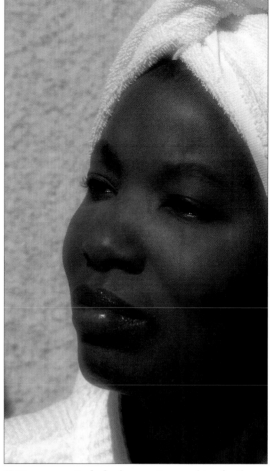

■ **Be open minded** *when you're searching for the right makeup for you – you may be surprised with the results you can achieve with some products that you might normally scorn.*

Trivia...

Although humans have used lip color for hundreds of thousands of years, the swivel-up cosmetic we now call lipstick was only created in 1915.

Just the basics: creating an everyday look

NOW THAT WE'VE ESTABLISHED *your likes and dislikes, I'm going to show you how to create a basic look for daytime wear. Remember, these are suggestions only – if you can't stand foundation, ignore the bit about foundation; if you hate lip color, ignore the information on lip color. And yes, choose whatever colors you like – the following is about application only.*

Applying foundation

Foundation can be applied with the fingers or with a makeup sponge – or both. Dot liquid foundation on your T-zone and, using your fingers or a makeup sponge, blend the makeup out toward the hair line, cheeks, and jawline. If using a cream or wet-dry foundation, glide a makeup-coated sponge along the T-zone and blend outward.

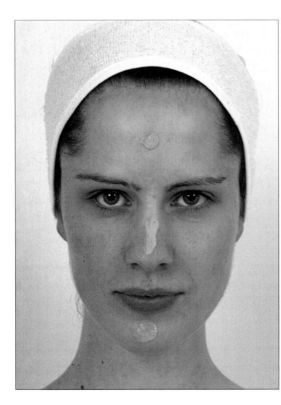

If your foundation looks heavy or blotchy – regardless of whether it was applied with a finger or a sponge – run a makeup sponge across the skin to soak up any excess product.

Concealer can be dotted on skin that's either clean or foundation-prepped. Using a makeup brush or finger, apply a generous coat of concealer to pimples, broken blood vessels, dark spots, scars, under eye circles, dark eyelids, or other skin glitches you'd like to camouflage.

■ **If you prefer liquid foundation,** *dot a tiny amount of the product on your forehead, nose, and chin before blending it in.*

COLOR SELECTOR

How should you choose makeup colors? An often-repeated guideline is to look for colors that have the same undertones as your skin. In other words, if your skin is naturally warm-toned, you should always choose warm-toned colors. If your skin is cool-toned, however, you should opt for cool-toned colors.

WARM COLORS

While this is good general advice, I find the best way to know what looks good on you is to hit a cosmetic counter and start trying on shades. Often, you'll find that a color that is "not supposed" to look good on you is terrifically flattering. Other times you'll find colors that "are supposed" to look good on you make you appear green, yellow, or washed-out. Trying on a color is really the only way to know if it will or won't work for you. Make sure you also take the opportunity to try new products as they become available.

COLD COLORS

Gently tap the area with a clean finger to blend the product and remove excess. Be careful not to rub concealer onto skin – this wipes off makeup and creates a smeared, messy finish.

Contour and highlighters come in cream, gel, stick, liquid, and powder formulas. Keep in mind that if you are using powder contour and highlighters, they go on after face powder. Contour should be dabbed on features you want to diminish, such as the chubby area below cheeks or on a jowly jaw line. Highlighter should be applied on those areas you'd like to stand out, such as the tops of cheekbones or the brow bones. When using either, dot a small amount on the area, and blend using a makeup sponge.

Trivia...
In the early 1900s, it was common for barbers to put rouge and lip color on clients after shaving them.

Using face powder

Face powder should be used after all cream products. This means that if you use cream blush, contour, highlighter, and/or eye-shadow formulas, these need to be applied before you reach for the face powder. Why? Because it is nearly impossible to get cream products to blend well on top of a powdered surface.

This is because face powder creates a barrier between creamy products and powder-based cosmetics, which are often streaky when they are applied, and have a tendency to be absorbed if you put them directly on top of a foundation or a concealer.

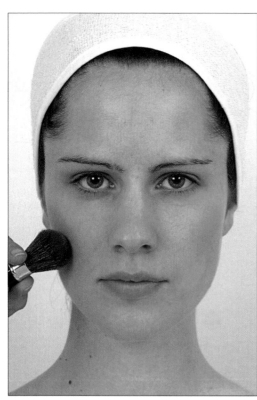

■ **Use a large blush brush** *and apply a small amount of color at a time. You can always add more color if you need to, but it's difficult to remove color if you start with too much – unless you take your makeup off and start again!*

Applying blush

Blush comes in cream, gel, stick, or liquid formulas (in which case it should be applied before face powder), as well as powder formula. Here, I'm going to assume you're using powder blush. A good-sized blush brush – not the dinky plastic one that comes with many powder blushes – is essential for creating a natural-looking result. Run the brush gently over the blush powder, then hold the brush at the apple of your cheek. Using small strokes, softly sweep the brush up the cheekbone, toward the hairline. For an especially realistic look, sweep a bit of blush across the top of the forehead, the chin, and the bridge of your nose.

Where does a natural blush come from? Blood vessels, which lie directly under the skin. When we're aroused, embarrassed, excited, or active, these blood vessels enlarge, allowing a greater amount of blood to flow to the skin. The result of this is visible as flushed cheeks.

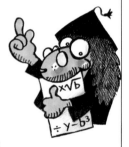

Applying eye makeup

Eye shadow stays on longer if your eyelids have been prepped with a bit of foundation or concealer, and a dusting of face powder. Many makeup artists use three, four, or five colors when making up the eye, but you need only two: a pale neutral that will look good on both the browbone and the lid, and a deeper neutral that can be swept into the eye's crease. Sweep the paler shade across the lid and browbone. Next, brush the darker shade in the crease of the eyelid.

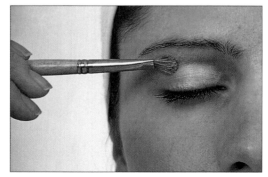

■ **Using an eye-shadow brush** *or your finger, cover the area of your eyelid up to the browbone with a pale neutral shade.*

Applying Mascara

Mascara is often applied after eye shadow, but it can be applied before. In fact, I like to apply mascara before shadow simply because I always spatter mascara everywhere – which can ruin a painted eye. Whichever you choose, if you curl lashes, it should be done before applying mascara. After you curl your lashes, you can make lashes look lusher, and help mascara to adhere better, if you lightly dust lashes with a bit of face powder. Next, close one eye and paint the upper side of the upper lashes. Then, open the eye and apply mascara to the inner side of the upper lashes. Yes, I know this sounds weird, but trust me – applying mascara to both sides of your upper lashes gives you an amazingly luxurious look.

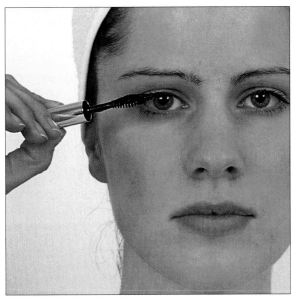

■ **Mascara is best** *kept to the upper lashes. As you apply mascara to your lashes, keep your eyes wide open and try not to blink too vigorously until your lashes are completely dry.*

Lower lashes are strictly optional. I know makeup artists that won't do them, saying it gives the eye a droopy, overly made-up look. Mascara is also especially prone to smudging when applied on the lower lashes. That said, if you like wearing mascara on your lower lashes, hold the wand vertically and apply a light coat to lashes. Let all lashes dry for a minute or two, and then comb through them with a lash comb to unclump them and create a more realistic-looking finish. Clean up any errant bits of mascara with a cotton swab dipped in a small amount of foundation, makeup remover, or moisturizer.

INTERNET

www.beautynewsletter. gq.nu

This web page, updated monthly, features quizzes, product reviews, extensive links, articles, and information for professional makeup artists.

Don't get stuck in a rut. Every once in a while, experiment with your look by trying a new makeup product or playing with new ways to apply old favorites.

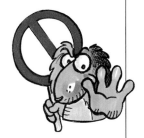

Using eyeliner

Eyeliner comes in pencil or liquid forms, or as a powder that you can apply with an eyeliner brush. Regardless of which you use, apply the product as close to the lash line as possible. The prettiest way to line eyes is to stick to the top lid; if you have droopy or round eyes, liner on the lower lid can exaggerate the eye's shape. However, if you like the look of eyeliner on the lower lash line, stick as close to the lashes as possible and concentrate the color on the outer half of the eye – getting eyeliner too close to the tear duct makes eyes appear smaller and more closely set.

Trivia...

More than 50 percent of lipsticks manufactured in the US contain substantial amounts of castor oil. Castor oil helps lipstick form a shiny film when it dries.

A damp eyeliner brush dipped in your favorite eyeshadow will achieve the same effect as a regular eyeliner – and in a color of your choice.

TIME TO RETIRE

Makeup doesn't last forever. While I'm sure you know that, I'm also pretty sure you probably have a 3-year-old tube of lipstick or 5-year-old eyeliner somewhere in your makeup kit. Unfortunately, makeup does begin to deteriorate after a while. Here are the average cosmetic lifespans for products once they are opened:

- All liquid and cream products, including cream foundation, rouge, bronzer, eye shadow, contour, and highlighter: 1 year.
- All powder products, including loose powder, pressed powder, blush, contour, and eye shadow: 2 years.
- Mascara and liquid eyeliner: 6 months.
- Eye pencils, brow pencils, and lip pencils: 3 years.
- Lipstick, lip color in pots, lip gloss: 2 years.

To prolong makeup's life, keep items stored in a cool, dry place away from direct sunlight. Capping products tightly after use helps further extend your makeup's life. Some products benefit from being manufactured with fresh plant extracts, making them more perishable than other brands. These products often have a "use by" date printed on the label.

APPLYING LIP COLOR

Lip color should be applied to moist, flake-free lips. If your lips are rough and dry, try "brushing" them with a toothbrush dipped in moisturizer, petroleum jelly, or lip balm, before prepping your lips with a light layer of foundation – this will give you a good base to work from. Remember that while you can glide on lipstick straight from the tube, using a lip brush will give you greater accuracy. A handy tip for longer-lasting results: After blotting off excess lipstick with a tissue, give your lips a light dusting of face powder. This will help set lipstick and keep it from migrating onto surrounding skin.

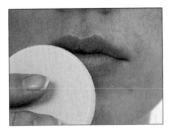

1 **Preparing lips**

Smooth a little foundation over your lips with a makeup sponge or your fingers.

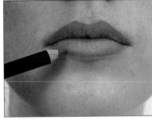

2 **Defining lips**

Use a lip liner in a natural shade to outline your lips. Then use the pencil to fill in the line.

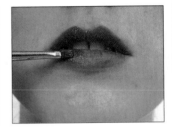

3 **Applying color**

Use a lip brush to apply your chosen lip color. Apply a little color at a time.

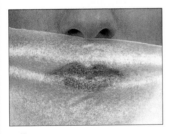

4 **Blotting lips**

Remove any excess color with a thin layer of tissue. Be careful not to smudge the color.

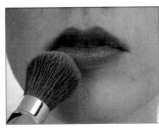

5 **Setting the color**

A little face powder will give your lip color staying power. Add a slick of gloss if you wish.

■ **Taking the time** *to prepare your lips will give impressive and long-lasting results.*

Face shape

WHILE YOUR PERSONAL TASTE *influences what makeup you like, your face shape may (or may not) influence how you wear makeup. Are you happy with the shape of your face? If so, there is no need to change its appearance with cosmetics. However, if you'd like to make your face look less square, round, oblong, triangular, or whatever, cosmetics offer an easy way to create the suggestion of a different face shape. If you haven't yet read the section in Chapter 8 on face shapes, now is the time to do so.*

■ **Oval is considered** *the perfectly balanced face, making it a beauty ideal. If you've got an oval face, don't worry about trying to change its shape.*

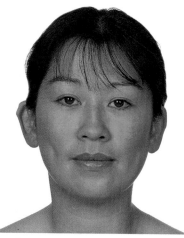

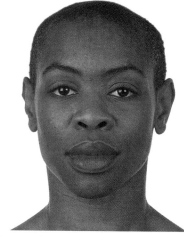

■ **If you have a round face,** *create a more chiseled shape by applying contour to the hollows of the cheeks, and highlighter on the browbone, down the length of the nose, and on the tip of the chin.*

■ **Balance a heart-shaped face** *by applying highlighter along the jawbone, chin, and the tops of the cheekbones. Contour should be applied sparingly at the temples where the forehead is wide.*

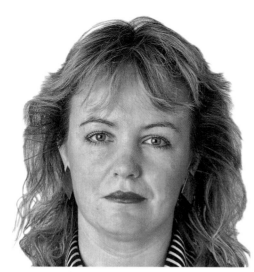

■ **Square faces can be** *"ovalized" by applying contour to the outside corners of the jaw and to each side of the forehead; and applying highlighter on top of cheekbones and down the nose.*

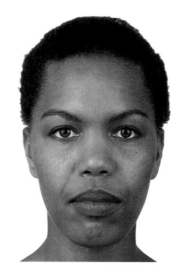

■ **The oblong, or rectangular,** *face can be shortened by applying contour to the base of the chin, and along the hairline. Highlighter at the temples, jaw line, and the top of the cheekbones creates width.*

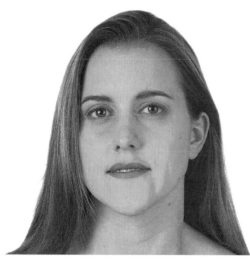

■ **A diamond-shaped face** *can be "ovalized" with a bit of contour at the top of the forehead, tip of the chin, and in the hollows of the cheeks. Highlighter should go at the temples, browbones, and jawbone.*

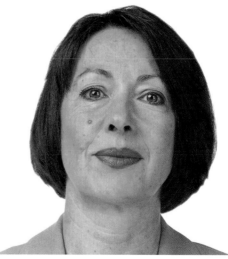

■ **The triangular face** *can benefit from highlighter at the temples and top of the cheekbones, and contour along the outer sides of the jaw.*

If you're using a brown eye shadow, a bronzer, or a brownish blush as a contour, be sure it has no sparkles in it. Sparkles draw attention to an area, defeating contour's purpose.

Evening glamour

FOR MOST OF US, *evening is a time to play with our beauty. We're not governed by those invisible constraints to look professional, or understated, that seem to exist during the day. Don't ask me why this is – I'm still trying to figure it out myself. I suggest, however, you simply enjoy it.*

The hallmark of evening makeup is drama. Note that there is a difference between drama and trying too hard: Putting every makeup product you own on your face will not create drama, it will just make you look like you're wearing every makeup product you own. For some of us, drama means creativity (an arty application of eyeliner); for others, it means seductiveness (smoldering lip color), or boldness (glittery orange, yellow, and green eye shadow), or trendiness (the latest fuchsia blush). Regardless of what drama means to you, the most effective way to create it is to practice the *one-feature rule*. By playing up a single feature, you guarantee that whatever look you create appears planned and gorgeous rather than like some slap-dash look created because you didn't know what to do with your face.

Focusing on a feature

Concentrating color on one feature also ensures that you'll look glamorous instead of tacky, which often happens to a face when there is too much going on. To create your own evening look using the one-feature rule, choose a feature you want to emphasize: your eyes, cheeks, or lips. Go ahead and prepare skin as you normally would – whether that be with foundation, concealer, or both, and a dusting of face powder. Next, concentrate your most attention-getting colors – whether dark or bright – on the chosen feature, downplaying the remaining facial features with neutral colors or no makeup at all. See how great you look?

■ **Evening looks** *work best when one feature is emphasized. Here, the eyes have been emphasized while a neutral shade flatters the lips.*

LASH OUT

There was a time when every Hollywood starlet wore false eyelashes. Today, most of us rely on mascara to pump up lashes and give our eyes a defined look. However, there are times when you might want the old-fashioned glamour of false eyelashes – say for a special evening out, or for your wedding. So you'll know how to use them when the time comes, here are some simple instructions:

1. Gather your supplies: You'll need a pair of tweezers, a pair of false eyelashes, eyelash glue, and liquid eyeliner. You can get false eyelashes and eyelash glue in makeup artist boutiques and in some drugstores.

2. Make sure your natural eyelashes are clean and free from moisture or oil. With clean tweezers, pick up one strip of false eyelashes and dab a bit of eyelash glue along the inside of the strip's base. Wait 15–30 seconds for the glue to dry slightly.

3. Close your eye and position the false eyelashes over the top of your own lashes. Press the strip of false lashes as close as possible to the roots of your own lashes. Make sure you secure both the inner and outer corners of the false lashes against your own lashes. Keep the eye closed for up to 60 seconds, gently pushing the false eyelashes against your own lashes' roots.

4. To hide the false eyelashes' seam, run a thin line of liquid eyeliner over their base.

5. Open your eyes and brush on a light coat of mascara on the underside of the upper lashes. This will blend your own and the false lashes, creating a more natural-looking result.

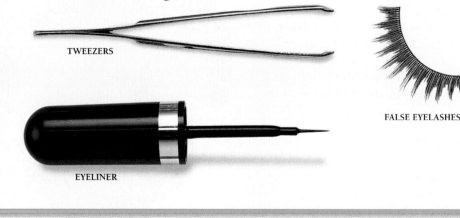

TWEEZERS

FALSE EYELASHES

EYELINER

DAY TO NIGHT DRAMA

Many of us work and can't run home to wash our faces and create an evening look from scratch. Instead, we must duck into our workplace's women's room and attempt to change our day look into an evening look. Actually, there's nothing wrong with this approach and it can be very simple. Try the following steps:

1. Blot your face with a damp paper towel.

2. With a cotton swab, clean up any migrating mascara, eyeliner, or eye shadow.

3. Apply concealer to those areas that need a bit of camouflage.

4. Lightly dust your face with face powder.

5. Choose the feature you are going to emphasize. If it is eyes, go ahead and put on fresh eye shadow (hopefully in bright or smoldering shades), eyeliner, and a new coat of mascara. If lips are what you are going to emphasize, line them with your chosen lip pencil, fill in with a bright or dark lip color, blot, then reline with lip pencil, and dust with powder. Finish by dipping a lip brush in colored gloss and applying a small amount to the center of your lips. If cheeks are what you are emphasizing, apply a bright shade on the apples of your cheeks. Lightly apply a small amount of blush across the nose, on the chin, and over the forehead.

6. Fix your hair in your chosen way, mist yourself with your favorite scent, and change into any special nighttime gear.

7. Do one last mirror check to make sure everything is blended and you have no lipstick on your teeth. Have a great night!

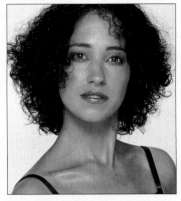

■ **With a little help,** *daytime makeup can easily be adapted for the evening.*

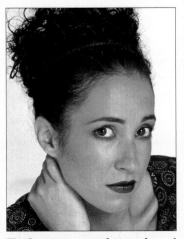

■ **Changing your hairstyle** *and emphasizing one feature, such as the lips, can transform your look.*

Makeup for special situations

SOMETIMES OUR EVERYDAY MAKEUP
just isn't enough and nighttime makeup is too much.
Perhaps we need help to correct a situation, want
something special to get married in, or something
that won't make our eyes look bug-like behind
glasses. The great thing about makeup is it is
adaptable and helpful – if you've got a beauty
situation, makeup can be of assistance.

Looking good in photographs

You're going to have your picture taken and you want to look your best. What do you
do? Focus on creating the most flawless skin possible. After smoothing on foundation,
pat concealer onto discolored areas, and then blend everything before powdering to
make sure there are no lines of demarcation. If
you don't normally wear eyeliner and lip liner,
try putting some on – they'll help define your
eyes and lips and keep them from "looking lost"
in photographs. While you can afford to go a
bit brighter with the blush and lipstick, don't
go overboard – overly heavy makeup will look
overly heavy in pictures. Choose clear colors.
Murky mauves, brown-burgundies, and
grayed roses don't translate well on film
and can make you look ill and washed out.
While an extra coat of mascara is a good
idea, keep the eye shadow lightly applied,
medium to light in tone, and neutral
in color; too much dark eye shadow
(or overly bright eye shadow) can
make eyes look small in photographs.

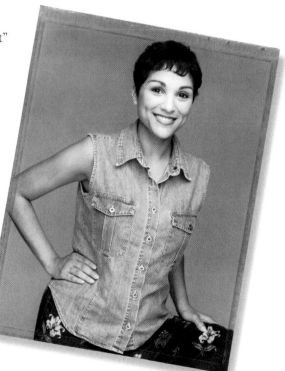

■ **For black-and-white** *photography, you*
can afford to be a little more dramatic with
your makeup. Stronger lip and eye colors
will define your features without making
you look unnatural.

Eyeglass and contact lens wearers

Eyeglasses can distort the eyes, making them look smaller or larger than they really are. Fortunately, makeup can counteract the effects of glasses.

When you're farsighted, you have trouble seeing things that are near you, therefore your glasses make objects appear farther away. They also make your eyes seem a bit smaller, so play up your eyes with an extra coat of mascara. If you like bright eye-shadow shades, you can afford to experiment with bold colors, as long as you blend makeup well. Eyeliner drawn along the top lashes will help further define the eye.

When you're nearsighted, you have trouble seeing distant objects, therefore your glasses help magnify these. They also magnify your eye area, which means unblended makeup, clumpy mascara, and smudged eyeliner is more noticeable to people around you. If you're nearsighted and wear glasses, opt for subtle eye-makeup colors, and be scrupulous about blending eye shadow, cleaning up smudges, and combing out any clumps of mascara.

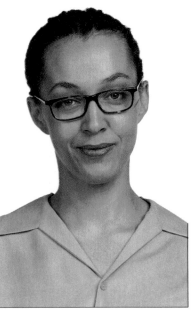

■ **Eyeglasses** *can emphasize any smudges and smears around your eyes, so take extra care when you apply your makeup. Clean up any glitches with a little eye-makeup remover if necessary.*

A special warning for contact lens wearers: If a mascara flakes, don't wear it; the flakes can become trapped between your contact and the eye.

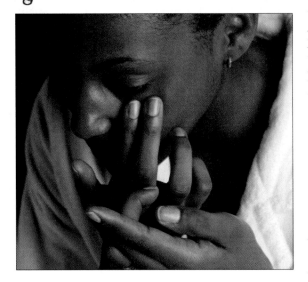

If you're a contact-lens wearer, put your contacts in before putting on your makeup. As for eye makeup, go easy on the eyeliner – or avoid it altogether – and do not use lengthening mascaras, which often contain fibers that can get in your eyes and cause irritation.

■ **Contact-lens wearers** *should avoid using products that flake or shed. Check the labels and opt for products designed specifically for people who wear lenses.*

Makeup for brides

Conventional wedding wisdom recommends soft, pink-tinted makeup. Yet, pink is more girly than womanly, and many brides do not want to look girly. I know I didn't, so I wore a lipstick that was both bright and deep – a dark red touched with a bit of brown. And instead of the peach or pink or lavender eye shadow so many bridal magazines were pushing, my makeup artist covered my eye with a neutral beige, smudged a smoky brown in the crease, then gave me winged black eyeliner, heavy black lashes, and just-dramatic-enough brows. I looked strong and glamorous – which is exactly the way I wanted to appear. Why am I telling you this? To show you that there is more than one way to face your wedding day. Ignore the wedding planners, those relentless wedding magazines, the makeup artist in the salon where you get your hair done, your mother, and your cousin. Instead, think about what you find beautiful and don't be afraid of makeup that is strong or sexy. After all, marriage is a very adult step – it's nice to look like an adult when you walk down the aisle.

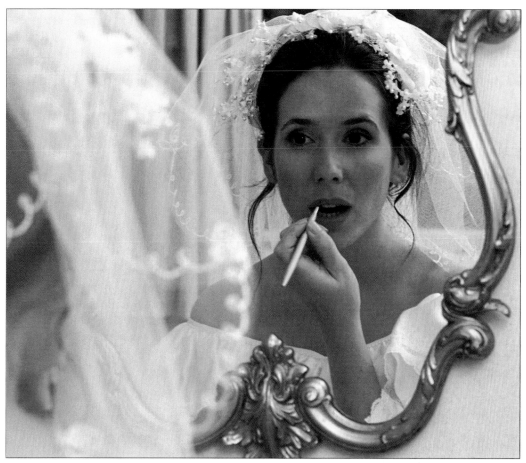

■ **It's important to feel comfortable** *in your wedding makeup. You may prefer to adapt your usual style rather than going for a typical bridal makeup. After all, you still want to look like you!*

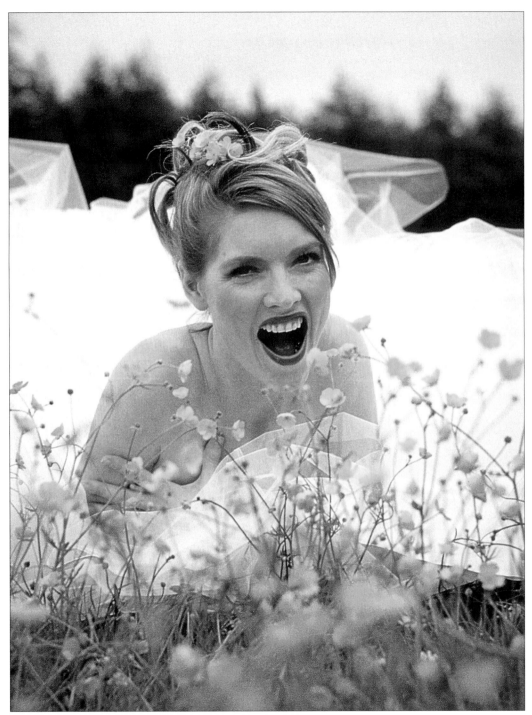

■ **Once your wedding makeup has been applied,** *you shouldn't need to worry about it for the rest of the day. Have your maid of honor or a friend carry your lip color and powder compact for quick touch-ups.*

Regardless of what makeup shades you choose, or how you decide to wear them, you'll want your skin to look perfect. Not only will all eyes be on you during the ceremony and after, there are wedding pictures to worry about – if your skin looks blotchy, it will look more so in those wedding photographs. Spend time applying foundation, use a brush to apply concealer where needed, and use a good pressed powder.

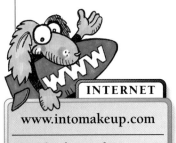

If you're wearing mascara on your special day, make sure it's waterproof! You never know when an emotional moment may strike.

Staying power

Furthermore, your makeup has to last through hours of tears, kisses, dancing, champagne drinking, and more. A good way to ensure makeup stays put is to use both cream and powder versions of everything. Apply foundation and concealer, then use cream blush and eye shadow. After dusting on face powder, apply powder blush and powder eye shadow. If you use pencil eyeliner, go over it with an eyeliner brush dipped in a similar shade of eye shadow. This double-teaming is a great technique to use any time you need budge-proof makeup.

INTERNET

www.intomakeup.com

This fun site features reviews, features such as "The 50 best cosmetics," advice, trend reports, and homemade recipes.

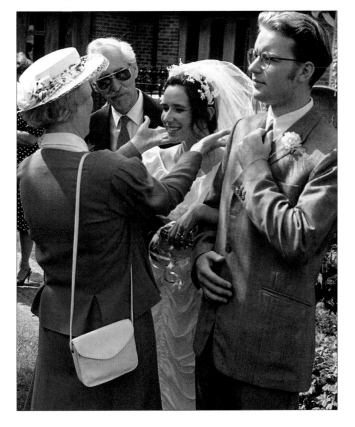

■ **Your wedding makeup** *has to go through a lot of kissing, touching, and the occasional onset of emotion, so make sure it has plenty of staying power.*

Creating even features

Very few people are blessed with perfectly symmetrical features. Eyes and lips are often uneven and one side of a face can be quite different from the other. Luckily, we have makeup, which is great for giving features a more balanced look.

Balancing your eyes

Many people have one eye that is lower, larger, or rounder than the other. One of the easiest ways to "fix" this is to get a medium taupe, tan, brown, or gray eye shadow and an eyeliner brush, and then gently "redraw" the eye. If one eye is higher than the other, you can line each eye at the lower lashes, making the line slightly thicker on the eye that is higher.

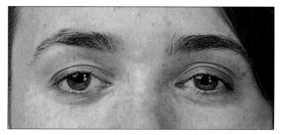

■ **If one eye is** *less round than the other, line both eyes at the upper lashes; pay attention to the flatter eye by making the line thicker at the eye's center.*

A thinner lower lip can look fuller if you use a slightly lighter shade of lip color than the shade you use on the upper lip.

Perfecting lip shape

Uneven lips are common. To create a more even outline, find a medium-to-dark, neutral lip liner, such as a natural spice or rose-brown shade. Use it to "beef up" the thin part of the lip by drawing slightly outside the lip's natural line. Fill the entire lip in with the pencil, then apply the lipstick of your choice. Be aware that light and frosty colors don't have the coverage necessary to pull off this effect, so stick with medium-to-dark, non-frosty shades.

Trivia...

No human face is perfectly symmetrical and many of us would look rather strange if this were the case. You can test your symmetry by holding a mirror side-on to your face, then looking in another mirror opposite you to see the effect!

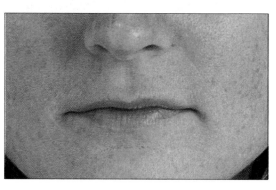

■ **Apply a slick of gloss** *to the center of the lips over the top of your lip color, to help make thin lips look fuller.*

Makeup looks by age

I AM LOATH TO PRESCRIBE certain looks for certain ages. Yes, I've heard those rules that say teenagers should wear only lip gloss and grandmas should stick to subdued shades, but I think a lot of what makes each of us beautiful is our uniqueness, and this often comes through in the makeup we like to wear. That said, I will give you a few general age-related guidelines, which you can choose to follow or ignore depending on your tastes.

Your teens

From a makeup standpoint, the teen years are difficult. Teens are naturally gorgeous – so gorgeous, in fact, that you don't need makeup. Moreover, too much makeup can literally cover right over your natural beauty. Yet, the teen years are also a time of trying to figure out who you are, so it is natural to want to experiment. My advice is this: Skip the foundation and get a good concealer to mask blemishes, and a powder to help sop up excess oil.

Go ahead and buy all the outrageous colors and sparkly stuff you want – but don't wear it all at once. A bright fuchsia lip is much more dramatic when it doesn't have to compete with a heavily shadowed eye, and a glittery chartreuse eyeliner will draw much more attention if it doesn't have to compete with bright orange blush.

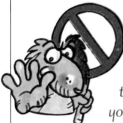

Avoid the temptation to try heavy foundation in your teens. Be as bold and bright as you like, but take advantage of your youthful complexion.

■ **Teenage skins** *may benefit from a little concealer and powder to even out any imperfections. Use bright, modern colors on lips and eyes and don't be afraid to experiment.*

Your 20s

The 20s are different for everyone. Some people spend a good part of this decade earning university degrees, some get married and start families, some embark on high-powered careers, and still others drift a while, searching for just the right way to live. Whatever you are doing with yourself and however your life may be changing, this is a terrific time to learn how to use makeup. If you don't know how already, spend a little time experimenting at home, let your makeup-savvy friends help you, or find a makeup artist whose work seems in sync with your own beauty thinking. Most 20-somethings are very busy during the day, so looking good quickly is important. If you feel you need foundation, by all means find yourself a product that suits you perfectly, but most people can get by with a good concealer and a dusting of face powder. Finish the look with mascara, lip gloss, and a quick application of blush. When the sun goes down, you may have more time to spend on your face, just don't go overboard – you want to look intriguing and very stunning, not obvious and very cheap (as my grandmother would say).

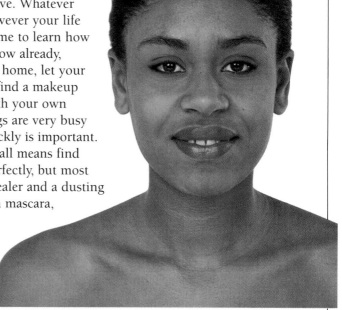

■ **In your 20s,** *you will probably begin to settle on a look you feel comfortable with. Don't be afraid to go crazy now and again with stronger colors and more products.*

After applying lipstick, close your mouth around the middle knuckle of your index finger, and then slowly slide the finger out of your mouth – any potential teeth-staining lipstick will end up on your finger.

Your 30s

During your 30s, your life gets crazy-busy and your looks begin to mature. Combined, these factors emphasize the need for simple, flattering makeup. If you have noticed a bit of discoloration, broken blood vessels, or scars, a good foundation is a practical solution that can save you time and angst. If you want to do full makeup – with eye shadow and lipstick – for day wear, keep in mind that subtle colors tend to be the most youthful. For nighttime, subdued brights are especially flattering.

Sheer lip and eye colors are becoming increasingly popular and most product lines carry some of these colors. They are very flattering in your 30s.

You will probably be feeling more comfortable with the way you look now than you did in your teens and your 20s. If you haven't done so already, now is a good time to start working on your "signature style" where your makeup is concerned. You can still try out new products as you come across them, but hang on to the makeup staples that you know work well for you. Your skin may start to feel a little drier and you may start to see some lines around your eyes and mouth so alter your foundation and powder products to accommodate this.

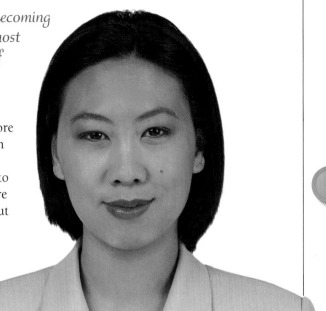

■ **In your 30s,** *you can still try out new looks but do avoid extreme fashion trends as these can have an aging effect. With the right makeup you can look much younger than you are.*

Your 40s

As women enter their 40s, it's common for their skin to become drier and finely lined. For this reason, dewy makeup, such as moisturizing-formula foundations, loose powders, cream blushes, and cream eye shadows, are smart choices. Subtle colors on the eyes and cheeks are generally more flattering than bright colors. If you love bold shades, however, find yourself a gorgeous, strongly colored, moist-finish lipstick – the lips are one area that can take unabashed color without aging the face, as long as that color flatters your coloring.

Look for foundations with skin-firming properties to pump up your skin and even out dry lines.

■ **In your 40s,** *indulge your passion for color, but restrict bright shades to your lips. Keep eyes and cheek colors as natural and neutral as possible.*

Your 50s

How a woman looks in her 50s depends on her genetics and how she's cared for herself. Some women are so youthful-looking that the makeup they wore during their 40s still works during their 50s. Other women may notice a distinct lack of firmness, deep folds between the nose and mouth, pouches under the eyes, dry skin, fine lines, and splotchy discoloration. Makeup can help camouflage these signs – but only if applied lightly. Too much makeup settles into the creases of your face, making you look decades older than you are. Opt for a moisturizing foundation, applied with a sponge. Follow with cream formula cosmetics, which are better for your dry skin than powder. A light dusting of face powder helps set makeup and a finishing mist of water from an atomizer helps keep makeup from looking heavy or cakey. As for colors, subtlety is most flattering for the eyes and cheeks, but if you'd like a shot of color somewhere, put it on the lips. Just be sure the lip color you choose flatters your complexion and has a moist finish. Anything that clashes with your skin can look aging, as can makeup with a matte finish.

■ **Mature looks** *benefit from having the character and personality that life has bestowed upon them. Make the most of your positive features.*

Your 60s and beyond

For a lot of older women, a full face of makeup can look aging. There are a few reasons for this: The color of our hair, eyes, and complexion all grow more subdued as we age, and makeup often competes with, clashes with, or totally overpowers our natural coloring. Gravity and collagen breakdown can leave our skin slack, making makeup placement – especially blush and eye shadow – difficult. Finally, our skin grows dry and lined, which in turn affects the way makeup sits on our skin. For these reasons, I suggest older women skip foundation and powder, and instead find a good concealer to pat on broken veins, brown splotches, and other skin glitches. Instead of trying to define cheekbones with blush – something that can be difficult if skin is slack – aim for a very subtle touch of color in the cheek area, the temple and the chin. This helps create a soft glow to older skin, which – thanks to slowed circulation – often lacks color. Lip color should also be subtle – and don't forget the lip liner, to keep color from migrating to the skin around the lips. As for eye shadow, I'd skip it. That doesn't mean ignoring eyes outright.

Our lashes often grow skimpy as we age, so mascara is a great way to keep eyes looking youthful. Black is too harsh against older skin. Instead, opt for mascara in brown-black or brown. Speaking of eyes, many older people's brows become unruly and gray. For this reason, keep a close eye on them, trimming long, curly brow hairs and plucking stragglers. You may also notice crazy hairs sprouting in other areas too, such as the top of the nose, the chin, or the jaw. Get a magnifying mirror and once a week position yourself in an area with strong light so you can remove these hairs with tweezers.

■ **Older skin** *needs special care and will often suffer from dryness. Counter this by using moisturizing makeup products.*

A simple summary

✔ Create a flawless canvas with foundation or concealer and everything that follows will look better.

✔ If you hate certain colors, don't wear them – even if people say they look good on you.

✔ Daytime makeup can be as easy or as complicated as you want.

✔ For evening glamour, follow the "one-feature rule."

✔ Even out asymmetrical features with clever makeup application.

✔ The teen years are for experimentation. Create "statement makeup" by using unusual colors on a single feature.

✔ In your 20s and 30s, try to create your "signature" makeup.

✔ If you are older, limit bright makeup to the lips.

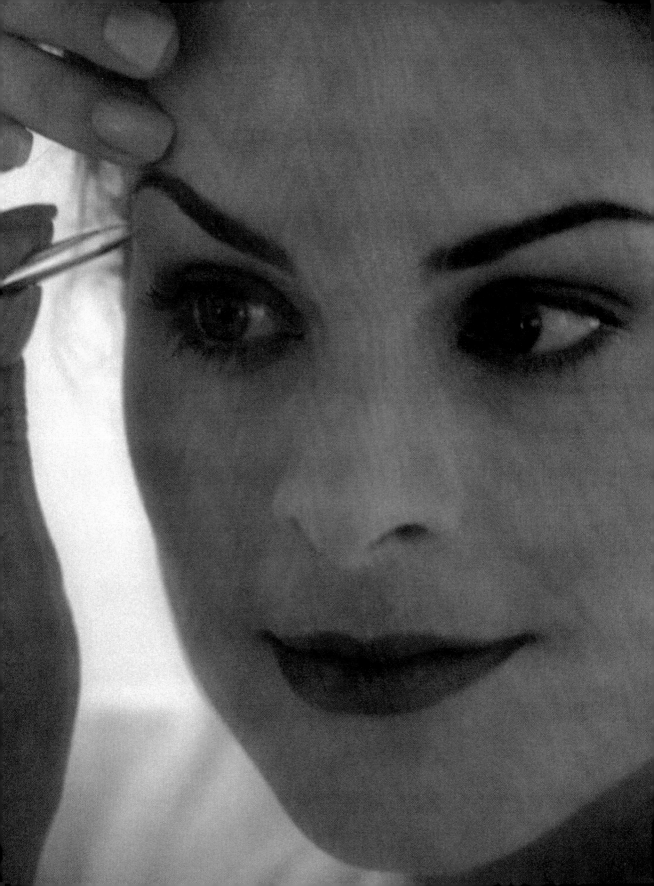

Chapter 13

Brow Know-how

BROW TRENDS CHANGE CONSTANTLY. In the 1930s and 1940s, women tended to imitate Hollywood's leading ladies, plucking their brows into the same slim crescents worn by Bette Davis, Marlene Dietrich, and Mae West. The 1950s saw boldly shaped brows popularized by Sophia Loren, Elizabeth Taylor, Ingrid Bergman, Audrey Hepburn, and Marilyn Monroe. During the 1970s, Brooke Shields and other natural beauties favored a full, almost bushy look. Conversely, 1990s superwaif models barely had brows at all. Fortunately, you don't need to go to extremes; you can be in fashion by simply working with what you've got!

In this chapter...

✓ *Natural is best: the most flattering shapes*

✓ *Other options in shaping*

✓ *Finishing touches: brow color*

WELL-SHAPED BROWS COMPLEMENT AND DEFINE YOUR EYES

Natural is best: the most flattering shapes

DEFINITION

Beauty insiders use the term tadpole or "pollywog" to describe what is perhaps the most common of bad brow shapes. A tadpole features a thick tear-drop or wedge shape at its inner corner. This lobe-like appendage resembles a tadpole head and is connected to an overly plucked, wispy "tail." Tadpoles are also referred to as hooks (as in fish hooks or crotchet hooks) apostrophes, or commas.

EYEBROWS CREATE a flattering frame for the eyes and lend balance to the face. A well-shaped brow can also deflect attention from what you consider a flaw, such as close-set eyes or a wide nose.

First, consider what you don't want: patchy, over-tweezed brows; *tadpole* brows with a thick inner corner and nearly nonexistent line; or brows tweezed into an unnatural half-moon shape. Such misshapen lines create an unfavorable frame for the eye and diminish your good looks. For instance, too-thin brows can make your nose seem wider, tadpole brows lend a furrowed expression to your face, and half-moon brows give your face an appearance of permanent fright.

Limit your hair-removal activities to between, underneath, and at the outer edges of the brows. Shaping above the brow can lead to a flat, archless, unnatural-looking line.

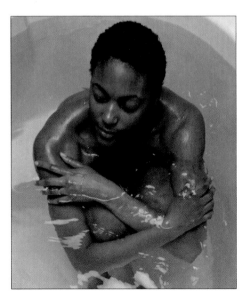

Now consider what you do want: a realistic line following your natural brow shape. After all, when it comes to flattering shapes, nature has probably done much of the work for you.

Preparing to pluck

Ready to shape up those brows? Always bear in mind that your aim is to make the most of what you were born with. The best time to tweeze brows is after a shower or bath, when your hair is at its most pliable; this will make for easier and less painful plucking.

■ **A soak in the tub** *will make you feel relaxed and the steam and hot water will open your hair follicles, making your eyebrows easier to pluck.*

If you have especially sensitive skin, consider numbing the brow area with a topical analgesic such as *Anbesol®* before plucking.

Tweezers at the ready

Stand or sit in front of a mirror. Natural light is ideal, but bright artificial light will also work. Identify obvious stray hairs between brows, under brows, and at brows' outer corners. Using a good-gripping pair of tweezers, grasp individual hairs near their roots. With swift, sharp movements, pluck hair in the direction it is growing.

TWEEZING

When it comes to at-home brow shaping, tweezing rules. It's fast, easy, cheap, effective, and precise, allowing you to work with one hair at a time. Tweezers come in several styles, each with its own virtues:

a **Needle-nose tweezers** These feature thin, needle-like tips. Their slimness allows you to maneuver easily in patches of dense hair, so you can target only those hairs you want to remove. Needle-nose tweezers are ideal for grasping short, hard-to-pluck hairs and ultra-fine hairs. They are a favorite of makeup artists and aestheticians, and can be purchased in cosmetic boutiques and beauty supply stores.

Avoid tweezers with weak grips, which make it hard to grasp single hairs. You need to have a firm hold on a hair before you tweak.

b **Blunt-edged tweezers** These are the tweezers most often sold in drug stores. Their blunt ends provide a firm grip, making this the ideal tool for anyone who suffers from coarse, hard-to-pluck hair.

c **Slant-edged tweezers** Terrific general purpose tweezers, they offer a slightly tighter grip than needle-nose tweezers and more precision than blunt-edged tweezers. Found in cosmetic boutiques and beauty supply stores.

■ **Blunt-edge tweezers** *are ideal for plucking coarse hair because they offer a firm grasp.*

Styling tips

If necessary, do minor reshaping. Unless your eyes are close-set or wide-set, brows should start at the inner corner of your eye and end slightly beyond the eye's outer corner. Removing hair judiciously along the underside of the brow creates more lid space, making small eyes appear larger and more open.

If your eyes are close-set, consider starting brows a few hairs farther from the eye's inner corner. Creating a wider space between the brows mimics the look of average-set eyes. If you have wide-set eyes, create the illusion of average-set eyes by starting brows closer to your nose, and then removing a few extra hairs from your brow ends. With a brow brush or an old toothbrush, brush brows vertically. Trim any individual hairs that are noticeably longer than the rest. As we age, our brow hairs often grow longer and more unruly. In other words, when you are 30, your brows may look tidy with no trimming, while at age 50 you may find numerous hairs in need of snipping!

Trivia...

During the late 16th century reign of the English Queen Elizabeth I – known as the Elizabethan era – it was fashionable to go completely brow-less.

Other options in shaping

TWEEZING IS THE MOST POPULAR *method of brow shaping – but it certainly isn't your only option. There are a number of other methods available at professional salons.*

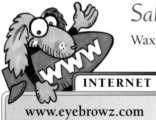

INTERNET

www.eyebrowz.com

This web site features a mix of products and information, including several different brow-shaping essentials, stencils of celebrity brows, and pictures of brow makeovers.

Salon treatments

Waxing wins fans for its clean finish and quickness. Warm, liquid wax is applied between and under eyebrows. After the wax cools and hardens, it is ripped off, whisking brow hairs with it. Brow waxing is best left to a salon professional, because it isn't as precise as tweezing. In other words, it is easy to remove too much brow – and bear in mind that brow hair can take 3 to 6 months to grow back!

Many people initially visit a salon to have their brows waxed, then maintain their brows with at-home tweezing. If you have sensitive skin, are pregnant, take oral hormones, or use a retinoid or alpha hydroxy acid product, avoid waxing: your skin may be too thin for this rough procedure.

Threading is an ancient form of hair removal used in Israel and the Middle East, and is becoming increasingly popular in urban centers such as New York, London, Paris, and San Francisco. Ultra-precise, it boasts the same long-lasting results as tweezing and waxing (with less pain, say some brow-shaping veterans). How's it done? A skilled practitioner uses a length of thread to quickly lasso and pull individual brow hairs.

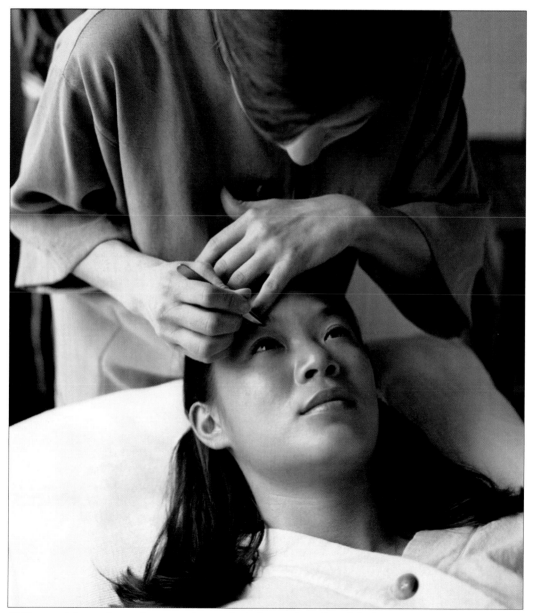

■ **If you visit a salon** *to have your brows plucked, waxed, or threaded, the practitioner will be able to offer you styling advice and then meticulously shape your brows for you.*

Finishing touches: brow color

MAYBE YOUR BROWS are so pale they seem invisible. You could have a brow that is thicker than its mate, or perhaps you've overplucked. Fortunately, there are ways to augment what you've got.

Brow definition

Eyebrow pencils are best for defining existing brows and creating subtle shape changes, such as adding an arch or making the brow look thicker. Apply color where needed using light, feathery strokes. Alternatively, cream brow color is a waxy, water-resistant cream packaged in small pots or compacts. Easier to apply than eyebrow pencil – and with a more natural-looking finish – cream color can be used to reshape brows and is a good choice for filling in patchy spots. Most cream brow color comes with a sponge-tip applicator; or try a small, tapered cosmetic brush. Cream color's slightly waxy consistency does not adhere well to oily skin – it's best for normal or dry complexions.

BROW POW

If you are uncertain about how to add color and shape to your brow, here are some helpful pointers:

a For the most natural results when using a brow pencil, brow powder, cream brow color, or brow mascara, select a color the same shade or a shade lighter than your own eyebrows. To extend the brow, simply apply color to eyebrows' outer corners.

b Creating a subtle arch is easy using a brow pencil, cream color, or brow powder. Stand facing a mirror. When looking straight ahead, the area of brow directly above the outer edge of the iris is where the arch should be placed.

c For thicker-looking brows, lightly trace above eyebrows with an eye pencil, cream color, or brow powder. Use a brow brush or an old toothbrush to blend color and create a natural-looking finish.

■ **Eyebrow pencils** *should be kept well sharpened so that you can achieve good definition.*

Although there are special eyebrow powder colors on the market, a tan or brown eyeshadow in a shade close to your brow color will work equally well. Apply powder in the same way you would cream color, using a small, tapered cosmetic brush. Powder's dry consistency makes it a great, stay-put option for oilier complexions. Brow mascara, also called wand color or brow color, is the product to use if you'd like to temporarily change the color of your brows.

Bleaching and dyeing

Eyebrows can be bleached or dyed to match hair color. Permanent brow color should be performed in a salon by an experienced hair-color technician who will take precautions to prevent chemicals from running into your eyes. Ask your hair colorist if he or she offers the service; in some states, permanent brow-coloring is illegal.

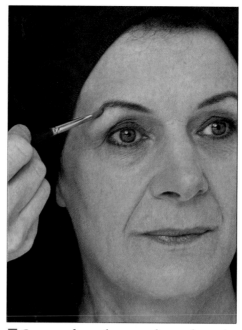

■ **Cream color** *or brow powder can be used to subtly reshape or thicken brows, or to enhance their tone and color.*

Cosmetic tattooing

Hormonal imbalances, stress, immune-system disorders, heavy plucking, and chemotherapy can all cause lasting brow loss. Brows can be temporarily fashioned with cosmetics, but tattooing, carried out by a dermatologist or a trained aesthetic tattoo artist, offers an alternative. However, because this method is essentially permanent, think long and hard about this option before undergoing the needle.

A simple summary

✔ Work with the eyebrows you have – your natural shape is always best.

✔ Sometimes you're better off going to a professional for brow shaping and color.

✔ When shaping brows, go slowly so that you don't make mistakes.

✔ After brows are shaped, brow color can help add definition.

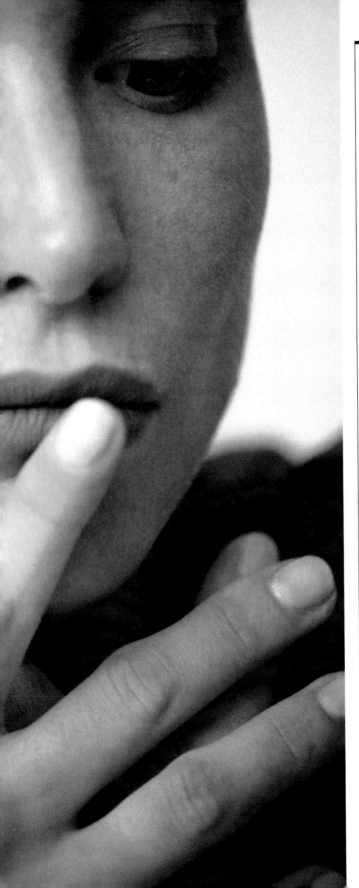

PART FOUR

Chapter 14
About Nails

Chapter 15
Caring For Your Nails

NAIL CARE

HUMANS HAVE BEEN PLAYING with their nails for centuries. In 4000 BC, Egyptians were buffing their nails with henna; in 1500 BC, Chinese royals were *painting their nails* red, black, or white, and as early as AD 100, Romans were applying "fingernail polish" made of animal fat and blood.

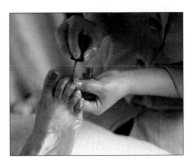

While our choice of nail cosmetics may have changed, we humans remain as *fascinated with fingernails* and toenails as we've ever been. How else can you explain the plethora of products, salons, and books devoted strictly to nail care? Fortunately, you don't need a lot of time, products, or money to have *gorgeous nails*. Just keep them healthy and they'll be fabulous. In this section, you'll discover how to achieve just that.

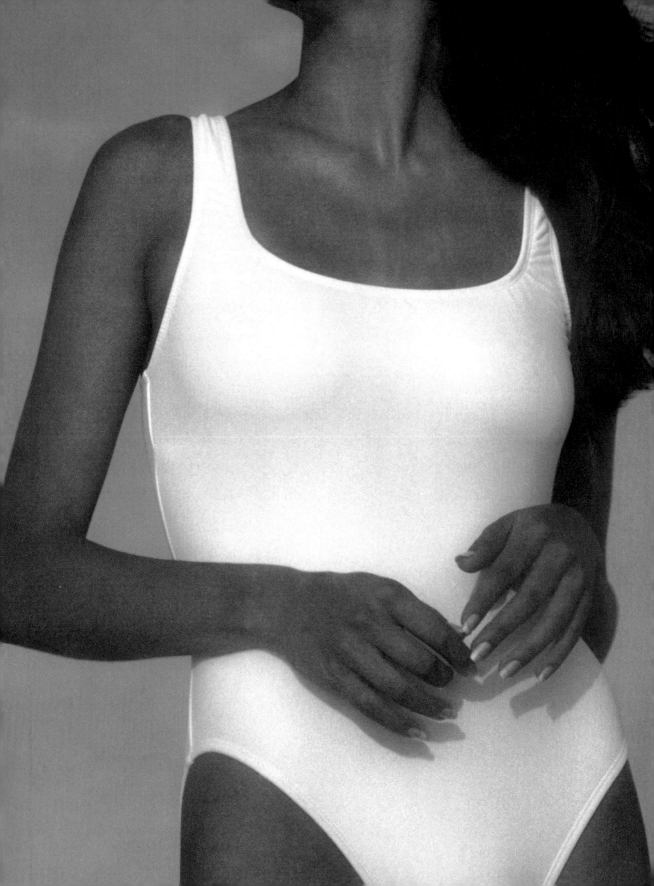

Chapter 14

About Nails

ONCE UPON A TIME, before humans looked like they do now, both hair and nails were essential to an individual's survival. Back then, hair protected delicate skin against environmental elements, while nails served as a kind of combined weapon-tool. Today, nails are still functional, yet modern humans tend to view nails less as a necessity than as an accessory. After all, the way you wear your nails is as telling as your clothing, your makeup, and your hairstyle. No matter what your preferences, however, your nails will be healthier and easier to work with if you take care of them.

In this chapter...

✓ **What are nails and why do we have them?**

✓ **How nails grow**

✓ **Nail enemies**

✓ **Nail health**

WELL-KEPT NAILS ARE A REAL BEAUTY ASSET

What are nails and why do we have them?

IF YOU'RE LIKE ME, you don't think much about your nails. Perhaps you wonder how you can grow them longer, keep them from chipping, or whether they'd look better painted a muted claret or a blush pink. However, you may not consider all the reasons why you have nails. In fact, fingernails and toenails serve several purposes: to support the tissues of the fingers and toes, to safeguard the fingertips and the tips of the toes from injury, to assist us in picking up small objects, to help us manipulate objects, and, quite simply, for scratching. Another interesting tidbit: like hair, nails are made of keratin.

Nail structure

Our nails are made up of several components, some of which are visible, some of which are not. What we see when we look at our nails is called the nail plate. A plate is hard, smooth, rectangular in shape, and slightly convex.

If you need medical attention for a toenail problem, a podiatrist or a dermatologist can usually help you. If a fingernail is troubling you, visit a dermatologist for advice.

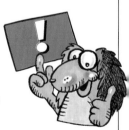

Nails are translucent in color, but they take on a faint pink cast thanks to the network of blood vessels located beneath them. This color is variable. It may become paler, for example,

■ **A healthy nail** *is smooth in texture and has well-formed cuticles.*

when you're feeling cold and the blood vessels in your fingers and toes have constricted.

Half moons

The whitish, half-moon area visible at the base of the nail is the lunula. Its shape and pale color come from nail cells that are not fully mature; these cells will mature and turn translucent as they grow toward the nails' tips. The size, shape, and brightness of the lunula varies from person to person and even from finger to finger – for some reason, lunulas are often most pronounced on thumbs. Should you happen to notice your lunula isn't as bright as it once was, don't worry: the lunula often fades with age.

Trivia...

Nails grow faster on a person's dominant hand. They also grow more quickly during pregnancy, and in the summer. The middle finger nail grows fastest, with the growth rate progressively decreasing on the fourth, second, and fifth fingers and finally the thumb. Also, fingernails grow faster than toenails.

Cuticles and nail beds

The cuticle is the thin tissue that grows from the finger to overlap the nail plate and form a rim around the base of the nail. Its purpose is protective: to keep out debris and microorganisms that can harm the matrix and nail bed.

The nail bed is the finger tissue directly under the nail plate; its network of small blood vessels provide nutrition for the nail. While the nail bed does support the nail, it does not contribute to the nail's growth.

INTERNET

www.waningmoon.com

This easy-to-navigate site features nail care aimed at those pale-skinned, black-clothed people known as Goths. Anyone, however, can benefit from the site's comprehensive information, which includes such offerings as how to remove black hair dye from nails, the pros and cons of acrylic nails, and nail care for men.

If you've ever wondered how the nail sticks to the nail bed, here's the answer: both the nail bed's surface and the nail plate's underside feature vertical ridges and depressions that fit together like puzzle pieces, locking the bed and plate together.

Also known as the nail root, the matrix is the area hidden beneath the cuticle. It is here that nail keratin is created. Nail cells divide in the matrix, thereby lengthening the nail plate, and pushing it forward over the nail bed. The folds of skin at the nail's base and sides are known as the nail folds. These folds frame and support the nails.

How nails grow

THE MATRIX IS WHERE THE NAIL'S keratin cells are created – one way to think of the matrix is as a fingernail and toenail birthing room. As new cells are "born," they are pushed past the cuticle, into the lunula. From the lunula, they keep traveling toward the nail's tip, where they take on a white opaque finish, a normal result of being separated from the nail bed and coming in contact with air. Once they reach the nail's tip, nail cells are broken off, filed down, or cut away.

Because nails can only grow so fast, I suggest a relaxed attitude toward growing them. Although individual nail growth depends on age, time of year, activity level, and heredity, the average growth rate for nails is 0.1 millimeter each day. At this speed, it takes from 5 to 7 months for a nail to completely regenerate itself.

Healthy nails are generally smooth nails. Yet there are times when a nail grows out ridged, pitted, or deformed. Vertical ridging – which is generally permanent – occurs in some people with age, or with injury to the nail. Horizontal ridging or pitting – which is usually temporary – can appear a few weeks after an illness and will grow out with the nail. When a nail is injured and falls off, it is usually replaced by a normal nail. However, if the nail matrix or nail bed has been injured or destroyed, the new nail will grow back deformed or not at all.

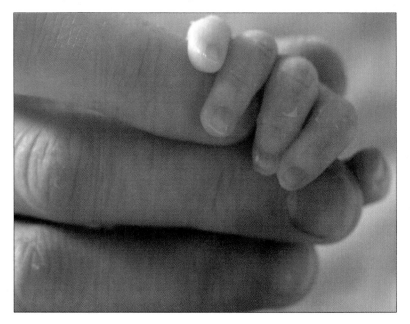

■ **When babies** *are born, they already have hair and nails. Their nails grow quickly and must be kept carefully trimmed so that they can't scratch their face with them.*

Nail enemies

WHEN YOU CONSIDER how rough humans are on their fingers and toes, you realize why nails have to be tough. Nails are the barrier between our skin and hard surfaces, hot water, chemicals, and physical trauma. Yet nails are also vulnerable. You may not realize this, but many everyday activities and situations can weaken, dehydrate, break, or even cause infections in nails or the nail bed.

If you experience separation of the nail from the nail bed, crumbling or splitting of the nail, redness and swelling of the skin around the nail, or discoloration of the nail, talk to your doctor. You may have psoriasis — a chronic skin disease.

Nail infections

Infections not only undermine nail health, they can make nails downright unattractive. When present in and around the nails, infections can cause redness, swelling, pain, blistering, oozing puss, discoloration of the nail, and deformation of the nail. Should you experience any of these symptoms, see a dermatologist or podiatrist immediately!

Bacterial infections occur when bacteria enters the skin around or under the nail. The nail is usually well-fortified to keep out the many types of bacteria we are exposed to each day. However, flaky skin, a cut, or an injury either to the cuticle or the area underneath the nail (perhaps from aggressive grooming with a sharp, metal instrument) is just the portal bacteria needs to enter your body. Once under your skin or nails, the bacteria attack healthy tissue. Bacterial infections almost always feature pus, and often involve blisters, redness, swelling, separation of the nail from the nail bed, and pain. An antibiotic ointment can clear things up; in severe cases, your doctor may also prescribe an oral antibiotic.

■ **If you have a nail infection,** *visit your dermatologist or podiatrist immediately. The sooner an infection is treated, the less chance there is of lasting nail damage.*

ABOUT INGROWN TOENAILS

Ingrown toenails occur when one or two corners of a nail – usually the big toe's nail – grow into the surrounding skin. They are painful, common, and surprisingly preventable. Here are some simple hints to help you avoid them:

a As unattractive as long toenails are, you shouldn't trim your nails too short. Aggressively cut nails often become ingrown – be moderate when you trim your toenails, and, if necessary, cut them more regularly.

b Keep toenails square in shape. Rounding the corners may look prettier, but this will encourage nails to grow into surrounding tissue.

c Don't wear toe-pinching shoes. Cramming toes into tight shoes often leads to nail problems.

d If you do find yourself with a mild ingrown toenail, you can try to remedy it yourself. Fill up a basin or tub with warm water, add a tablespoon of salt, and soak your foot for 15 to 20 minutes. Next, gently wedge a tiny bit of dry cotton, such as part of a cotton ball, under the ingrown corner or corners of the nail. This will need to be repeated nightly for 2 or 3 weeks until the nail has grown out.

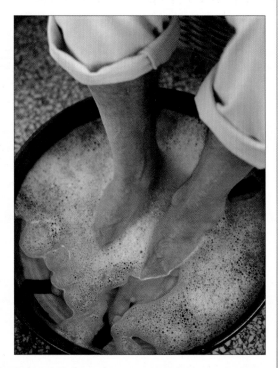

e If strong pain, swelling, redness, or infection develops around an ingrown toenail, visit a podiatrist, who will remove the ingrown portion of the nail.

■ **If you are suffering** *from an ingrown toenail, soak your feet in warm water – this will help to soften the nail and the skin, and the problem nail will be easier to treat.*

Fungal infections

A form of microscopic plant, fungus can attach itself to a variety of surfaces. Fungal nail infections occur when these small plants take up residence in your nails' keratin. The best way to treat fungal infections is prevention. Fungus breeds in dark, damp, warm environments, so avoid walking barefoot in locker rooms, through mud, or in swampy areas. Furthermore, fungus loves dark, damp shoes and socks, which means toenails are more frequently plagued than fingernails. If you should get a fungal infection, your doctor will prescribe an antifungal ointment or oral antifungal medication. Fungal infections are particularly vexing since they must grow out with your nail. This means that even with care, an infection can take up to 7 months to cure. If left untreated, fungus-infested nails will become yellowed and deformed.

The majority of nail problems are caused by improper trimming, minor injuries, or repeated nail trauma.

Aggressive handling

I can't think of anyone who actually wants to ruin their nails. Yet in an attempt to keep our nails looking groomed, many of us go overboard. We gouge dirt from under the plate, stab at cuticles with a sharp implement (or worse, cut cuticles away), file nails down to the quick, or pull at ugly *hangnails*. In short, our good intentions can actually damage our nails.

> **DEFINITION**
>
> A hangnail isn't really a nail at all – it's a snag of skin near the cuticle or at the sides of the nails. Hangnails occur most often in dry, flaking, or cracked skin.

You may pine for perfect-looking nails, or perhaps you couldn't care less how your nails appear. Either way, listen up: The less you do to nails – and the gentler you do it – the prettier they will look, the healthier they will be, and the better able they will be to protect your fingers and toes.

Don't manicure or pedicure your nails more than once a week. Throw away anything with a sharp point – this includes metal nail files and metal cuticle pushers. Instead of digging at the dirt under your nails, use soap and a nail brush to keep nails clean. Do not file your nails so short that you expose the area where the nail bed and nail plate come together.

You mustn't be tempted to pull at hangnails, because if you do you risk removing long strips of healthy skin. Not only are these raw areas painful, they are unsightly and vulnerable to infection. A better way to remove hangnails is to clip them away with a pair of fingernail clippers.

■ **Invest in a good nail brush** *with firm bristles, and use it to gently scrub your nails clean of dirt.*

Misusing your nails

Nails can do so many things: open soda cans, pry off stickers, twist in small screws, dig into an orange's peel. Of course, those of you who want strong, unbroken nails wouldn't use your nails for any of these tasks. You know that – as convenient as they are – nails should not be used as a household tool. Doing so traumatizes nail's keratin, causing small or large fissures that lead to breaking and splitting. Fortunately, you needn't spend your days wearing kid gloves. For strong nails, simply try adopting the following habits:

- Dial the telephone with the end of a pen or pencil.
- Instead of using your nails to pry things open or scrape things off, reach for a butter knife, bottle opener, or a small screwdriver.
- Use a letter opener, not your fingernail, to open envelopes and packages.
- "Start" an orange or banana by cutting into its peel with a knife.

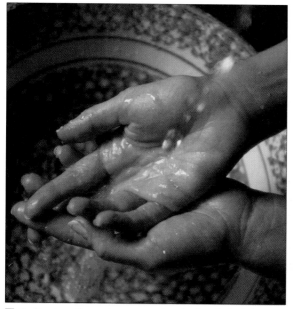

■ **Protect nails against water** *and other liquids by coating nails with hardener or polish. Limit the time your hands spend submerged in water, or wear gloves.*

Nails and water

Ask your favorite nail technician what nail enemy number one is, and there's a good chance she'll say "water." Before I explain why water is the bad guy, let me offer this anatomy lesson: to create a strong barrier, nail cells must fit tightly together. Without this tight fit, nails grow weak and are easily bent, torn, chipped, split, peeled, or broken.

At the same time, the keratin that forms nail cells behaves a bit like a sponge; when exposed to water, the keratin soaks up the liquid, swelling to several times its size. It is this swelling that disrupts the tight fit of nail cells. Try to keep your contact with water to a minimum – you should even consider taking shorter baths and showers!

It is estimated that 15 percent of Americans bite their fingernails. If you're among them, consider one of the "no-bite" products available from dermatologists and pharmacies. These terrible-tasting liquids are painted on the nails. Try to nibble and you're left with a bad taste in your mouth.

Drying chemicals

While overabundant moisture damages nails, so does a lack of moisture. That's why drying household chemicals, the oil-zapping ingredients in some face products, rubbing alcohol, and some nail products are so damaging to nails – they dry nail keratin out. When moisture is taken from nails, the nail cells shrivel. The result? The smooth, tight interlocking of nail cells becomes disrupted; in its place is a bunch of ruffled, barely joined cells, which lead to nail weakness, brittleness, and breaking.

If there's one thing that really dries out nails, it's nail-polish remover. In fact, nail-polish remover is the reason most dermatologists recommend that you manicure nails no more than once every 7 to 10 days. Nail polish remover works by dissolving nail polish. There are two types of remover: *acetone* and non-acetone. Acetone removers have a reputation for being especially drying. Non-acetone removers, usually formulated with a chemical called acetate, are billed as gentler to the nails. Yet, despite the claims of many nail technicians and cosmetic companies, both remover types are drying.

DEFINITION

Acetone is a colorless liquid that evaporates easily, is flammable, and dissolves in water. It is also known as dimethyl ketone, 2-propanone, and beta-ketopropane.

COLOR CHANGES

There are a number of outside influences that can affect nail color. Chemicals, medications, medical conditions, and pollution can temporarily alter the nail's natural color. Here are some of the most common "nail-changers":

- **Anemia** This condition can cause pale nail beds.
- **Antibiotics** Taking antibiotics can produce a tan or gray tint to the nail bed.
- **Antimalarial medications** These drugs can cause a yellow tint to the nail bed.
- **Chemotherapy** This treatment may result in a nail bed with a tan or gray tint.
- **Cigarette smoke** Smoking can cause a yellow or tan discoloration of the nail.
- **Dark nail polish** This can produce a yellow or orange discoloration.
- **Diabetes** This may produce a yellowish nail bed with a blue cast at the base.
- **Hairspray, gel, mousse, and other hair styling products** If you use these products regularly, you may notice a yellow or orange nail discoloration.
- **Heart Conditions** These can produce a reddish nail bed.
- **Kidney diseases** Sufferers may notice pink and white areas on their nail beds.
- **Liver disease** The disease can produce a whitish nail bed.
- **Lung Diseases** These conditions can cause yellow, thickened nails.

Nail health

HEALTHY NAILS ARE PRETTY NAILS – *something worth considering if your nails never seem to look good. Fortunately, nails don't need a lot to be healthy. The most important thing is to avoid those activities and substances that damage nails. There are also a few pro-active things you can do to help foster good health. No, I don't mean costly supplements, exotic-sounding nail creams, or expensive salon treatments. What I'm talking about are easy, common sense types of things that don't take a lot of effort, thought, or money.*

Cuticle massage

Massage has a reputation for being a frivolous, feel-good kind of thing we treat ourselves to on birthdays or Mother's days. And that's too bad, because massage can stimulate blood flow, encourage oxygen to reach body tissues, and help us relax, placing it firmly in the realm of everyday health care.

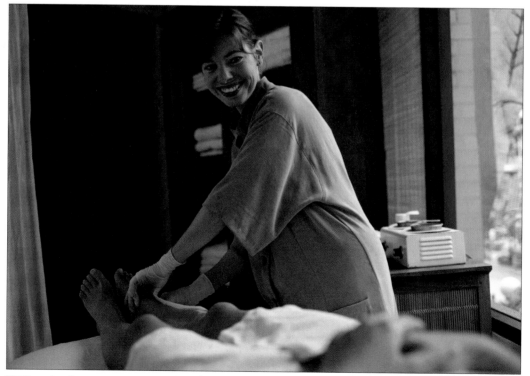

■ **If you're having a massage,** *don't forget your hands and feet. They need as much care as the rest of your body, and your nails will benefit from the increased blood flow a massage brings.*

If you need further convincing, massage can also help our nails. Dermatologists have long known that nails on a person's dominant hand grow faster and stronger than nails on a person's nondominant hand. The reason? The busier hand enjoys an increase in blood supply, which nourishes and prompts nails to grow faster.

Massage also encourages increased blood flow to the fingers and toes. To massage your nails, reach for some heavy hand cream, massage oil, baby oil, or even olive oil. Place a drop or two of the product at the base of the nail, and rub it into the cuticle, up the nail folds, and onto the nail plate itself. Nail massage has a secondary benefit: the massage lotion or oil moisturizes the nails, cuticles, and surrounding skin so that nails stay strong and flexible enough to fend off breaks and the surrounding skin remains supple and hangnail-free.

INTERNET

www.1st-spot.com/ topic_nailcare.html

This web site is packed with information about nail care and nail products. Visit and learn everything you want to know about nail health and beauty.

Nail-loving nutrients

For centuries, women have swallowed *royal jelly*, eaten liver, and drunk gelatin concoctions to get longer, stronger, faster-growing nails. In a way, all this supplementation makes sense. Nails are living tissue, which means they are affected by what you do – and don't – put into your mouth. Yet unless you are severely malnourished, you probably get what your nails need from either your daily diet or whatever vitamin supplements you take. Keep that in mind as you peruse the following list, comprised of nutrients that contribute to healthy nail growth:

DEFINITION

Royal jelly is a jelly-like substance made by bees and fed to a hive's queen bee.

a Studies have shown that biotin, also known as vitamin B-7 and vitamin H, strengthens nails by aiding in nail-cell growth. Good sources of biotin are brewer's yeast, broccoli, cheese, nuts, soy, sunflower seeds, sweet potatoes, and whole grains. Aim for 30 to 100 mcg a day.

b Vitamin B-12 is also known as cobalmin. It benefits nails by helping the body absorb protein and by aiding in nail-cell formation. Good sources include brewer's yeast, dairy products, eggs, and sea vegetables such as kelp, nori, or arame.

c Calcium is the most abundant mineral in the human body. It contributes to the growth and maintenance of teeth, bones, and nails. Good sources of calcium are bitter leafy greens such as arugula, broccoli rabe (a vegetable, sometimes called rapini, easily found in large metropolitan areas, which is just loaded with calcium), dandelion, dairy products, tofu, and nuts. Aim for 800 to 1,200 mcg daily.

(d) Protein is essential to healthy keratin formation. However, before you start downing protein shakes, consider that the body needs only 1½–1¾ oz (45–50 g) of protein a day. A bowl of oatmeal, one large egg, a glass of cow's milk or soy milk, a bean burrito with cheese, a 6 oz (170 g) carton of yogurt, and a 4 oz (113 g) serving of tofu all equal 1¾ oz (50 g) of protein. Also consider that because all foods (even vegetables, fruits, and grains) contain protein in some amount, most people who follow a healthy diet get more than enough each day.

Nail disorders of some form comprise about ten percent of all skin conditions.

(e) Silicon helps the nails use calcium effectively and is necessary for healthy nail formation. The mineral is found in alfalfa sprouts, beets, brown rice, bell peppers, soy, leafy green vegetables, and whole grains. While there is no established daily requirement for silicon, one or two daily servings of silicon-rich food is enough to provide benefits for your nails.

(f) Sulfur accounts for nearly 10 percent of a healthy body's mineral content and is vital to hair, nail, muscle, and skin cells. Good sources of sulfur are Brussels sprouts, cabbage, dairy products, eggs, garlic, legumes, onions, turnips, and wheat germ. While there is no established daily requirement for sulfur, one or two daily servings of sulfur-rich food is enough to provide benefits.

(g) Zinc is a mineral that contributes to cell growth and function and is essential for healthy skin and nails. Good sources of zinc are brewer's yeast, egg yolks, legumes, pumpkin seeds, pecans, sunflower seeds, wheat bran, and whole grains. Aim for 15 to 30 mcg a day.

Don't waste your money on gelatin capsules. Despite the old wives' tale, there is no evidence that gelatin makes nails grow faster or stronger.

Trivia...

Nails and hair share several characteristics: both are composed of keratin, both are direct outgrowths of the skin, and both are formed in interior pockets of the skin (a nail fold, and a follicle).

The importance of gloves

No one I know wears gloves while cleaning or gardening. I don't know why this is, although I suspect it may be a generation thing. My reasoning? My grandmother and her friends were harder on their hands than our generation is on ours: those ladies pulled weeds, harvested vegetables, picked apples, pitted cherries, peeled peaches for preserves, made minor repairs around the house, did hand laundry, washed dishes without the aid of a machine, and scrubbed floors. Yet, unlike me and my friends, those ladies never

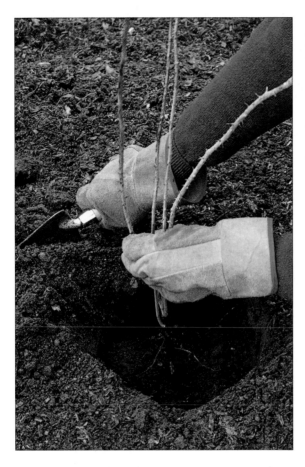

got professional manicures. Also unlike me and many of my friends, those ladies had strong, healthy nails.

So what was their secret? Many dermatologists and nail technicians point to the gloves that the older generation wore. Gloves provide a barrier that protects nail keratin from the weakening affects of water; collisions with hard surfaces; corrosive household chemicals; and more. Fortunately, glove-wearing has nothing to do with your generation and everything to do with habit. To develop the glove-wearing habit yourself, get several pairs for dishwashing and indoor cleaning, and a pair or two for gardening – then wear them!

■ **If you wear gloves** *while gardening, you can prevent dirt from lodging in your nails, and protect your nails and skin from nicks, cuts, and drying elements.*

A simple summary

✔ Nails are comprised of a hard substance called keratin.

✔ Nails protect sensitive fingertips and toe-tips from chemicals and physical trauma.

✔ Nails are vulnerable to a variety of substances.

✔ Infection, misuse, and aggressive grooming can damage nails.

✔ If you want gorgeous nails, get into the habit of wearing gloves when you're doing housework.

✔ If you eat healthy foods, you'll see the results in your nails.

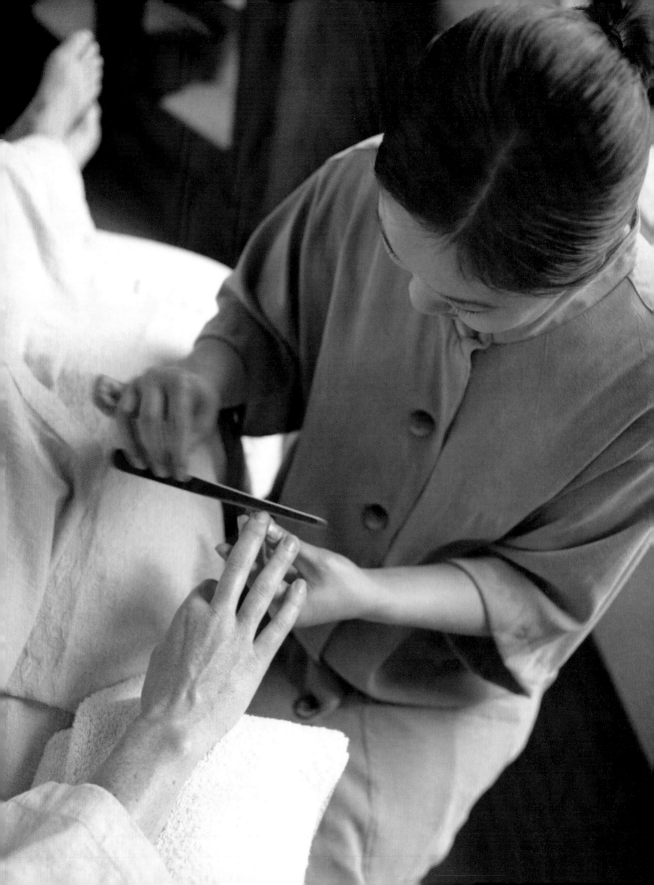

Chapter 15

Caring For Your Nails

A LOT OF WOMEN, AND SOME MEN, are fanatical about nail care. These folks carry nail glue in their bags, dial their cell phones with pencils, and don't appear to have cuticles. Conversely, many people couldn't care less what their nails look like. The closest these people come to a manicure is a fast snip with a pair of fingernail clippers. Neither approach is good for your nails. Moderation is your best option: just enough grooming to keep nails and cuticles looking healthy, but not so much that you cause irritation or infection. A simple approach to nail care makes your life easier, and it also produces beautiful results.

In this chapter...

✓ Assembling a nail tool kit

✓ The do-it-yourself manicure

✓ The do-it-yourself pedicure

✓ Salons: sanitation counts

✓ Enhancing your nails

TREAT YOURSELF TO A PROFESSIONAL MANICURE ONCE IN A WHILE

Assembling a nail tool kit

WALK INTO ANY DRUGSTORE, *head toward the nail-care aisle, and what do you see? A lot of stuff! So many products that you may not even know what half of them are. Do you really need all this paraphernalia to keep your nails looking good? No, not really. However, a well-stocked nail kit does make home nail care simple – and anything that's easy is more likely to get done.*

Trivia...

The Ancient Egyptians are said to have dipped their fingernails into henna, which not only colored nails, but acted as a moisturizing and strengthening agent.

Nail files

You shouldn't use a metal nail file because it can rip nails, creating a jagged, tear-prone finish. Coarse-grade wood files are not good either, for the same reason. You want finesse in a file, a type with a fine-grade grit that can glide over nail tips – something that puts you in control and that gently sands nails to the perfect finish. There are a number of fine-grade wood files – sometimes called emery boards – available at drugstores, department stores, and nail salons. Some come stuck on a wood board opposite a coarser grit; some cover both sides of a wood or foam board; and some are sanitizable (can be washed).

Polish remover

Polish remover dissolves the chemicals in nail polish, breaking them down so polish can be swiped off the finger. Acetone polish remover is the stronger of the two types and a better choice for especially resistant nail polish. If you wear any kind of artificial nails that can be melted by acetone, non-acetone polish remover is the only choice.

The acetone found in some nail-polish removers is the same substance used to make plastics, fibers, drugs, and some chemicals. It is also used to dissolve other substances, and is present in vehicle exhaust fumes, tobacco smoke, and landfill sites.

■ **Make sure that your** *nails are completely dry before you use an emery board – filing wet nails can cause tears and splits.*

To use nail-polish remover, dampen a cotton ball with remover and swipe over each finger, taking care not to saturate nails and cuticles in the solution. In fact, if you can avoid getting polish remover on your cuticles and skin, you'll be better off for it, since both types of remover are drying and irritating.

Cuticle cream

Cuticle cream, cuticle lotion, cuticle oil, cuticle softener – these are all names for a moisturizing product that is applied to your nails. What's the purpose? To soften cuticles enough so that you can easily push them back off the nail plate. There are some lovely cuticle moisturizers on the market that contain everything from alpha hydroxy acids to delicious-smelling essential oils – however, you don't need anything fancy. Petroleum jelly, olive or almond oil, thick hand cream, or baby oil are all just as effective as any cuticle products you can buy.

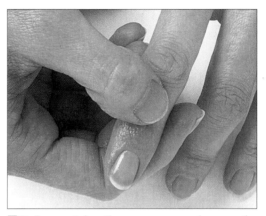

■ **Rub a cuticle oil or cream** *around your nails before you manicure. This will soften your skin and make your cuticles easier to manipulate.*

Cuticle pushers

Repeat after me: I will not buy or use metal cuticle pushers! Metal cuticle pushers can damage cuticles and lead to infection! Instead, go with orangewood or birchwood sticks, which are gentler. You can find these wood sticks in drugstores or nail salons.

CUTICLE ALERT

Avoid anything labeled cuticle remover, cuticle solvent, or alkaline cuticle solution. These contain an aggressive alkaline ingredient called potassium hydroxide, which works to dissolve the cuticle. First of all, dissolving your cuticle is not a good idea – you need this layer of skin to keep out marauding microorganisms. Secondly, when ingested (and this could happen, for example, if you put your finger in your mouth), potassium hydroxide can cause mouth pains, breathing difficulties, intense abdominal pain, diarrhea, a drop in blood pressure, and collapse. If potassium hydroxide gets in the eyes or nasal membranes, it can cause burning and tissue damage. If in doubt about a product's ingredients, read the label.

When using a cuticle pusher, work gingerly. You don't want to shove the cuticle so far back that it disappears into the nail fold. You also don't want to remove the cuticle outright. Your goal is to clear any bit of skin that has crept onto the nail plate. Do this by shimmying cuticles back toward the area where the nail fold and nail plate meet.

Here's a surprising fact: The nail polish we use today is a refined version of car paint.

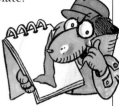

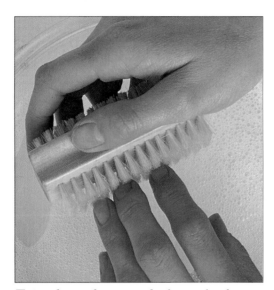

■ **Gently scrub your nails** *clean with a firm nailbrush. Use warm, soapy water to help dislodge dirt from underneath the nails.*

Nailbrushes

A nailbrush is a great thing to have. You can use it to scrub away dirt, clean off oily vestiges of cuticle cream or hand lotion, rub away callused or dry foot skin, and even to gently nudge back cuticles. A nailbrush needn't be expensive; all you need is something that feels comfortable in your hand and that features slightly flexible plastic or natural boar bristles.

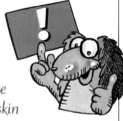

A tip on choosing a nailbrush: Bristles that are too soft don't have enough resistance to work well, while bristles that are too stiff can damage the skin under and around nails.

Buffers

Buffers are used on bare fingernails, bare toenails, and polish-coated nails. These tools usually come in the form of a rectangular block or a two-sided board, with a different strength of buffer on each of the block's or board's sides. The buffing material can be fiberglass, rubber, fine-grit sandpaper, chamois, or even leather.

Here's the origin of that pink glow that appears when you buff your nails: buffing removes the top layers of the nail plate, which in turn makes the nail more translucent. You also generate heat by way of friction. This heat encourages blood to flow to the nail bed's surface. The newly thinned nail plate makes it easier to see the blood below.

A buffer is not an essential piece of nail-care equipment. If you decide you can't possibly live without a buffer, go ahead and get one – I don't recommend using it on bare fingernails, where it can cause thinning of the nail plate. Buffers are best used on bare toenails (which are thicker than fingernails) or to give a gleaming finish between manicures to polished fingernails and toenails.

Clippers

Clippers are handy for large jobs, such as eliminating a half-inch worth of fingernail (either real or fake) or shortening toenails which, because of their thickness, don't yield easily to nail files. They're also good for trimming hangnails. The most important quality in a pair of clippers? Sharpness. Depending on the brand of clippers, what you use them for, and how often they are used, a pair should remain sharp anywhere from 6 months to 2 years.

If you notice that your clippers have lost their edge, head to a drugstore or nail salon and buy yourself a new pair. Your nails will thank you.

Nail masks

Nail masks fall into the "nail care extra" category. While not necessary, they are an effective way to draw moisture to dry, parched, peeling nails, and to soften stubborn cuticles. Not all cosmetic companies make nail masks, but there is a lot of variety on the market. A nail mask can be done immediately before a manicure.

■ **Use a sharp pair** *of nail clippers so that you can achieve good, clean cuts – a dull pair of clippers can mangle nails instead of cutting them.*

MASKING AT HOME

Fortunately, you can create an easy nail-mask treatment at home by warming up a little olive or almond oil, and then massaging it onto your clean nails. Allow it to sit for at least an hour.

If you're done before bedtime, why not go a step farther and slather your hands and feet with your favorite cream, put a pair of clean socks on your feet and cotton gloves on your hands? When you wake up the next morning, remove the socks and gloves – you'll be amazed at how youthful your hands and feet look.

Nail antiseptic

A base coat needs a clean, oil-free nail surface to adhere to; if there's even a trace of oil on the nail, the base coat will begin peeling as soon as it dries. If a scrub brush and soap aren't removing all the oil, cream, or cuticle softener you've used, you could try a nail antiseptic – this is a kind of a toner for nails. Nail antiseptics typically come in nail polish-style bottles and are brushed on. *Seche Prep®* is a particularly effective one.

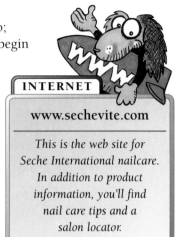

INTERNET

www.sechevite.com

This is the web site for Seche International nailcare. In addition to product information, you'll find nail care tips and a salon locator.

If you don't want to go out and buy nail antiseptic, you can use rubbing alcohol, witch hazel, white vinegar, or a strong skin astringent.

All about base coat

If you were to ask me what my personal favorite nail product was, I'd have to say base coat. I love the smooth finish base coat creates, the extra layer of strength it imparts to my nails, the way it keeps dark nail colors from staining my nails and – when I don't feel like wearing nail color – the clean, well-groomed look it lends nails when worn alone. There are several types of base coat available and this can lead to confusion. I have stood in a drugstore aisle, eyes bleary from reading labels, trying to figure out which base coat to buy. For those of you who've ever done the same thing, I offer this short base-coat primer:

a) **Base coats:** These are standard, no-frills nail primers. They provide some strengthening, but they are primarily used to help nail color glide on smoothly and to keep darker colors from staining nails. When a base coat features ingredients that create an extra hard finish, it is called a nail strengthener.

b) **Ridge fillers:** These are base coats that contain silk, talc, or other types of particles to fill in depressions. If your nails have any kind of depressions, ridges, or peeled-away layers at the tip, ridge fillers can provide a smooth finish.

c) **Anti-microbial or anti-fungal base coat:** These products are formulated with ingredients that help kill harmful microorganisms that can cause infection.

d) **Nail fortifier or nail-growth formula:** These are growth formulas and consist of clear polish infused with epoxy or formaldehyde resins and polyvinyl butyral (some also contain things like calcium). They are meant to be painted on nails daily for 7 to 10 days. Nail fortifiers can be used under and over your favorite nail colors, or they can be worn alone. Why do they work? Supposedly, the products' resins and polyvinyl bind with nails' keratin, actually creating stronger nails. Of course, I have heard plenty of people say that nail fortifiers are useless – but you know what? I've tried all kinds of base coats, and nail fortifiers are the only ones that strengthen my nails enough so that they can grow without splitting or breaking.

e **Matte-finish base coats:** Instead of the customary shiny finish, these offer a non-glossy, natural finish, and give added strength to nails.

Nail color

For many people, nail color – also called nail polish, nail paint, nail lacquer, and nail varnish – is what manicured nails are all about. Nail color is fun, it's sexy, it's eye-catching and, if you choose trendy seasonal colors, it can be a cheap way to update your overall look. Although there are perhaps a hundred different companies that manufacture nail polish, most of it is pretty much the same. Sure, some brands are thinner, some thicker, some dry more quickly than others, or wear better. Some companies include nail hardeners in their products, while other nail colors omit irritants such as formaldehyde and toluene.

There are numerous types of nail colors to choose between. One-coat formulas feature a concentrated amount of pigment, which gives you full coverage in one coat.

A polish with an opaque, high-gloss, non-sparkly finish is often referred to as a cream or gloss color.

Frost colors or pearl colors are another alternative. They come in a variety of gorgeous pearlescent shades and are formulated with ingredients such as iron oxides or mica to create a frosty finish. Nail glitters are colored or clear polishes formulated with a generous amount of colored glitter for a fun, fleck-toned finish – perfect for special occasions.

■ **A brightly colored nail polish** *can change your whole look. Choose a color that you're comfortable wearing and, like your favorite fragrance, it may become your signature style.*

Top coat

Top coats are a type of clear polish designed to protect nail color from the chipping, flaking, and peeling that comes with wear. They are similar to base coats, but most dry faster and feature a glossier finish. Standard issue top coats form a barrier that protects your manicure from chips and other "contact injuries." To keep a manicure fresh-looking and long-wearing, many nail technicians suggest painting on a fresh layer of top coat every day or every other day.

Alternatively, fast-dry or quick-dry top coats are designed to help rapidly dry the nail polish below. Within 2 minutes of painting on a fast-dry top coat, your manicure should be dry to the touch; within 7 to 12 minutes, the manicure should be completely (or near-completely) dry. UV-protective top coats that contain a sunscreen are also available – these protect nail color from the shade-changing effects of sunlight.

COLOR TROUBLE

With the exception of color additives and a few prohibited ingredients, the Food and Drug Administration cannot keep a cosmetic manufacturer from using almost any raw material as a cosmetic ingredient. It can, however, set limits on how an ingredient is used. This explains why an ingredient that is poisonous when swallowed may be banned from food items, but can be used in a nail polish. (This is another good reason not to bite manicured nails!) Although legal, many nail product ingredients are irritating. If you're sensitive, you may experience a rash after getting nail polish or nail-polish remover on your skin.

There are a number of common allergens in cosmetics. The solvent benzene is found in many nail polish removers. It causes redness, swelling, or an itchy rash in some people. Because it is toxic, avoid getting any in your mouth. Formaldehyde, a preservative and disinfectant, is a suspected carcinogen, and some people experience itchy rashes and redness upon physical contact with it. Toluene is a solvent found in some polishes, where it helps keep color pigment from hardening into a rock-solid blob. Contact with this highly toxic ingredient causes itchy rashes in sensitive individuals; if ingested, toluene can lead to convulsions, coma, or even death. Many nail-product manufacturers make nail-care items without these ingredients, so always check a product's label before purchasing.

INTERNET

www.cir-safety.org

Visit Cosmetic Ingredient Review's site to learn more about cosmetic ingredients and their uses, as well as possible allergic reactions and signs of poisoning.

The do-it-yourself manicure

THERE'S NOTHING LIKE A MANICURE to create a polished, well-groomed appearance. Yet for many of us, manicures are something to be had in a salon. Unfortunately, traveling to a salon, receiving a manicure, then waiting for your nails to dry can take 1 to 2 hours. Who has time for such luxuries?

You do, if you do it at home. "I can't give myself a manicure," you say. "There are so many steps, so many products. It's all so confusing." It does seem difficult, but with guidance, an at-home manicure is not only easy, it's quick and very enjoyable.

Assemble your tools

Here are the materials you need in order to carry out your at-home manicure:

- Nail-polish remover
- Cotton balls
- Fine-grained nail file
- Hand cream
- Nail mask (optional)
- Cuticle oil
- Orangewood or birchwood stick
- Nailbrush (optional)
- Bowl of warm, soapy water with a few drops of lemon juice and a few drops of olive oil or your favorite essential oil
- Nail antiseptic (optional)
- Base coat
- Nail color (optional)
- Top coat (optional)

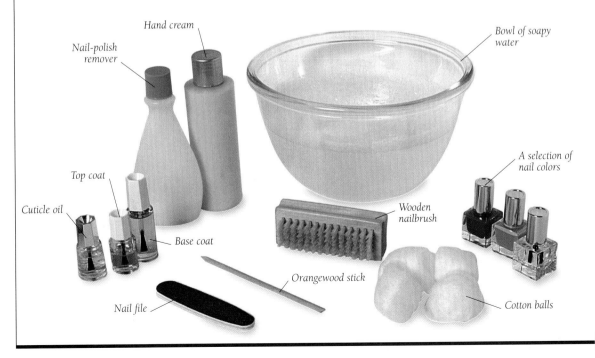

Hand cream

Nail-polish remover

Bowl of soapy water

A selection of nail colors

Top coat

Cuticle oil

Base coat

Wooden nailbrush

Orangewood stick

Nail file

Cotton balls

DO-IT-YOURSELF MANICURE

Choose a moment when you'll be uninterrupted for an hour or two. Put on some soothing music and sit comfortably next to a table or some other flat surface – it may be wise to cover this with a cloth, in case of any spills. Then you're all ready to begin your at-home manicure. Enjoy!

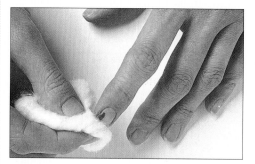

1 Removing old polish

To remove any remaining old nail color, apply polish remover to a cotton ball, and gently rub from the nail base toward the nail tip.

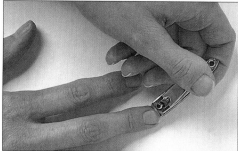

2 Clipping nails

If your nails are overlong, use a pair of clippers to remove excess length – be careful not to cut them too short, or down to the quick.

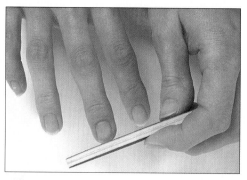

3 Filing down

Use a fine-grained nail file and file in one direction only – this will help to keep your nails strong. The most flattering shapes for nails are slightly square, oval, or squared-up oval. These are the healthiest shapes, too; pointy or talon-like nails are prone to tearing.

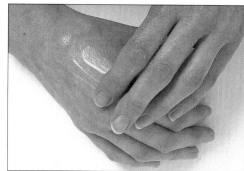

4 Hand care

Parched hands draw attention away from manicured nails, so give your hands a 2- or 3-minute massage using your favorite hand cream. Work cream up your fingers and into the nails. If you want to use a nail mask, apply it now and leave it on for an hour.

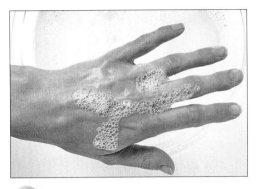

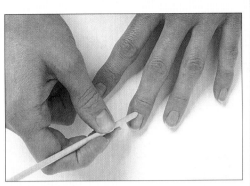

⑤ Cleaning nails

Soak fingers for 2 or 3 minutes in a bowl of soapy water to help clean under the nails and soften the cuticles. Dry thoroughly.

⑥ Cuticle care

Using an orangewood stick, gently clean any remaining dirt away and nudge back overgrown cuticles. If you like, apply nail antiseptic.

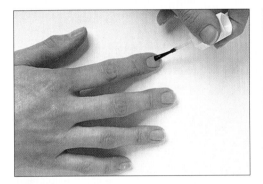

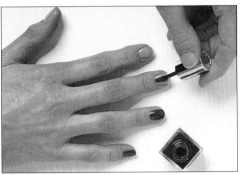

⑦ Applying base coat

To create a smooth surface, ready for nail color, apply a base coat. Rest your right hand on a flat surface and spread fingers apart. Paint a thin layer of base coat on each finger. Switch hands. If you prefer a natural look, end the manicure here.

⑧ Adding color

Apply polish in the same way you applied the base coat. When dry, apply a second coat.

⑨ Finishing touches

Clean any excess nail color off your fingers, using an orangewood stick wrapped in cotton wool and dipped in polish remover. When nail color has dried, apply a protective top coat.

The do-it-yourself pedicure

WHEN MOST PEOPLE THINK OF NAIL CARE, *it's fingernails that come to mind. Yet, in cities like New York and Paris, pedicures outrank manicures as the current beauty "must-haves."*

I'm not sure why this is. Perhaps it's the hoseless legs, bare feet, and strappy shoes ladies wear with no regard to the season – although it could be something else that I have no knowledge of. Regardless of the reason, however, urban sophisticates have gorgeous toes: smooth, moisturized, and dressed with subtle nude, classic red, or some seasonal shade of nail color. You too, can have lovely feet – in fact, good-looking toenails are easier to create and maintain than attractive, well-cared-for fingernails. That's because your toenails need in-depth attention only every 2 to 3 weeks, while fingernails need a fresh manicure every week or week-and-a-half.

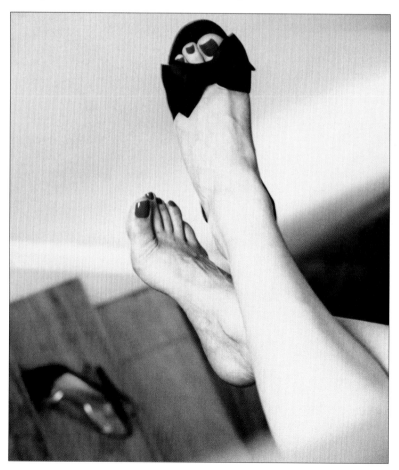

■ **A vibrant nail** *polish can complement a pair of open shoes, and add a stylish, colorful touch to your look.*

Assembling your tools

Your pedicure accessories should include nail-polish remover and cotton balls; hand and cuticle cream; a buffer; an orangewood or birchwood stick; a nail brush; nail clippers; and nail antiseptic. Have a bowl of warm, soapy water with a few drops of lemon juice and a few drops of olive oil to hand. An antimicrobial base coat is a smart option for those of you worried about fungal infections, while a foot pumice, nail mask, nail color, and top coat are optional extras for your pedicure. Now that you have got all the equipment together, you can get to work on your toenails.

Preparing your toes

With nail-polish remover and a cotton ball, remove any traces of old polish. If you have any thick, ridged toenails, or calluses on your toes, use a buffer to gently smooth these. Work gently and conservatively! Too little buffing is safer and healthier than too much.

Soak your feet for 2 or 3 minutes in a basin of warm, soapy water to help clean under your nails and to soften nails and cuticles. Use a nailbrush to dislodge dirt and exfoliate any dry skin, and dry

■ **Gentle rubbing**
with a foot pumice will leave your feet feeling smooth and supple – the perfect accompaniment to your pedicure.

thoroughly. Using an orangewood or birchwood stick, GENTLY clean away any remaining dirt under nails. Now would be a good moment to treat your feet to a gentle exfoliation with a foot pumice.

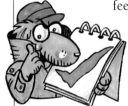

Trim your nails with nail clippers, taking care not to clip them too short, or to curve nails in at the corners.

Moisturizing your feet and toes

Dry, cracked feet steal attention from well-tended toenails. Moisturize feet with a 2- or 3-minute massage using your favorite hand or body cream. If using a nail mask, apply it now and allow it to remain on for an hour. Not everyone has heavy cuticles on their toenails. If you do, massage a bit of cuticle cream into cuticles and gently nudge back overgrown skin with an orangewood stick; if you are particularly sensitive, wrap the end of the stick in cotton.

To remove any oily residue, swipe nails with nail antiseptic. Prime nails for polish with a base coat. To apply, place your foot flat on a level surface and spread your toes out – if your toes are particularly bunched, separate them with cotton balls. Paint a thin coat of base coat on each toenail. Those who prefer a natural look can end the pedicure here.

You should apply polish in the same way that you applied the base coat. When the polish is dry, apply a second coat. Remove any stray traces of nail color with an orangewood stick wrapped in cotton and dipped in nail-polish remover.

When nail color has dried, apply a top coat. Do nothing, touch nothing, put on nothing, until your toenails are dry.

Trivia...

In the royal courts of the Ming Dynasty, the Chinese wore red and black nail polish made from vegetable dyes, beeswax, egg whites, and gelatin.

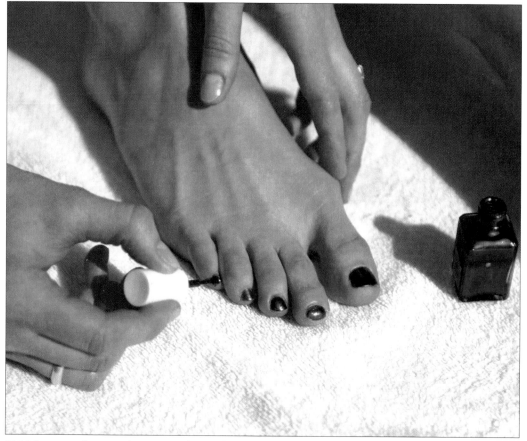

■ **Make sure that you leave** *enough time for your nail color to dry between each coat of polish, so that you can achieve a silky, smooth finish.*

CUTICLE CARE

Despite all the admonitions from doctors about the dangers of cutting cuticles, I have never (never!) been to a nail salon or spa where the nail technician HAS NOT moved toward my fingers and toes with her cuticle nippers. In fact, cuticle clipping appears to be so common in the nail industry that whenever my friends and I talk about professional manicures we always end up comparing cuticle-cutting stories. What we've found: It helps to sweetly say to the technician at the start that you'd prefer to have your cuticles nudged back instead of cut. (This way, you still get to have well-shaped half moons without losing your cuticles). Most nail technicians are nice about doing what you want – still, don't be surprised if you get a strange look and perhaps some attitude: my friends and I have gotten both. If you experience something similar, you can always stand up and walk yourself out of that salon and into one that serves your needs.

Salons: sanitation counts

FIRST, THE SCARY NEWS: All manner of fungi, viruses, and bacteria can be transmitted in salons – everything from staph and salmonella, to influenza and the hardy pseudomonas bacteria, which love to breed under the nail plate in cuts. Some of these cause minor nail or skin infections, some lead to infections so serious that you may lose a nail, while others waylay you with the flu, a cold, or conjunctivitis. Before you vow to never again step into a salon, I've got reassuring news.

INTERNET

www.epa.gov

The US Environmental Protection Agency's mission is to protect human health, and it is one of the agencies responsible for regulating salon conditions. Its site includes information on laws and regulations affecting all businesses, including salons.

If a salon practices proper sanitation, harmful microorganisms don't have a chance to infect clients. Whether you are trying to find a salon you like, or have been going to the same place for years, there are some sanitation measures that can help keep you safe.

Salon sanitation

Everyone must wash their hands! Not only your nail technician, but you. Instead of making you trek off to the bathroom to do this, many nail techs will squirt a bit of germicidal, no-rinse hand sanitizer onto your hands and their own hands.

Sanitized instruments prevent the spread of germs from one client to the next. Some tools – such as nail files and cuticle pushers – can't be sanitized, which means your nail technician must use fresh ones on you. To decrease waste, some salons ask you to bring your own nail file, cuticle pusher, and buffer; if you don't supply these, you can purchase them at the salon and take them home after the service. All hard surfaces must also be wiped down between clients with disinfectant, so make sure that this happens.

Trivia...

Some nail technicians use small tabletop ultraviolet lamps to dry nail polish more quickly or to finish nail enhancements. These lamps typically use UVA light, the same type of aging UV light used in tanning salons. Ask any dermatologist: UV light is not good for your health or your looks. When searching for a nail salon, play it safe and ask whether it uses UV light.

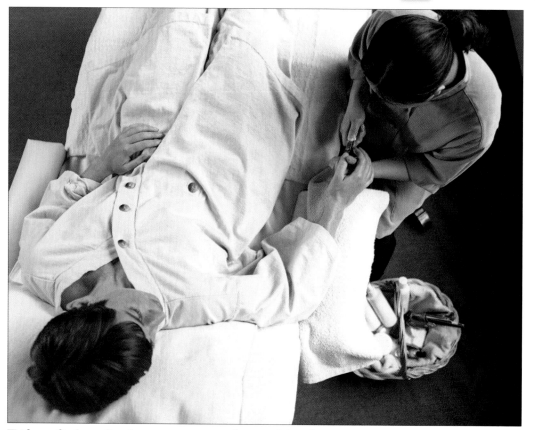

■ **If you find a nail salon** *you can trust, and are confident that it practices good hygiene methods, lie back and enjoy the luxury of a professional manicure.*

Enhancing your nails

NAIL ENHANCEMENT IS A BROAD TERM that encompasses several methods of augmenting your natural nail. Actually, in some instances, enhancements have less to do with enhancement and more to do with faking it, hence the commonly used term "fake nails." Personally, I am not a fan of nail enhancements. Every time I see an unnaturally thick, 2-inch (5-cm) talon, aggressively squared at the tip and curving unnaturally away from the nail bed, words like "cheap," "tacky," and questions like "how does she type, make bread, tie shoes, button a shirt, put on face cream, play catch with a kid or a dog?" creep into my head. Still, I realize that each of us has different tastes and lifestyles, so I'm more than happy to offer information about the following enhancements:

If you get nail enhancements, you'll be returning to the salon every 2 to 6 weeks — depending on your nail's growth and your own vigilance — for a "fill" or "touch-up." This is nail-speak for getting your nails' newly grown area enhanced so that it matches the rest of the nail.

Wraps

Nail wraps use sheets of fiberglass, linen, or silk to add a strong, protective layer to the nail, which in turn helps nails grow longer without breaking. To create nail wraps, your nail technician takes small pieces of fabric mesh and affixes them to your nails with an adhesive – typically one of those nail glues that reminds everyone of Crazy Glue or Super Glue. After buffing the enhancement a bit to create a smooth surface, your nail technician applies a sealant to help keep out moisture and discourage the wrap from *lifting*.

Acrylic nails

To create acrylic nails, a nail technician mixes together two ingredients called powdered polymer and liquid monomer. When combined, the powder and liquid react to form a plastic-like paste.

DEFINITION

In nail-care circles, the word lifting *has nothing to do with picking up heavy objects. The term refers to any type of nail enhancement partially coming loose from the nail plate. These loose spots create gaps between the enhancement and the natural nail where moisture and microorganisms can enter, breed, and infect the natural nail.*

This paste is smoothed onto the nail, where it cures, or hardens, at room temperature. Acrylic nails are a good choice for anyone who wants long nails that are virtually indestructible.

If you are sensitive, you should avoid acrylic or porcelain nails. The monomer used in acrylic and porcelain nails is an irritant that can cause allergic reactions in people with sensitive skin.

Porcelain nails

Porcelain nails are similar to acrylic nails, except that they use a finely ground, glass-like material in the powder. They are applied just like acrylic nails and are good for creating a hearty, long nail. The finish is a bit more natural-looking than acrylic nails, making them a better choice for those of you who like to wear pale, sheer nail colors.

Gel nails

Gel nails, or gel systems as they are also called, are a newer type of nail enhancement that are created by applying layers of resin to the nail; these layers combine and harden to form a solid nail. Depending on the formula a particular nail technician uses, nails are hardened with an ultraviolet curing light or under ordinary room lighting. Gel nails are among the most natural-looking of the nail enhancements – something to keep in mind if you want nails that look like your own, only longer and stronger.

Using nail tips

Nail tips are one of the oldest forms of nail enhancements. Preformed plastic nail shapes are applied to the natural nail plate with nail glue. Sometimes they cover the nail from the cuticle to the end, but more frequently they are applied midway down the nail plate. To get a smoother finish, some nail techs may apply acrylics, gel, or wraps over either the natural "untipped" nail or both the natural nail and the newly affixed nail tip. The entire shape is then sanded and filed into the length and shape you want.

■ **You can buy** *nail enhancement do-it-yourself kits. However, because of the chemicals involved in their application, the best option is to visit a nail technician.*

Trivia...

Some nail technicians believe that nail enhancements can be worn continually, while many dermatologists feel it is important to take several 2-week to 1-month "rests" a year from nail enhancements. Why? Nail enhancements trap the natural nail underneath, causing the nail plate to atrophy. These rests allow the weakened natural nail to grow stronger.

Nail art

Perhaps you're a showy type, someone who loves to express herself through her appearance. For you, a shockingly bright, trendy-colored nail isn't enough. You want to set yourself apart from the manicured crowd. From the sound of it, you are a nail art kind of gal. Nail art is not so much a way to augment nails' length as it is a way to enhance their appearance.

There are several ways you can dress up nails. Decals – much like the decals you got from boxes of sugared cereal, and stuck on windows or your own body as a kid – are an easy way to add whimsy to your nails. Most nail salons have a selection of seasonal (jack o'lanterns, snowflakes) as well as standard (roses, stars) designs. These are embedded in slightly sticky nail color. When nail color is dry, a swipe of top coat keeps decals secure.

Decorative nails

Nail jewelry can be expensive 14-karat gold, but it is usually made of cheaper silver- or gold-colored metals. Most nail jewelry comes in simple designs, such as initials, stars, and hearts; it is applied just like nail decals. For those with very long nails, there is another type of nail jewelry: earrings for nails. If you're interested, your nail technician will actually pierce one of your nails and install a stud or a small hoop. Nail detailing, sometimes simply called nail art, uses extra-fine paintbrushes and several colors of nail polish, which your nail technician uses to paint scenes onto the nail. The finished product depends greatly on your nail technician's skill as a fine artist.

A simple summary

✔ Having the right tools makes home nail care easy.

✔ It's not difficult to give yourself a manicure or a pedicure.

✔ Many nail-product ingredients are strong allergens. Always read the labels!

✔ When visiting a salon, pay attention to its sanitation practices.

✔ If you can't grow your own nails, you could try nail enhancements.

✔ For the adventurous, nail art and jewelry are an option.

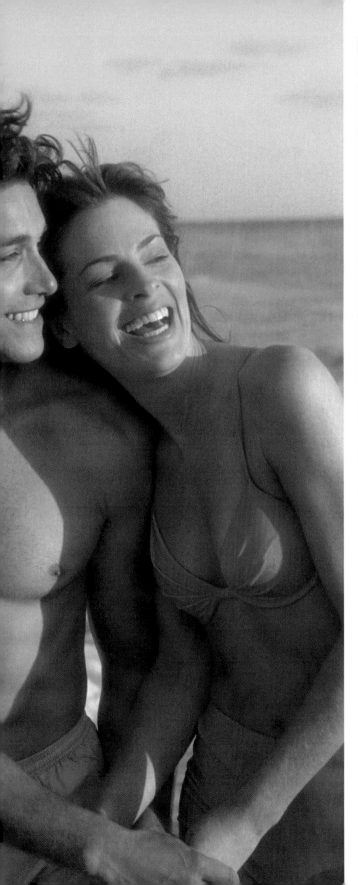

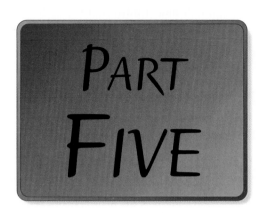

PART FIVE

BEAUTY AND BEYOND

NOW IT'S TIME TO TACKLE all those extras – such as body care, cosmetic surgery, and emotional states of mind – that can help you look and feel even better about yourself. Anyone who has worn a bathing suit in public knows that your body (and your feelings about it) affects *your self-esteem*. But if you take care of your body, you will feel confident and, in turn, *look beautiful*.

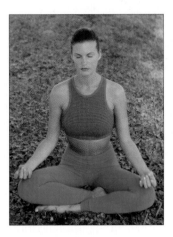

Being troubled about a part of your face or body can make you feel and look less attractive. If you cannot find a way to appreciate a specific feature, you may want to consider cosmetic surgery. We'll also explore the way our lifestyles, actions, intellect, and countenance affect our beauty. After all, total beauty is about more than your hair or face – it's about all of you.

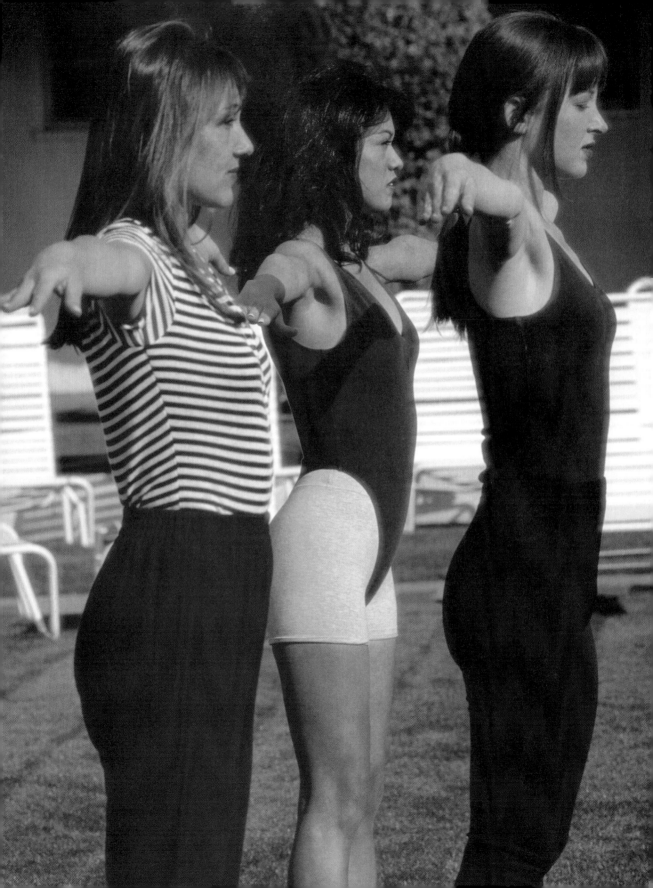

Chapter 16

Body Care

IN OUR QUEST FOR BEAUTY it's easy to be fixated by the face. Yet a well-treated body adds to a person's total beauty. Notice that I did not say flawless, voluptuous, slim, or any other word that describes a minority of figures. I said well-treated. This is important – it truly doesn't matter what kind of body you have if you look after it and treat it with respect.

In this chapter...

✓ Posture

✓ Exfoliation

✓ Body lotions and creams

✓ Sunscreen

✓ Fragrance

✓ Body glitches

✓ Hair removal

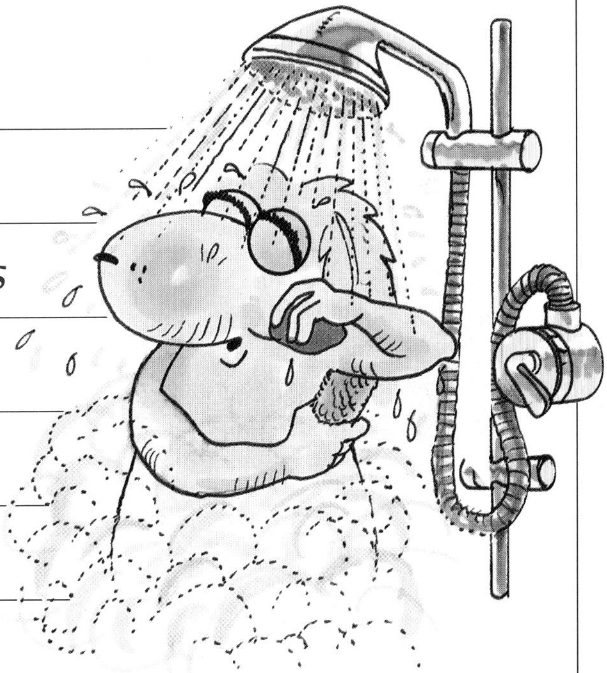

REGULAR EXERCISE WILL IMPROVE YOUR POSTURE AND BEARING

Posture

NO MATTER what your weight, color, or level of fitness, you'll look better if you stand up straight. I sound like your mother, right? But it's true: Good posture helps you look fit, strong, energetic, and healthy – all important facets of personal beauty. Compare that with the message you give out by slouching, which can make you look weak, ineffective, or mousy. Furthermore, posture affects your health. If it's good, you'll find yourself strong enough to meet a day's – and a life's – challenges without unnecessary fatigue or aches. If it's bad, you'll be more prone to tiredness, poor circulation, back problems, neck aches, and weak stomach muscles.

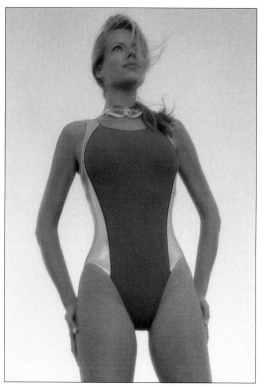

■ **If you have good posture** *you will exude confidence and self-assurance, as well as an air of natural elegance and grace.*

To determine if your posture is good, stand as you normally do but with your heels against a wall. Your calves, buttocks, shoulders, and the back of your head should touch the wall. If your posture is good you should be able to just barely slip your hand through the space between the small of your back and the wall. Do you need help in developing good posture? Keep reading:

1. When you are sitting, push your navel back toward your spine, and hold your torso upright. Yes, you should do this even (especially!) when you're spending those long hours at the computer.

2. To put yourself in touch with your body, try some form of stretch-intensive exercise, such as yoga or *Pilates*.

3. When standing for long periods of time, check that your abdominals are pulled in and your hips are slightly tilted forward. Your knees should be relaxed.

DEFINITION

Pilates is a form of exercise – some people compare it to yoga – created by Joseph Pilates. It uses careful stretches, calisthenic movements, and workout machines to help stretch, lengthen, and strengthen muscles.

(4) If you find it painful to straighten your posture, a form of body work – such as *rolfing* or the *Feldenkrais method* – can make standing up straight more comfortable.

(5) Exercise regularly, because inactivity is the most common contributing factor to poor posture.

(6) This quick back-strengthening exercise can be done several times a day and is a good way to stretch the back after an hour at the computer: Squeeze your shoulder blades together and hold for 10 seconds. Repeat ten times.

(7) If you spend more than an hour a day at the computer, it's important to find a chair that supports your lower back and allows you to put your feet flat on the floor. If your legs don't reach the ground, find some kind of platform (even a telephone book) to rest your feet on.

DEFINITION

Rolfing involves deeply massaging the connective tissue that encloses muscles. This in turn provides the body with greater mobility, making it easier to stand up straight. It usually involves ten 1-hour sessions. The Feldenkrais method revolves around discovering improper movement habits. These are then replaced with proper movement techniques. Most people need at least two to five 1-hour sessions.

Exfoliation

IN CHAPTER 3, we discussed how regular exfoliation helps maintain a healthy complexion; we also discussed types of exfoliators. But exfoliation is not for faces alone – regular exfoliation of the body helps remove dead skin cells and scaly patches, and it also helps prevent ingrown hairs. The type of exfoliator you use is up to you and your skin – the important thing is to exfoliate every time you bathe or shower.

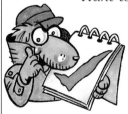

Want to turn your favorite liquid soap or shower gel into a body exfoliator? In your palm, mix a dollop of the soap with a tablespoon of coarse salt, turbinado sugar, or sea sand.

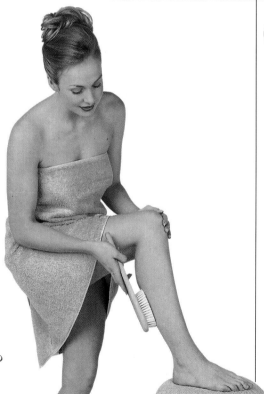

■ **Some people prefer** *to use a dry brush to exfoliate their skin before bathing or taking a shower.*

265

Body lotions and creams

THE SKIN ON YOUR FEET, *legs, belly, breasts, hands, arms, and shoulders is typically drier than the skin on your face. This means a once-daily – or even twice-daily – application of body lotion is a must for combating – and preventing – scaly patches. The great thing about body lotions today is that many are formulated with special active ingredients, such as retinol, alpha hydroxy acids, antioxidants, or sunscreens – all of which help fight visible signs of age. (Yes, you can tell a person's age by looking at body skin.) Furthermore, body lotions also come in a range of intensities, from light lotions to rich creams.*

When choosing a product, keep in mind that the lighter the consistency of the lotion, the less moisturizing power it has. Heavy creams are best for super-dry skin and seemingly always parched areas of your body, such as feet and elbows, while light lotions may be enough for your torso. Another thing to keep in mind: If you break out on your back, chest, or buttocks (don't feel bad, many people do), choose a light lotion that contains blemish-blasting ingredients such as alpha hydroxy acid or salicylic acid.

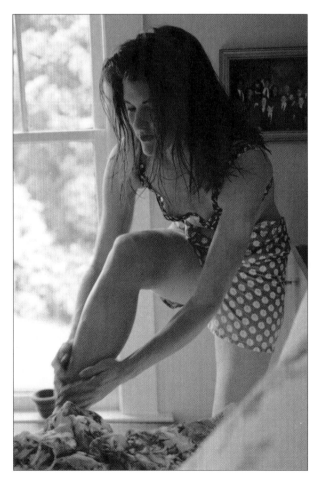

Can you use hand lotion on your body? Of course! In fact, hand lotion and body lotion are simply two different names for the same product.

■ **Get into a regular** *routine of applying body lotion after a bath or a shower.*

Thigh creams

If you suffer from cellulite, you've probably been tempted to buy one of those thigh creams, also known as cellulite creams, toning creams, or firming creams. Most firming products contain one or more ingredients such as caffeine, or algae extracts, which temporarily tighten the skin, thus making your thighs appear more toned and your cellulite appear less obvious.

While some products claim that regular use can permanently tone thighs, I know no skin-care expert or dermatologist who agrees with this. You can expect results to last from 4 to 12 hours. Note that these creams are not for the thighs only – all can be used any place where skin is dimpled or slack, including the hips, buttocks, tummy, breasts, and upper arms.

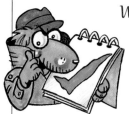

In the United States, endermologie® was the first medical treatment for cellulite to be approved by the Food and Drug Administration.

Décolletage creams

On your next trip to a spa, cosmetic boutique, or department store, you may encounter a décolletage cream – also known as bust cream or breast cream. As its name implies, this product is for the chest and breasts. But what exactly does it do?

These creams moisturize and temporarily tighten the skin. There are parts of the world where no well-tended woman is without her bust cream – but as far as I can tell, I am not living in one of those places. Instead, I use the same products on my chest that I use on my face; other women use body lotion of various intensities, or even thigh-toning cream.

While makers of some décolletage creams claim that regular use can permanently boost your bust, this is another beauty world fallacy – the truth is that a décolletage cream's effects last from 4 to 12 hours.

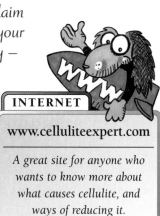

INTERNET

www.celluliteexpert.com

A great site for anyone who wants to know more about what causes cellulite, and ways of reducing it.

ABOUT CELLULITE

For you lucky people who have no idea what cellulite is, let me tell you: it's that dimply fat found on the back of many people's legs and buttocks. However, despite the large number of people who suffer from cellulite, doctors can't agree on what it is made of. The most oft-repeated explanation is that cellulite is composed of deposits of fat that are caught between skin fibers. There are a number of treatments, ranging from the completely ineffective to the slightly effective. Read on.

a **Exercise:** This is one of the most effective – and most permanent – treatments for cellulite. By shedding excess weight and building muscle, you not only remove excess fat, which is prone to dimpling, you also create a smooth, taut surface to your skin.

b **Liposuction:** This treatment can improve the appearance of cellulite by removing excess fat, which is prone to dimpling.

c *Endermologie®*: A patented technique involving a mechanized device that has two motorized rollers and regulated suction. Along with firm massage, it is used to "work up" thighs. It is said that this increases circulation, which in turn boosts skin's firmness and makes skin smoother. The procedure needs to be performed once or twice a week for an average of ten to 30 times. While *Endermologie®* does not totally eliminate cellulite, it does greatly reduce cellulite's appearance. Results last anything from 3 months to a year.

d **Body wraps:** These cause the body to sweat away water, which in turn makes skin lie flatter against the underlying muscles. The effect on cellulite is strictly temporary and usually lasts from 8 to 12 hours.

e **Vigorous massage:** This can temporarily soften the appearance of cellulite by increasing circulation, making skin look firmer. It also encourages the body to release the excess water that it is holding in the massaged tissues, thereby reducing the look of cellulite. Results last on average from 8 to 12 hours.

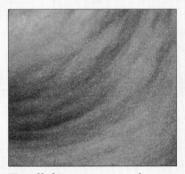

■ **Cellulite occurs** *mainly around the legs and buttocks – it affects slim and overweight people.*

Sunscreen

THERE WAS A TIME when we didn't know tanning was bad for us.
Back then, we'd lie in the sun for hours, slathering ourselves with homemade
concoctions such as baby oil mixed with iodine, in an effort to increase that tan.
Today, we absolutely know better – there is no such thing as a healthy tan!

In Chapter 2 we discussed the importance of sunscreen for the face – what many people forget, however, is that sunscreen is just as important for the body. Daily sunscreen is a must. Opt for a product with high UVA and UVB protection, such as a formula with zinc oxide or Parsol 1789 (also called avobenzone).

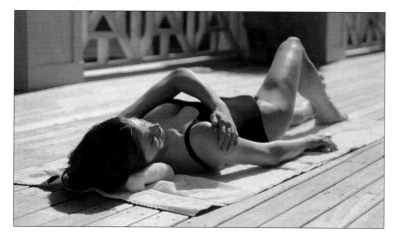

■ **Body skin** *ages in the same way as facial skin and should be protected when you are exposed to the sun.*

FAKE 'N' BAKE

Self-tanners are an easy way to give yourself some color without damaging your skin. They contain a chemical called dihydroxyacetone (DHA) – a nontoxic, chemical sugar that reacts with your skin to create a toasty color. To use, exfoliate your skin, dry yourself off, and apply self-tanner thickly to the chosen area – you can apply the product a bit more sparingly on elbows and knees, which seem to soak up color. Wash your hands and don't let anything touch your "self-tanned" skin for at least 30 minutes, which is how long it takes most self-tanners to develop their color. You can use a cotton ball dipped in nail polish remover to wipe away any stray orange color that may remain on the palms of your hands.

Fragrance

WHEN I WAS A TEENAGER, *I had a number of different drugstore scents in my collection. Each morning, I chose a scent according to my mood and my outfit – a sporty ensemble required a crisp, lemony fragrance; a ruffly shirt needed a cloying jasmine-based scent; and so on. It wasn't until I was 20, during a visit to France, that I even considered a "signature scent." After a week there, it became apparent to me that the women – and men – I was with wore the same scent every day. What's more, I could tell who was near me just by their scent; I could use my nose to "see" people just as much as my eye.*

The idea of a personal scent fascinated me so much that I wanted my own. After visiting several parfumeries to try on scents, I found one – which I still wear today and which the people in my life have come to associate with me.

Splurging on one well-made, gorgeous scent that suits your personality is much easier and much more satisfying (I find) than having a dresser littered with numerous bottles of less expensive fragrances.

FRAGRANCE FORMULAS

Ever wonder what the difference is between perfume and cologne? Here's a rundown of fragrance formulas, from the strongest-smelling to the weakest:

- Perfumes contain the strongest concentration of fragrance oils, giving them a long-lasting fragrance and a high price tag.
- Eau de parfum contains a percentage of fragrance diluted with alcohol and water. It is weaker than perfume, and has shorter staying power.
- Eau de toilette, also called toilet water, contains a higher percentage of alcohol and water than fragrance ingredients.
- Eau de cologne, also called cologne, contains mostly alcohol and water and has very little lasting power. It is the least expensive of all fragrance products.

Choosing a scent

To choose a signature scent, go to a department store or fragrance boutique and try on a few perfumes. I realize that magazines offer all kinds of quizzes that tell you whether you should be wearing a spicy fragrance, a floral scent, a herbaceous perfume, and so on – but in reality, you won't know what will work until you try it on. That's because perfume reacts differently on each person's skin, depending on that person's body chemistry. In other words, a scent you love in the bottle – or on your cousin or friend – may smell putrid on you. When testing, don't spritz yourself with more than four scents a day. (Yes, it might take a month or more of this before you find a scent you love, but take your time; you get no prize for rushing.) Allow the fragrances to develop for 3 hours, 7 hours, 10 hours – noting how they develop with time. The fragrance you like throughout its development is most likely the fragrance for you.

Body glitches

FEW OF US MAKE IT TO ADULTHOOD WITHOUT *a few surface imperfections – perhaps a scar from a teenage cycling accident, a strange mole caused by past sun exposure, or broken veins brought on by birth control pills, pregnancy, or just plain genetics. If you're like me, these skin glitches make me dread summertime, when I have to decide between the comfort of sundresses, shorts, and sleeveless shirts, or the camouflaging ability of long skirts, pants, and sleeved shirts. Fortunately for women like me, there is a host of new treatments available to reduce the appearance of surface flaws. Most scars cannot be eliminated completely, but they can be softened.*

Scars

Like many of you, I have quite a number of scars on my legs, thanks to childhood bicycling accidents, teenage clumsiness, and an adult run-in with an adorable yet feisty kitten.

I've found that exfoliating ingredients such as glycolic acid and salicylic acid help soften the appearance of scars, as do pigment-lightening ingredients such as kojic acid and hydroquinone.

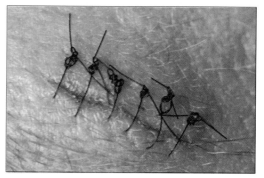

■ **Skin heals remarkably** *quickly after a cut or injury, but small scars can remain.*

For bad scars, onion extract (also called *cepium allium*) has been found to soften the appearance of all types of scars when used two to four times a day for 1 to 4 months. Topical gels or bandages containing silicone have also been shown to soften the appearance of all types of scars. You either use the gel two to four times a day or wear the bandage continually for 4 months. A dermatologist can also soften the appearance of scars through microdermabrasion, or laser resurfacing.

A scar is the skin's healing response to an injury or wound and is composed mostly of inelastic collagen fibers. Scar tissue is disorganized and appears distinctively different from the normal tissue surrounding it.

Mole check

Moles are not inherently dangerous. It is only "irregular" moles – or a mole's sudden "irregular" behavior – that may indicate you've got skin cancer. To catch a potential problem while it is still small, examine your entire body monthly, carefully studying each mole. Contact your dermatologist if you find any of the following signs:

- A mole that has changed color, size, or shape.
- A mole that itches, bleeds, or has a crusty surface.
- A mole with an asymmetrical border.

Stretch marks

Stretch marks, known medically as *striae gravidarum*, are fissures in skin's middle layer. They occur when the body grows faster than the skin can accommodate, which makes adolescence, pregnancy, sudden weight gain, or quick muscle-building all prime times for stretch marks to develop. While stretch marks do fade with time, they often remain visible enough to make you self-conscious.

Perhaps no other skin glitch seems to cause such dissension among dermatologists. Some say stretch marks are treatable, some say the marks are mildly treatable, and others say there is nothing you can do to make them better. Daily applications of a trentinoin cream, or a product containing glycolic acid or onion extract, have been shown to soften the marks in some people. So have microdermabrasion, intense pulsed light treatments, and laser resurfacing. And there are people who swear by pure vitamin E or jojoba oil. If you have stretch marks and want them gone, you may have to experiment with several types of treatments to get results.

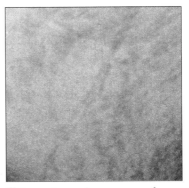

■ **Stretch marks** *appear as fine lines or wrinkles on the skin.*

Vein troubles

Broken veins – also known as spider veins, thread veins, or broken capillaries – are threadlike veins that have become stretched out and distended. These unnaturally dilated veins fill up with an abundance of blood, making them extremely visible beneath the skin. At one time, dermatologists cauterized these small vessels with electric current. Cosmetic lasers soon replaced cauterizing. *EpiLight*® (also called *PhotoDerm*®) is a modern treatment which produces good cosmetic results on spider veins, using pulses of intense light.

> **Trivia...**
> *Varicose comes from the Latin root word* varix, *which means twisted.*

Varicose veins – which occur most often on the legs – have a dark blue, green, or purple cast. They occur as a result of a malfunction of the vein's valves. Normally the valves help propel blood to the heart but they can be stretched due to pregnancy, obesity, blood clots, or a hereditary defect. When this happens, the valve is unable to close normally, and blood pools in the vein. If the problem is mild, a saline solution can be injected into the vein, encouraging the vein to restrict. In moderate cases, your doctor can close off the vein at the valve. In severe cases, your doctor might remove the entire vein.

Hair removal

AT ONE TIME, removing body hair was a cultural thing – in some countries it was done, in others it was not. However, in the last decade an increasing number of us – regardless of our nationalities – are removing the leg and underarm hair we once kept.

Shaving

Shaving is a utilitarian, easy, quick, and affordable way to temporarily get rid of unwanted body hair. Avoid razor rash – an itchy, bumpy reaction some people get to shaving – by exposing hair to warm water for at least 5 minutes before shaving. This softens hair and makes it easier to remove.

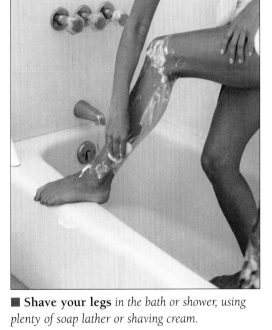

■ **Shave your legs** *in the bath or shower, using plenty of soap lather or shaving cream.*

A thick buffer of shave cream or soap lather further protects skin against shaving rash. If you frequently suffer from dry, itchy, red skin after shaving, you may find it less irritating to shave in the same direction as hair growth. Note, though, that you won't get as smooth a finish as shaving against hair's growth.

Creams

Depilatory, or hair removal, creams use thyiogylcolate – the same ingredient found in permanent waves – to melt hair. Depilatories are great for anyone who gets rashes from shaving, or who hates the coarse, blunt-edged way that shaved hair grows back. The downsides to depilatories are their intense chemical odor, and the way you must stand still for 5 to 10 minutes as the cream works. Furthermore, people with sensitive skin may find depilatories irritating.

Waxing

If you can get past the pain of having liquified wax poured onto your skin then swiftly ripped away, then you'll no doubt love the week or two of fuzz-free skin that follows. However, regular waxing does slightly damage hair follicles, causing them to produce finer, skimpier hairs. Another downside to waxing – besides the pain – is that it breaks hair off just below the skin, which appears to promote ingrown hairs.

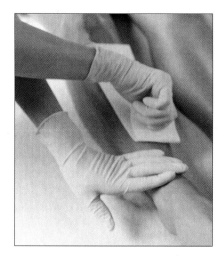

■ **Waxing can be** *carried out by a beautician, but there are also do-it-yourself kits available at drugstores and cosmetic boutiques, so that you can try it yourself at home.*

INGROWN HAIR

If you've experienced a red pimple-like bump on your leg, underarm, or bikini line, you've probably had an ingrown hair – this is a hair that has grown sideways, forcing the hair's tip to lodge into the follicle wall. To prevent the problem, try daily exfoliation with a grainy scrub or washcloth, followed by an application of body lotion that contains a high percentage of salicylic or glycolic acid. To treat an ingrown hair, don't pick! Keep up the exfoliation treatments and twice a day dab on an acne cream containing benzoyl peroxide, glycolic acid, or salicylic acid.

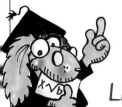

Sugaring works much like waxing. A sticky, sugar-based paste is painted onto skin, then rubbed off, pulling the hair away with it.

Light and laser treatment

Not only can intense pulsed light be used to treat sun damage, scars, and broken veins, it also works to remove hair by temporarily inactivating the follicle, leaving you hair-free for 2 to 6 weeks.

You may have heard of eflornithine cream, a new product that slows the growth of facial hair. It is believed to work by blocking an enzyme in the follicle that is necessary for hair growth.

Laser hair removal systems use a laser to disable hair's follicles and once a follicle is destroyed, it is believed to stop producing hair. However, some research indicates that with some medications or hormonal imbalances, dormant hair follicles can be stimulated to regrow hair. Two to four treatments carried out at 4- to 6-week intervals are required. Many dermatologists are also advocating long term control of hair growth using lasers, rather than advocating permanent hair removal.

Hair removal with electrolysis

Electrolysis directs electric pulses into hair's follicles where they shock the hair's root and inhibit hair growth. It is done one follicle at a time, so it's impractical for large areas – but it is perfect for hairy chins or upper lips. It must be performed by a skilled practitioner, because electrolysis can cause slight scarring in some people.

A simple summary

✓ A lovingly tended body is a powerful facet of beauty.

✓ Your posture sends people signals about you.

✓ Regular exfoliation keeps your skin healthy and beautiful.

✓ Can you boost your bust with creams? Not permanently.

✓ Sunscreen – it's youth serum for your body.

✓ Dislike body hair? You've got more treatment options than ever.

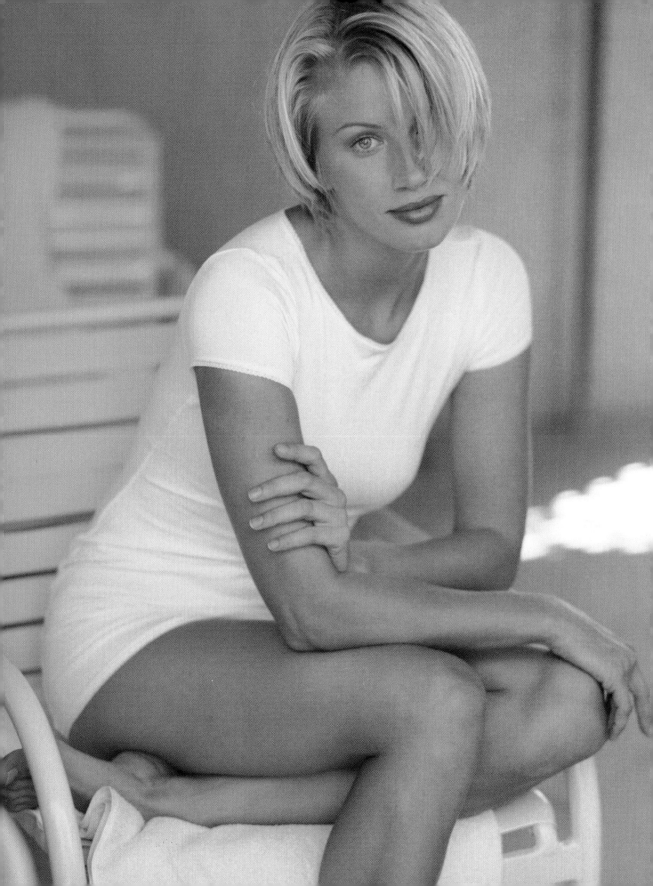

Chapter 17

Considering Cosmetic Surgery

COSMETIC SURGERY HAS GOTTEN A BAD REPUTATION. And rightly so: sometimes we're faced with a nose that doesn't look right, aggressive globelike breasts, or a strangely tight face that is at odds with the wearer's loose neck. That's unfortunate, because when used correctly, cosmetic surgery is about gently improving a feature you personally feel needs improvement, while at the same time maintaining your face's or body's integrity. After all, if you erase your natural features, you won't have any uniqueness to celebrate – and enjoying your uniqueness is what total beauty is about.

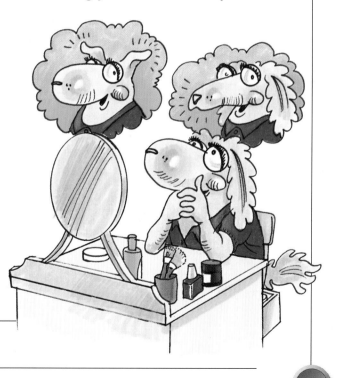

In this chapter...

✓ **Is cosmetic surgery for you?**

✓ **What's out there?**

CONSIDER COSMETIC SURGERY CAREFULLY BEFORE MAKING A DECISION

Is cosmetic surgery for you?

SHOULD YOU OR SHOULDN'T YOU HAVE *cosmetic surgery?*
Ultimately, only you can decide. But to help you determine whether cosmetic surgery is an option for you, ask yourself the following probing questions:

Things to consider

Why do you want cosmetic surgery? If your answer is to look like a model or celebrity, to win the affections of a certain person, or to have a happier life, you may be disappointed. Cosmetic surgery will not change your life – it will only change a certain feature, and it rarely can make you look like another person. The healthiest reason for wanting cosmetic surgery is to simply improve your appearance.

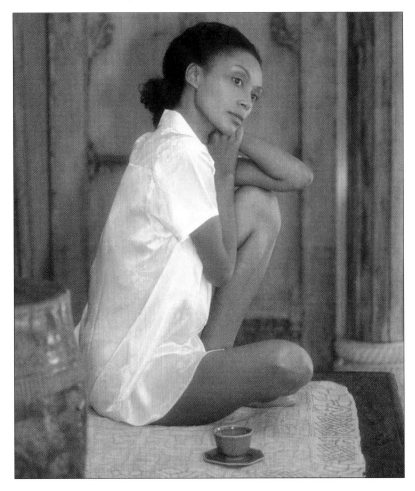

■ **Cosmetic** *surgery should not be rushed into. Think carefully about how you will feel after it has been carried out; how you will explain it to your friends and acquaintances; and in what ways it could affect your life – for better or worse.*

Your well-being

Are you in good health? Cosmetic surgery is serious surgery. Therefore, if you suffer from a pre-existing condition, you may not be a suitable candidate.

If you're a smoker, try to quit as far ahead of surgery as possible. Nicotine slows wound healing – sometimes severely. Many surgeons will not operate on smokers.

What is your threshold for pain? Cosmetic surgery is surgery, and as such involves pain – perhaps during the procedure and most certainly afterward during the healing process. How much pain you'll feel depends on the procedure and your tolerance level.

Ask your surgeon about the homeopathic remedy Arnica. Many doctors are now prescribing Arnica before and after surgery to reduce swelling and bruising and speed healing.

Considering the costs

Can you afford cosmetic surgery? Surgery fees vary widely depending on the procedure, the doctor, and the part of the country the doctor practices in. After researching surgery fees, ask yourself if you can comfortably afford to go under the knife. Furthermore, do you have time for surgery? Depending on the surgery and your age – the older you are, the longer you'll take to heal – you will spend from 5 days to a month healing. During this time, you are bandaged and swollen, and often bruised and uncomfortable – you remain indoors until you feel good enough to be seen by others.

Let's say you see a surgeon about a certain feature you'd like to improve and he or she responds by pointing out additional features that "need fixing." Leave his or her office immediately! An ethical doctor does not try to sell surgery by telling you that you have flaws.

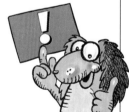

Finding a surgeon

Have you found a reputable doctor? When searching for a cosmetic surgeon, be prepared to visit several before deciding on one. When interviewing surgeons, ask about their educations, how long they have been practicing cosmetic surgery, what surgeries they specialize in, how many of a certain procedure they have performed in their careers, and whether or not they have ever been sued for malpractice.

What's out there

ONCE UPON A TIME, COSMETIC SURGERY *seemed limited to facelifts and nose jobs. But with time, other procedures were developed and now it is possible to change the appearance of almost any facial or body part. To give you an idea of what exists, I offer the following brief overview of today's most popular procedures. For more extensive information, contact your doctor, visit your local library or bookstore, or get on the Internet and research the topic.*

Lifts and tucks

Gravity, age, and weight gain cause some areas of the face and body to sag. Surgery can counter this by trimming away excess skin. Below are the most popular "lift and tuck" operations available:

(a) **Facelift:** As we age, the effects of gravity, sun exposure, smoking, and even genetics can change the way our faces look. Deep creases may form between the nose and mouth, our jawlines can grow slack and jowly, and our cheeks seem to hang lower and more loosely than they did when we were young.

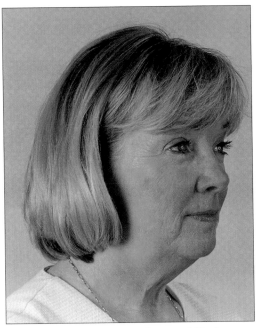

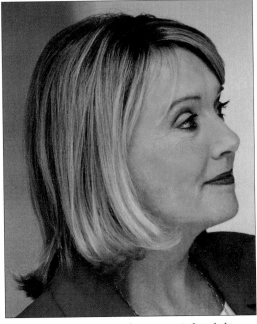

■ **As our skin ages,** *it can become difficult to hide loose skin and wrinkles.*

■ **Following surgery,** *this woman's facial skin has a tighter, firmer appearance.*

A facelift, known medically as rhytidectomy, can help improve the visible signs of aging by removing excess fat, tightening underlying muscles, and pulling up or redraping the skin of your face and neck.

b **Eyelift:** Are you unhappy with sagging skin around your eyes? An eyelift, or eyelid surgery, is known medically as blepharoplasty. It was designed to correct drooping upper lids and puffy bags below your eyes – glitches that can make you look older and more tired than you perhaps actually are. This is done by removing fat, excess skin, and muscle from the upper or lower eyelids. An eyelift can be done alone, or in conjunction with other facial surgery procedures.

c **Tummy tuck:** Abdominoplasty is major surgery designed to reduce a protruding abdomen by removing excess skin and fat from the middle and lower abdomen and tightening the muscles of the abdominal wall. However, it cannot always produce the results you hope for and you should be realistic in your expectations.

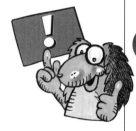

While before-and-after photographs can give you an idea of a surgeon's work, they can't show you how your surgery will turn out. That's because every individual responds differently to surgery.

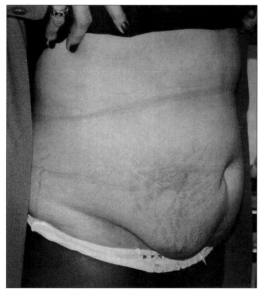

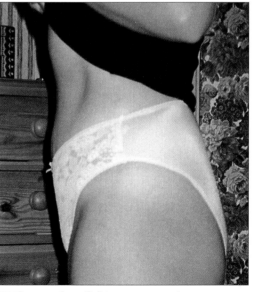

■ **A protruding stomach** *can cause you discomfort, and greatly reduce your self-esteem.*

■ **The results of this tummy tuck** *are exceptionally good: be realistic in your expectations.*

d **Breast lift:** If your breasts are average-sized or large, you may notice that they aren't as firm as they once were. That's because pregnancy, nursing, and the force of gravity cause breasts to sag. If this bothers you, a breast lift – known medically as mastopexy – can raise and reshape sagging breasts, as well as reduce the size of the areola, the darker skin surrounding the nipple. Breast lifts are often done in conjunction with breast implants or breast reduction.

Implants

There are several types of implants used in cosmetic surgery. Breast implants are perhaps the most commonly known, but there are others too:

a **Breast implants:** These are perhaps one of the most controversial surgeries today – they are used to make breasts look larger. The implants themselves are made of either a silicone gel or a saline gel. These implants are positioned behind the breast and are inserted through an incision made in the fold of the armpit, in the breast crease, or around the nipple.

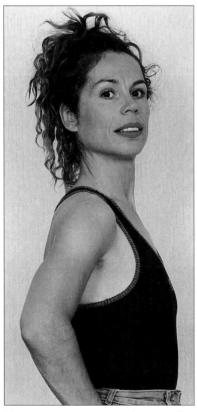

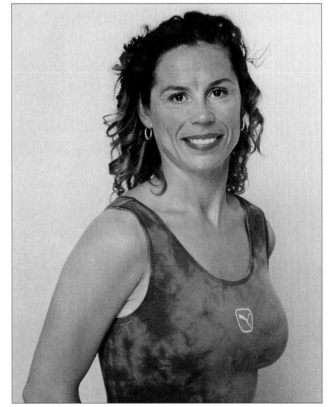

■ **Many women** *are not happy with the size and shape of their breasts.*

■ **Breast implants** *have dramatically altered this woman's upper-body shape and posture.*

b **Chin implants:** If you suffer from a weak chin, an implant – usually made of a hard, medical-grade silicone – can bring this area forward and give your face more definition. During the procedure, the surgeon places a small implant inside the mouth along the lower lip, or in the skin just under the chin.

c **Cheek implants:** If you were born without noticeable cheekbones, implants can provide the cheeky look you may crave and help improve the structure of your face. The procedure uses implants that are usually crafted of hard, medical-grade silicone. Typically, the surgeon inserts these implants through an incision in your lower eyelid or inside your upper lip.

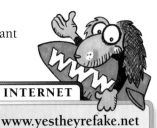

INTERNET

www.yestheyrefake.net

This pro-surgery site features in-depth and up-to-the-minute information on an enormous range of cosmetic procedures. There are also message boards to share your thoughts and experiences.

Filling indents and wrinkles

Dermatologists and cosmetic surgeons are able to inject or implant a variety of materials into the face to fill recessed areas such as acne scars, hollowed cheeks, wrinkles, and those deep lines that run between the nose and mouth, and mouth and chin. They can also add fullness to the lips. Popular plumpers include:

a **Collagen:** In Chapter 5, we talked about collagen, a temporary filler that can be used to fill indented scars and deep lines, and also to fatten lips. As you may recall from that chapter, collagen's effects are short-lived, lasting anywhere from 2 to 6 months.

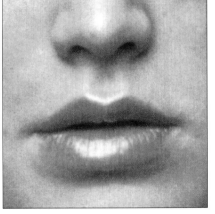

■ **If you have collagen** *injections to plump your lips, keep in mind that the effects are not permanent.*

If you are on blood-thinning medication, be sure to mention it to your plastic surgeon. Your doctor will have you stop the medication at least 2 weeks prior to surgery to prevent you from losing large quantities of blood during surgery. Be aware that garlic, vitamin E, and aspirin are also blood thinners, so if you've got a procedure planned, avoid these until after your operation.

b **Fat:** A small amount of your own fat can be harvested from an area of your thighs or buttocks, purified, then injected into deep lines, sunken depressions, or the lips. Fat lasts longer than collagen – often 6 months to a year – and does not cause the allergic reactions that collagen does in some people.

c **Fibril:** This is a gelatin compound that's mixed with your own blood and injected to plump up wrinkles and indented areas. The results typically last 3 to 6 months.

When it comes to post-surgery healing, every person is different. Although your physician will give you a general overview, don't be afraid to ask specific questions about how long you may need to heal. It's always best to plan ahead.

d **Gortex:** This is a permanent, threadlike material that is implanted beneath the skin to fill deep lines, depressions, and lips.

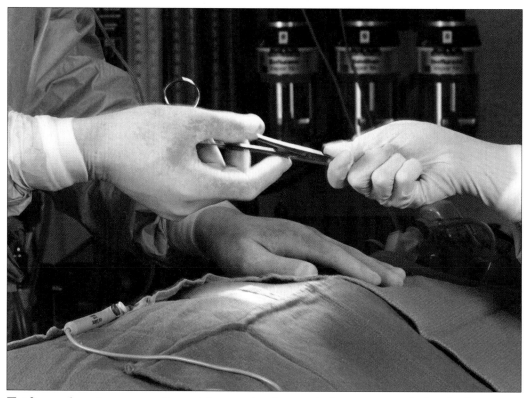

■ **After undergoing surgery,** *it may take some time for your body to recover – the length of time it takes depends on the procedure undergone, your age, and your general health.*

Liposuction

Liposuction, also known as lipoplasty or suction lipectomy, is the removal of fat from a specific area. It is performed with a small suction tube that is inserted just under the surface of the skin and used to literally vacuum fat away. However, don't expect the procedure to give you a perfect result. Liposuction is most often associated with the abdomen, hips, outer thighs, and inner thighs, but surgeons also use the procedure to reduce the appearance of double chins, jowly cheeks, and fatty upper arms, knees, and ankles.

Due to their tissue-healing powers, vitamin C, vitamin K, and bromelain (the enzyme found in pineapples) have been found in some studies to speed post-surgery healing. Talk to your doctor, however, before taking any supplements.

INTERNET

www.bodylanguage.net

The official web site for the British publication Body Language Magazine offers informative reports and features on the most up-to-date cosmetic surgery procedures available and casts an eye on cosmetic surgeons around the world.

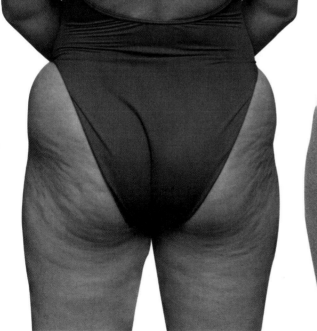

■ **As we grow older,** *we are generally prone to gain fat around our hips and buttocks.*

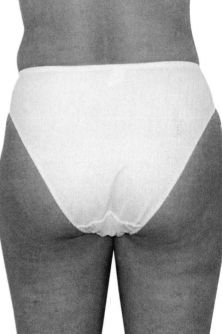

■ **Liposuction** *reduces areas of fat, although it cannot always produce such good results as this.*

Breast reductions

Some doctors are also experimenting with liposuction as a way to reduce breast size in women with very large, pendulous breasts. However, breast reduction surgery – medically known as mammaplasty – remains the most popular way to reduce breast size. The procedure removes fat, glandular tissue, and skin from the breasts, making them smaller, lighter, firmer, and more in proportion with the rest of the body. Breast reduction can also reduce the size of the areola.

Consult your doctor or cosmetic surgeon about the alternative breast reduction procedures open to you.

Nasal reshaping

Rhinoplasty is the medical name for a nose job, one of the most popular cosmetic procedures in the world. The procedure can change the shape of the tip or the bridge, reduce or increase the size of your nose, narrow the nostrils, or change the angle between your nose and lip.

> **DEFINITION**
>
> *The word* rhinoplasty *is derived from the Greek words for nose (rhino) and shape (plasty).*

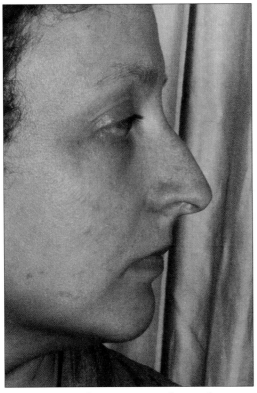

■ **The shape of a nose** *gives a distinct character and expression to a face.*

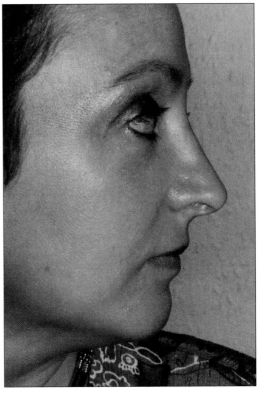

■ **With rhinoplasty surgery** *you can change the structure of your nose.*

Final thoughts

If you are seriously considering cosmetic surgery and have questioned yourself closely about your motives for considering it, it's always wise to gather as much knowledge and advice on the subject as possible.

There are a number of bodies and organizations that can offer you advice on different cosmetic procedures and after-surgery care, such as the American Society of Plastic Surgeons, and the Canadian Society of Plastic Surgeons.

Talk to your doctor for advice, and to decide whether you are a suitable candidate to undergo surgery. And remember, there is no need to rush into anything.

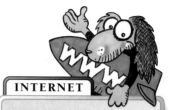

INTERNET

www.plasticsurgery.org

Run by the American Society of Plastic Surgeons, this site features in-depth information on a wide range of procedures, along with after-surgery care, complication possibilities, a physician's referral service, and more.

A simple summary

✔ The purpose of cosmetic surgery is to enhance your unique, natural beauty – not completely change your looks.

✔ Cosmetic surgery is about gently improving a feature you personally feel needs improvement, while carefully maintaining your face's or body's integrity.

✔ Don't rush into surgery. Instead, take time to ask yourself why you want surgery, and whether you are a suitable candidate.

✔ Interview several cosmetic surgeons before deciding on one – there is no need to rush.

✔ Ultimately you and your doctor are the only ones who can decide if cosmetic surgery is right for you.

✔ Today there are more cosmetic surgery procedures available than ever before.

✔ There are a number of organizations that can offer you advice on cosmetic surgery.

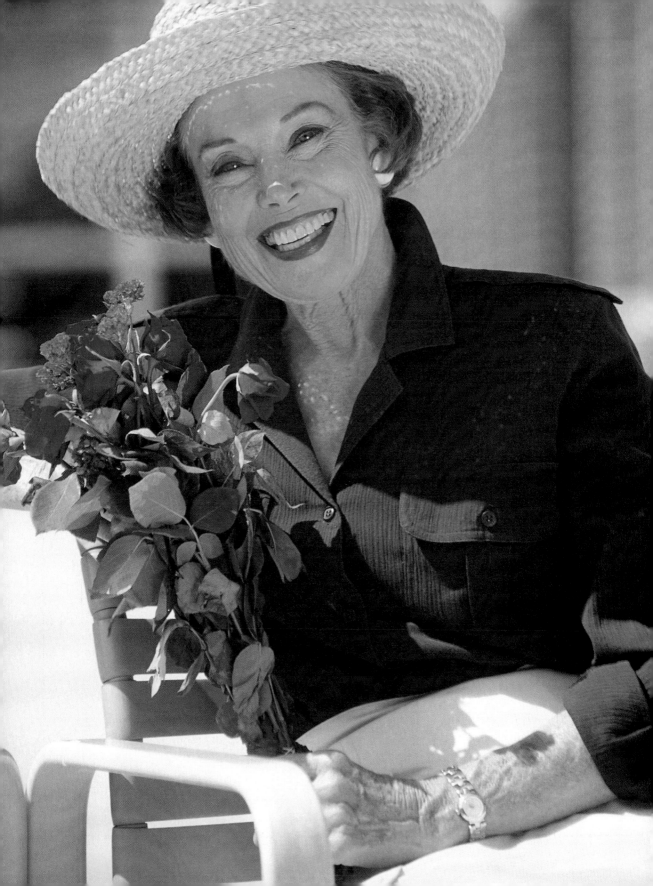

Chapter 18

Creating a Beautiful Life

LIVING BEAUTIFULLY has nothing to do with how your life looks and everything to do with how your life feels. What I mean is living vibrantly – which is another way of saying living with sound health and a vigorous spirit. After all, when health joins with spirit, the result is that irresistible kind of "there's something about her" quality that we've all seen and admired in women who are fit, smart, and excited by life. Beauty really is more than skin deep.

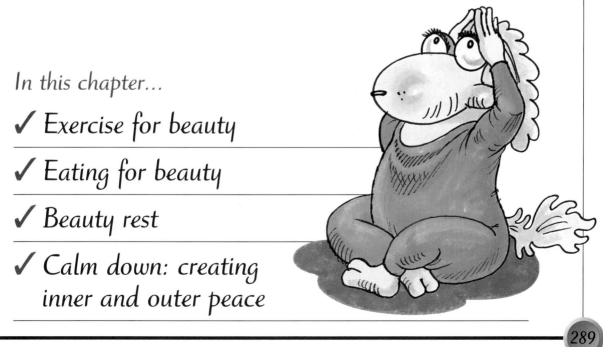

In this chapter...

✔ Exercise for beauty

✔ Eating for beauty

✔ Beauty rest

✔ Calm down: creating inner and outer peace

Exercise for beauty

ASK MEDICAL EXPERTS to name one stay-young beauty strategy and there's a good chance "exercise" will be the answer. And with good reason. Exercise, whether a gentle walk around the block or a full-tilt weight lifting session, strengthens the cardiovascular system, boosts circulation to the body and brain, revs up the metabolism, and burns calories. All of which give you vibrant skin, a toned body, graceful posture, and an attractive demeanor.

To be effective, exercise must be performed several times a week – a good workout won't work for you if you only get to the gym once or twice. In the recent past, experts claimed moderate *aerobic* exercise, when performed for 20 to 60 minutes, three times a week, was enough to maintain fitness. After further research, experts at the American Heart Association, the Surgeon General's office, and the Centers for Disease Control, now say aerobic exercise should be performed 5 to 7 days a week, along with at least two 30-minute strengthening workouts per week.

DEFINITION

Aerobic *is a Greek term meaning "with air" or "with oxygen." Any activity that uses large muscle groups, is maintained for 15 minutes or more, and is rhythmic in nature is considered aerobic.*

THE SECRET TO AGING GRACEFULLY

Think of the older adults you know. Among them there are probably sedentary types who are glued to the TV, and those whose lives are crammed full with volunteer work, errands, hobbies, and daily exercise. Regardless of their ages, I'll bet the go-getters are the most youthful looking.

There's a lesson here for all age groups: use it or lose it. The first "it" I'm talking about is your body; the second "it" is your health, your looks, your personality – in short, your vitality.

According to health research, inactivity makes your muscles atrophy, your bones frail and brittle, and your coordination and balance disappear. Other side effects include a dull complexion, slack skin, and more wrinkles. In the "beauty is as beauty does" department, lack of exercise affects your personality, making you prone to impatience, moodiness, confusion, forgetfulness, and irritability.

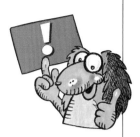

Exercise improves your complexion by boosting circulation and raising body temperature, both of which nudge blood to your skin's surface. This blood carries oxygen and nutrients that keep your skin healthy and glowing.

By slowing cell degeneration and collagen breakdown, exercise also helps slow signs of skin aging, such as slackness and wrinkles.

Exercising aerobically

Aerobic exercise, which includes dancing, jogging, and walking, should be the foundation of your beauty-health fitness plan. That's because aerobic exercise trains the heart, lungs, and cardiovascular system to process and deliver oxygen more quickly and efficiently to every part of the body, including those "appearance-enhancing" parts such as your skin, nails, and the roots of your hair. As the heart muscle becomes stronger and more efficient, a larger amount of blood can be pumped with each stroke. Fewer strokes are then required to rapidly transport nourishing oxygen through the body.

Wondering what type of aerobic exercise keeps you healthiest? Those that you like. When you enjoy an activity, you're more likely to get up off the couch, put on your workout clothes, and get moving. Ideally, you should aim for 5 aerobic workouts per week. A positive side effect of *weight-bearing* aerobic exercise is an increase in bone density, which keeps your bones strong.

DEFINITION

A weight-bearing exercise allows your body to come into direct, forceful contact with the ground. Swimming, for example, is a good form of aerobic exercise, but it is not weight-bearing. Running, jumping rope, and marching in place are weight-bearing exercises because the body is constantly striking the ground.

Wondering why weight-bearing exercise increases bone density? Every time your body impacts against the ground, your bones are gently stressed, which causes them to produce new cells to withstand the stress. It is these new cells that increase bones' density.

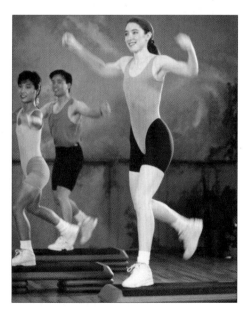

■ **Regular, weight-bearing aerobic** *exercise will strengthen bones and help reduce your chances of developing bone diseases such as osteoporosis.*

Strength training

Strength training – exercise such as weight lifting, push-ups, and pull-ups – is often an overlooked part of a beauty-health fitness plan. And that's too bad, because it's a great way to burn weight-making calories, keep your metabolism humming along at an efficient clip, give a pleasing firmness to arms, legs, tummies, and other muscles, and encourage good posture (slumping, slouching, and stooping can be the result of weak muscles). Furthermore, strength training helps maintain strong, dense bones, which, as already noted, is important if you want to avoid osteoporosis.

If it's been a while since you worked out, or if you are severely overweight, are pregnant, or if you have a medical condition, do not embark on any kind of fitness program without first contacting your doctor for guidelines.

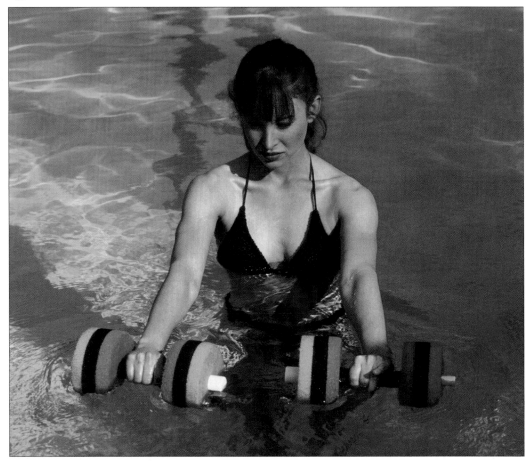

■ **Weight training doesn't have to be in a gym:** *Aqua-exercise classes allow you to take advantage of the resistance provided by water instead of using regular hand weights.*

Strength training helps you develop your muscles. The more developed your muscles, the easier it is for you to move heavy loads (this includes your body), whether they require carrying, pushing, pulling, or lifting. Strong muscles also allow you to participate in sports that require strength, and to physically withstand the rigors of day-to-day life. Aim to do two to four strength-training workouts per week, allowing at least a day between workouts to let your muscles rest. If you vary the types of workouts you do each time you go to the gym, you are more likely to stick with it. Doing the same routine each time can be boring and demotivating.

Trivia…

According to experts, many older people are 20 years older physically than they are chronologically. Inactivity is the main culprit, although diet and lack of mental stimulation are also factors.

Mind–body workouts

Mind–body workouts, as the name suggests, are workouts that exercise both your mind and your body. Tai chi, the various forms of yoga, and Pilates, are all examples of mind–body exercise that require you to train your thoughts on your breath, your posture, the individual moves you are making, and how your body feels as it makes each individual move. If you're jogging, stepping on a *Stairmaster®*, or cycling, you can simultaneously watch TV, listen to music, or think about a birthday gift for your mother. With a mind–body exercise, you must remain in the moment so you can focus on everything you are doing and feeling.

While mind–body workouts may sound mentally exhausting, they are actually soothing. When you've finished you will probably feel as refreshed and peaceful as you do after meditating; in a way, mind–body exercises are an active form of meditation. Mind–body workouts also help you develop an awareness of your body's signals and abilities.

■ **Meditation** *can have healing and calming effects on a stressed mind. For total relaxation, you must avoid all other mental stimulants and make time to empty your mind of all the mental clutter of your daily life.*

Flexibility work

You know the languid, willowy gait that dancers and yoga teachers have? The gait that prompts all heads to turn as one of these lithe creatures enters a room? That kind of physical presence comes with flexibility work. This form of exercise encompasses any movement that stretches muscles, such as yoga. Muscles act like springs. If a muscle is short and tight, it loses the ability to absorb shock, so there is more strain on the joints. Stretching, in fact, is essential for healthy joints – and healthy joints are essential for a youthful body that is free from a bowed, bent posture, or stiff movements.

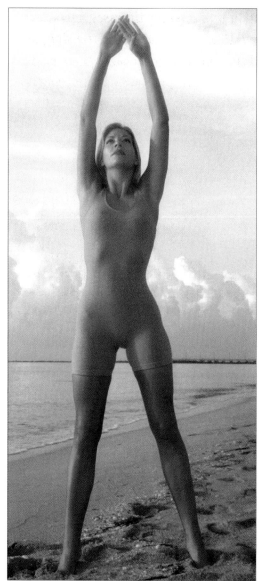

Stretching also helps to lengthen muscles, giving you more flexibility. Because we often lose our regular range of motion with age, stretching is especially important as we get older to help prevent sprains, strains, and falls – as well as to sustain a youthful-looking carriage. An easy way to incorporate flexibility work into your life is to perform 15 minutes worth of simple stretches before aerobic and strength-training workouts. Examples include bending at the waist and touching your toes, sitting with legs outstretched in front of you, and rolling your neck.

If you have trouble climbing out of a car or twisting to put on a coat, your joints are not flexible and the range of motion in your hips, neck, shoulders, and spine may be limited.

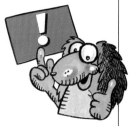

■ **Incorporate simple stretching** *into your daily routine. Reach up to the sky, taking a deep breath in. Relax your arms down and exhale slowly. Repeat as necessary.*

Eating for beauty

IT'S OFTEN SAID THAT GOOD HEALTH is the foundation of beauty. I'm willing to take that statement a step farther and claim that a balanced diet is the foundation of good health – and, therefore, beauty. For proof, just read the numerous medical studies that link healthy eating with disease prevention and disease reversal. These same studies connect high fat intake, high sodium consumption, and diets with too much protein to numerous illnesses, including obesity, cancer, cardiovascular diseases, diverticular diseases, hypertension, and kidney disease. And of course, there are all the looks-stealing side effects of a poor diet, such as thinning hair, scaly skin, breakouts, pale complexion, nail disorders, and excess weight. A nutrient-weak diet can also exacerbate existing skin conditions such as psoriasis and rosacea.

There are all kinds of health reasons to curb your salt intake to the recommended limit of 500 mg per day. For those prone to breakouts, iodine – a mineral found in iodized salt and seafood – is believed by many professionals to contribute to acne flare-ups.

But what exactly is a balanced diet? Generally speaking, it is a diet comprising carbohydrates, dietary fiber, fat, protein, water, 13 vitamins, and 20 minerals. More specifically, it is a diet built around a wide variety of fruits, legumes, whole grains, and vegetables. Animal protein, high-fat foods, high-sodium foods, highly sugared foods, sodas, and processed foods are consumed sparingly, if at all. Of course, there are several ways to get your daily allotment of nutrients. Here are several of the most common diets.

All about omnivores

How healthy is an omnivorous diet? It depends. Omnivores may eat cheese, eggs, meat, poultry, fish, or seafood every day, choose refined snacks, and get only one daily serving of fruits and vegetables. This is not the healthiest option for those on an omnivorous diet.

■ **An omnivorous diet** *includes plant-based foods, dairy products, eggs, fish, seafood, red meat, organ meats, and poultry.*

295

On the other hand, those omnivores who limit animal-based foods to two or three times a week, choose water over soft drinks, and get the recommended five or more daily servings of fruits and vegetables have a much healthier diet. The usual complaints about traditional omnivorous diets revolve around the diet's high levels of cholesterol and saturated fat (found in animal-based foods), which can increase the risk of cancer, diabetes, heart disease, and obesity. However, an omnivorous diet can actually be a healthy one, provided that thoughtful choices are made. To keep cholesterol and saturated fat to a minimum and nutrients to a maximum, omnivores should aim to eat five or more daily servings of fruits and vegetables, choose whole grains over refined grains, enjoy daily legume or soy food protein sources, and limit their consumption of animal-based foods.

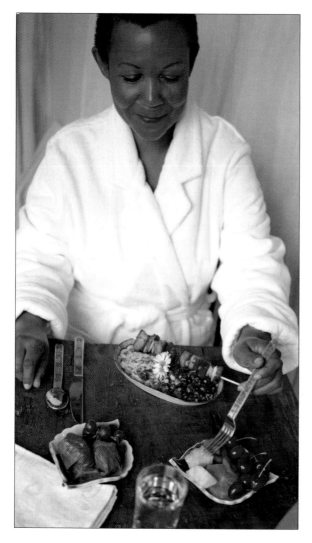

Macrobiotic eating

A macrobiotic diet includes plant-based foods, limited amounts of white-fleshed fish, limited amounts of fruit, and very limited amounts of salt. Dairy products, eggs, foods with artificial ingredients, hot spices, mass-produced foods, meat, vegetables from the nightshade family (such as peppers, potatoes, and eggplant), poultry, some fish, shellfish, warm drinks, and refined foods are not consumed.

Macrobiotics is based on a system created in the early 1900s by Japanese philosopher George Ohsawa. The diet consists of 50 percent whole grains, 20 to 30 percent vegetables, and 5 to 10 percent legumes, sea vegetables, and soy foods. The small remainder of the diet is composed of white-fleshed fish, fruits, and nuts. The diet's low amounts of saturated fat, absence of processed foods, and emphasis on high-fiber foods, such as whole grains and vegetables, may

■ **Macrobiotic** *foods are mostly grain- and vegetable-based, but include a small amount of fish and fruits.*

promote cardiovascular health. Because soy and sea vegetables contain cancer-fighting compounds, a macrobiotic diet is often recommended to help treat cancer. However, critics worry that the diet's limited variety of food can leave followers lacking in certain vitamins and important cancer-fighting and immune system-boosting *phytonutrients*.

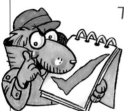

The more varied your diet, the less chance you'll have of missing out on important nutrients. That's why the Japanese government urges its citizens to eat 30 or more different kinds of food each day. To sneak more diversity into your diet, consider using your snack time as a chance to sample new, nutritious foods.

Piscatorial diets

This diet includes plant-based foods, dairy products, eggs, fish, and seafood. Red meats, organ meats, poultry, and foods made from these are not eaten. Like an omnivorous diet, a piscatorial diet is as healthy as a person makes it. Individuals who eat high-fat and highly processed foods, fail to get the recommended daily number of vegetables and fruits, and eschew whole grains for processed grains will not enjoy optimum health. That said, individuals who are conscientious about eating a balanced, varied diet and who limit fish and seafood intake to two or three times per week, can expect a lower risk of heart disease. Be aware, however, that oily saltwater fish, such as shark, swordfish, and tuna, have been found to carry mercury in their tissues; many health authorities recommend eating these varieties no more than once a week and avoiding them altogether if you are trying to get or are already pregnant, are lactating, or have a weak immune system.

Going vegetarian

A vegetarian diet includes plant-based foods, dairy products, and eggs. Fish, gelatin, seafood, red meats, organ meats, and poultry are not eaten. Vegetarians should concentrate on a wide variety of whole foods, including beans, fruits, grains, low-fat dairy products, sea vegetables, nuts, soy foods, and vegetables. A varied diet insures enough protein, calcium, and other nutrients for all vegetarians, including children, pregnant women, and the elderly. A well-chosen vegetarian eating plan has been shown to lower blood pressure, decrease the risk of breast cancer, and prevent heart disease. In addition, the diet's high fiber level cuts the risk of diverticular disease and colon cancer.

The vegan way

A vegan eats only plant-based foods. This means that dairy products, eggs, fish, seafood, red meats, organ meats, poultry, and novelty meats are avoided. Foods made by animals or processed with animal parts, such as gelatin and honey, are not consumed.

A vegan (pronounced VEE-gun) diet can be extremely healthy. Like the vegetarian diet, a vegan diet has been shown to lower blood pressure and prevent heart disease. In addition, the high fiber intake cuts the risk of diverticular disease and colon cancer. Some vegans may need to supplement their diets with vitamins.

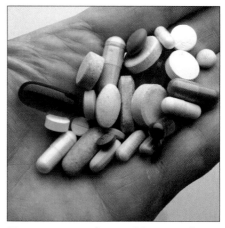

■ **Vegans** must be *careful to eat either plant foods with vitamin B12 and vitamin D, or to take supplements of these nutrients.*

FAT FACTS

We are so scared of fat these days that you may not realize that you need some fat in your diet. Fat helps the body assimilate skin-friendly, fat-soluble vitamins, such as vitamins A and E, and it is also needed to keep skin plump and resilient. However, when I say fat, I'm not referring to the saturated fat you find in animal products, nor the cheap hydrogenated oils found in mass-produced snack food. I'm talking about the healthy fats – which promote cell growth and assist in specific bodily functions. These are called essential fatty acids, which come in three "families":

1. **Omega-3 fatty acids:** These help in cell formation, assist in nervous system development and visual function, and contribute to the creation of hormone-like substances called prostaglandins. They are found in hemp seeds, pumpkin seeds, almonds, walnuts, dark green leafy vegetables, deep-water fish, flaxseed and flaxseed oil, sea vegetables, evening primrose oil, borage oil, and blackcurrant oil.

2. **Omega-6 fatty acids:** These help maintain healthy skin and hair. They are found in corn, soybean and other vegetable oils, seeds, seed oils, and milk.

3. **Omega-9 fatty acid:** This is a relatively new discovery. Studies indicate that it is a cancer-fighting agent. The best source of it is olive oil.

CLEAN LIVING

Exercise, diet, hair care, skin care, good sleep, stress-reducing measures – these are all essential to inner and outer beauty, not to mention overall well-being. But these aren't the only elements that make up a beautiful life. Clean living and compassion are also important. Here are some examples:

a **Go organic:** When you purchase organic produce and prepared convenience foods made with organic ingredients, you're getting food that was grown without synthetic fertilizers, fungicides, or pesticides. Not only is this important for your own health – many of these substances have been linked to skin, hair, and nail conditions, allergies, cancer, and lung conditions – but it's important for the environment. Many fertilizers, fungicides, and pesticides kill beneficial (not to mention beautiful) animals, such as ants, butterflies, and frogs, as well as causing air pollution and contributing to the Greenhouse Effect. Pesticides run off into wells, streams, and rivers. In fact, according to the Environmental Protection Agency, 40 percent of America's rivers, streams, and lakes are not fit for fishing or swimming due to runoff of agricultural chemicals.

b **Limit your exposure to chemicals:** It's nearly impossible to avoid all chemical toxins in today's world. There's ammonia in cleaning products, chlorine in the water, lead in old paint and pipes, dibromochloropropane in pesticides, carbon monoxide from auto exhaust, and toluene, trichloroethylene, and formaldehyde from printers, photocopiers, and fax machines. Many of these toxins have been linked to skin eruptions, watery eyes, thinning hair, nail conditions, allergies, breathing problems, cancer, headaches, infertility, lethargy, lung conditions, reduced attention span, and even violence. You can try to reduce your exposure to toxins by using environmentally-sound dry-cleaning, drinking filtered water, purchasing (or making) natural cleansers, limiting the amount of driving you do, and adding a few chemical-filtering plants – such as dracaena, florist's mum, and Kimberly queen – to your home.

c **Quit the junk:** Cigarettes, cigars, junk food, recreational drugs, too much alcohol – these all rob the body of nutrients and lower immunity. Enjoyed occasionally, some things, such as a cookie or glass of wine, have little effect on health. Others, like cigarettes or recreational drugs, cause disease and can make you dangerous to others. If you can't quit drinking, drugging, or smoking on your own, find a counselor or join a support group.

Beauty rest

BEAUTY NEEDS SLEEP. You may recall from Chapter 2 that sleep is the time when all your body's cells renew themselves and repair damage from environmental sources and toxins. Sleep is essential for overall health, muscle tone, efficient fat-burning, and radiant skin. It is also necessary for clear thinking, physical stamina, good posture (who among us doesn't slouch when we're tired?) and a pleasant mood – four often overlooked aspects of beauty.

Having problems sleeping?

If you're like most people, you've experienced one of the following: you crawl under the covers at 11 p.m. and lie there, eyes open, until 2 a.m. or 3 a.m. or 4 a.m; you wake up at some ridiculous predawn hour and never fall back to sleep; instead of deeply slumbering, you toss and turn all night and awake the following morning feeling tired and irritable; you repeatedly wake, then return to sleep throughout the night.

The side effects of sleeplessness are not pretty: studies have found that long-term insomniacs have 2½ times more car accidents than those who sleep well. Insomniacs also demonstrate reduced productivity, impaired memory and concentration, and get sick more often due to lowered immune-system function.

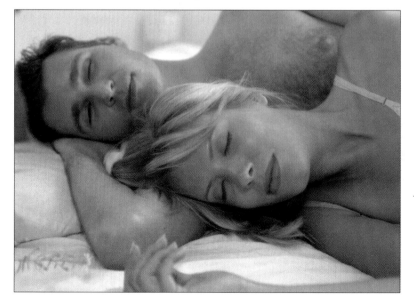

■ **Sleep is vital**
for your body to regenerate its cells and for your mind to recharge its batteries. Interrupted sleep can rob you of your feeling of well-being.

Dealing with sleeplessness

If you're like many people, you've also experienced any one or more of these just-described symptoms for more than several nights running. If so, you probably had (or have) insomnia, the medical name for inadequate sleep that occurs for at least one week.

Among the causes are a noisy environment, high caffeine or alcohol intake, recreation or prescription drug use, an existing illness, stress, a fidgety bed partner, or something else altogether. Yet, regardless of what causes insomnia, the results are the same: daytime tiredness, slowed thinking, slowed movements, moodiness, complexion changes (some people start breaking out, some look pale, others experience dry skin), and a haggard appearance. Fortunately, the occasional sleepless night and full-blown insomnia can be either prevented or banished with good *sleep hygiene*. If you're having difficulty sleeping, take note of some of these simple rules.

> **DEFINITION**
>
> *One definition for the word hygiene is "conditions or practices conducive to health." Sleep hygiene is a popular term among doctors and sleep researchers; it refers to environments and habits that help you sleep well.*

Dim the lights and draw the blinds

Many sleep experts believe exposure to bright light, either before bedtime or after retiring can hamper sleep. How? By tricking your body's internal time clock into thinking it is earlier in the day.

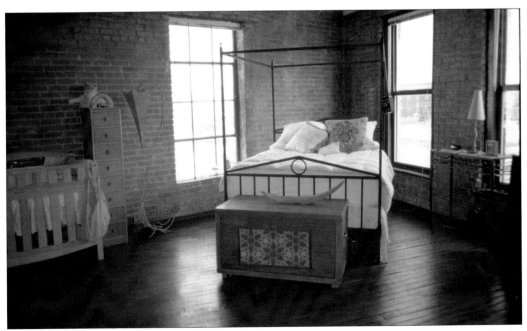

■ **A bright, airy bedroom** *won't help you if you have problems sleeping. Try installing black-out blinds behind your drapes to prevent the light from filtering through and waking you in the early hours.*

The pre-bed countdown

This is vital to a sleep pattern. Have you ever noticed that whenever you pick up a can opener, your cat comes running? Or that you can't pick up that old tennis ball without your puppy assuming it's time to play catch? As the cause-and-effect creatures we are, living things love a routine. That's why your body comes to view things like face-washing, teeth-brushing, and pajama-donning, as signals that mean sleep is near. Make a routine of these pre-bedtime chores and your body will react by slowing down and growing sleepy.

■ **Make a habit** *of brushing your teeth just before bedtime.*

Keep regular hours

Your body functions best on a schedule. Help your body maintain a healthy *circadian rhythm* by retiring at the same time each night and rising at the same time each morning – yes, this includes weekend nights and mornings, too.

> **DEFINITION**
>
> Circadian rhythm *is a kind of synonym for our bodies' internal clock; both terms refer to the internal timekeeper that governs our patterns of sleep and wakefulness.*

Exercise the right way

Daily exercise keeps your body running efficiently, and this helps promote regular sleep. However, vigorous physical activity energizes the body, making sleep difficult, so experts recommend that you exercise at least 4 hours before bedtime.

Avoid eating heavily before bed

While your first impulse upon finishing a big meal may be to nod off, the sleep won't last. That's because your bodily systems – such as metabolism, heart rate, and breathing – must begin speeding up to digest all that food sitting in your stomach. As soon as they start revving up, you're going to wake up.

INTERNET

www.holisticonline
.com

At this far-reaching site, you can find articles on everything from skin care, insomnia, body image, stress reduction, and more – all with a friendly holistic, New Age bent.

An empty stomach is detrimental to good sleep. Why? Your growling stomach may disturb you, and perhaps even your bed partner.

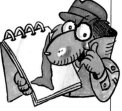

Limit your caffeine intake.

Because caffeine is a stimulant, it can upset your body's natural time clock. For that reason, don't consume caffeine after 2 or 3 p.m.

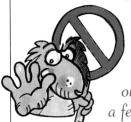

Be aware of hidden caffeine in cola and non-cola soft drinks, coffee-flavored ice cream, yogurt, and chocolate.

Avoid too much alcohol

Yes, a third glass of wine makes you want to fall asleep, but after spending 3 to 5 hours in your system, alcohol turns into a kind of stimulant that disrupts your body's deep sleep. And because it is dehydrating, this can also disturb your sleep.

Try a small portion of tryptophan

Tryptophan is an amino acid that helps the body produce the sleep hormones serotonin and melatonin. Bananas, milk, peanut butter, whole grains, and turkey all contain tryptophan. Take advantage of these natural sedative powers and eat a small amount of one or more of these foods an hour or two before bedtime.

> ## Trivia...
> *Most individuals spend one-third of their life sleeping.*

Get herbal help

Valerian root, kava, passionflower, chamomile, catnip, verbena, and skullcap all have tension-relieving and sedative powers. Try an herbal infusion brewed with one of these herbs.

If you're one of those small-bladdered types (no judgments here, I'm one too), avoid herbal teas or other drinks just before bedtime. After all, what's the good of being knocked out if you're going to be roused by a full bladder a few hours later?

Scented sleep

Essential oils have long been used by aromatherapists as natural sedatives. My personal favorite is lavender oil, which I sprinkle on my sheets and which never fails to knock me out. Other oils to try include chamomile and sandalwood. Try scenting your bedroom with oils, or try making yourself a scented sleep pillow like the ones you see in aromatherapy and gift boutiques, by stuffing a small pillow with a blend of relaxing dried hops, chamomile, and lavender.

■ **Aromatherapy oils,** *such as lavender, can be sprinkled on sheets or used in oil burners to scent your bedroom.*

Bath therapy

Warm water has a soothing effect on your body and mind. It can ease stress and lower the body's temperature, which in turn induces sleepiness. Avoid hot water (which can speed heart rate and respiration, as well as cause sweating) and time your bath to within an hour of bedtime. Throw chamomile tea bags into the water or add a few drops of relaxing lavender.

Trade mass media for a book

Instead of watching heart-pumping TV shows, listening to the radio, or reading newspapers and news magazines, opt for a relaxing book before bedtime. Violence, stimulating music, disturbing news – all these signal the body to produce adrenaline and won't help you get to sleep.

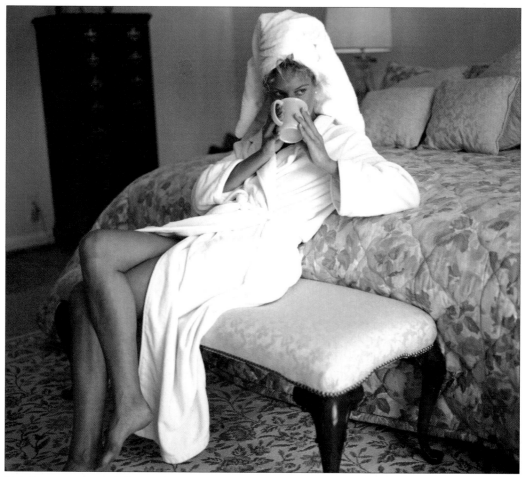

■ **Take time to wind down** *after your bath. Quietly relax and try to empty your mind of all the day's stressful thoughts. This will help prepare your mind and body for sleep.*

Don't just lie there!

If you find yourself wide awake, get up, go to another room, turn on a dim light, and read until you feel ready to fall asleep. According to sleep researchers, remaining wide awake in bed "trains" your body to associate your bed with wakefulness – not something you want to do.

According to a survey conducted by the National Sleep Foundation, the average American woman sleeps only 6 hours and 41 minutes per weeknight. The reasons for this? Small bladders, headaches, hormonal upsets due to menstruation, pregnancy, lactation, and menopause, as well as snoring or cover-hogging partners, and disruptions from children are all cited.

Trivia...

Some historians, anthropologists, and sleep researchers believe early humans did not get all their sleep in one stretch, but in two segments. It is theorized that our ancestors retired at dusk, slept 4 or 5 hours, spent a few hours awake doing quiet activities, then returned to sleep until dawn. As proof, experts point to writings by Virgil and Homer, which referred to "first sleep" and "second sleep."

HOW WE SLEEP

As the sun begins to set and the sky grows dark, a small gland in your brain called the pineal gland secretes melatonin, a hormone that prompts you to grow sleepy. As melatonin courses through the body, your breathing and heart rate slow, your muscles relax, and your body temperature slightly drops. The rapid beta waves that characterize your daytime brain activity shift into slower alpha waves. At this point, you may appear to be sleeping, but you are so aware of your surroundings, you may actually feel awake. Soon, the alpha waves are replaced by theta waves, which signal the onset of relatively deep sleep. Sleep researchers often call this theta-controlled sleep, or stage one sleep.

As the night progresses, your body and brain pass back and forth through different stages of sleep – all with varying degrees of deepness and all lasting anywhere from 5 minutes to an hour. Punctuating these stages are periods – usually two to four – of dream sleep, where your eyes move rapidly behind your shut lids. As morning nears, your brain waves move more quickly, your breathing and heart rate increase slightly, and your body temperature gradually increases. You slowly grow more alert until you are no longer sleeping at all, but lying in bed, half-awake with your eyes half-open, then open.

Calm down: creating inner and outer peace

RUSH-HOUR TRAFFIC, *bathing-suit season, a drill-sergeant boss, whining children, 5 minutes to find your already-boarding plane – regardless of the cause, stress does a number on your emotional and physical well-being. Common stress symptoms include sleeplessness, fuzzy thinking, pessimism, frazzled skin, body aches, an upset stomach, and much, much more.*

When you're feeling pressured, your personality and even your outward appearance may turn less than pretty: you don't feel like being generous with a co-worker, you may snap at a stranger who cuts you off in a supermarket aisle. Furthermore, you can't muster the enthusiasm to stand up straight, work out, get that haircut you had scheduled, or notice a cherry tree in blossom, a child's toothless smile, or your own inner gorgeousness.

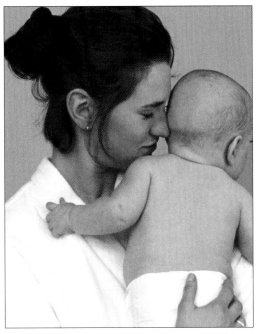

■ **Becoming a mother** *can be a very stressful time of your life, often compounded by sleeplessness.*

Stress's inner workings

When stressed, your body's 650 muscles tense, readying themselves for action. Your endocrine glands pump out adrenaline, cortisol, and other hormones. These in turn elevate blood pressure, quicken both breathing and heart rate, and release energy-giving sugar and fats into the bloodstream. Combined, all this activity is called the fight-or-flight response, or stress response, and it prepares your body for a momentary emergency. So, yes, your body's stress response is beneficial in times of trouble.

Stress is your body's reaction to anything your brain finds upsetting.

Effects of stress

It's when tension becomes long term – as it has for so many of us – that your mood, your body, and your beauty – suffers. The following conditions are common beauty-leaching reactions to stress. Fortunately, most disappear once you stop feeling frantic.

a **Spots and breakouts:** The stress response hormone, cortisol, causes the body to secrete extra androgen, a sex hormone that increases sebum production. This excess sebum clogs pores and leads to blackheads and whiteheads.

b **Pale complexion:** Have you ever looked in the mirror one morning during a particularly hellish week at work and wondered why you look so washed out? Blame it on a decrease in blood flow to the skin, because blood is what gives skin its rosy glow. A stressed body prioritizes its blood flow, sending the majority of blood to vital organs like the brain, heart, and lungs and, therefore, away from the skin.

Trivia...

Between 60 percent and 90 percent of all medical office visits in the United States are for stress-related disorders.

Stress is not a disease. It can, however, lead to numerous ailments and aggravate any existing health conditions.

c **Scaly skin:** The diminished blood supply that makes skin pale can also cause flakiness. That's because without a rich supply of blood, the skin's cells renew themselves more slowly. Keep in mind that when you're under stress, your skin may simultaneously break out, look pale, and display flaky patches.

d **Itchy bumps:** When your body is stressed, it often releases *histamines*, which in turn can create itching, inflammation, rashes, and hives in those of us who are prone to those kinds of things.

DEFINITION

Histamines *are chemicals present in your body's tissues. When released, histamines create an allergic reaction, which just happens to be your body's way of trying to scare off a perceived invader.*

If you tend to pick at your skin when you are under stress (don't be ashamed – lots of us do that), don't spend time standing in front of mirrors. You'll only end up staring at your face, searching for pimples to squeeze. This leads to infected cyst-like pimples and scars.

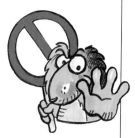

(e) **Body aches:** When tension persists, the primed muscles (remember the fight-or-flight response?) remain rigid and inflexible. Blood flow diminishes, starving the muscles' fibers of oxygen and causing them to shorten. The result: sore shoulders, stiff neck, tight jaw, and/or knotted back, plus enough discomfort to make life miserable. This can really have an affect on your posture and bearing.

Most heart attacks occur on Monday mornings. Why? Experts believe it's the stress of having to return to a pressure-filled job. Now what more motivation do you need to find work you love?

(f) **Tummy troubles:** You remember those nervous stomach aches you got as a kid before your first day of school – or you still get when faced with a week of insane work deadlines or some unpleasant relationship or family issue? When stress strikes, the brain douses the gastrointestinal tract with neurotransmitters and hormones. The gastrointestinal (GI) tract, in turn, responds in several ways – by going into spasms, slowing down or speeding up, or secreting more acids. The not-so-lovely result of all this is a churning stomach, waves of nausea, or an irascible bowel.

■ **Tension in the neck** *and upper body causes pain and discomfort and can lead to severe headaches.*

(g) **Headaches:** Clenched muscles in the neck, face, and scalp can lead to tension headaches. Also known as muscle-contraction headaches, these range from mildly irksome to severely painful. They feel like pressure, often described as a "vice grip," is being applied to the head or neck. For some people, the pain is so bad that shampooing, brushing, and styling hair is painful.

Trivia...
One study found that chronic worriers reduced their anxiety levels by reserving a half-hour each day to use solely for worrying.

Stress depletes the body of B-vitamins, especially vitamin B6. If you're undergoing a prolonged period of stress, consult your health-care provider about taking a vitamin B-complex supplement.

Feeling less frantic

The best way to deal with stress is to eliminate the cause. Easier said than done – after all, you can't get rid of your kids, your job, your mother-in-law, your thighs, or any of the other irritations that make you tense. The second best way to deal with stress is to minimize a stressor's power to aggravate you by learning how to deal with it in a relaxed, healthy manner. There are several ways you can do this.

Build a strong support system

Several studies have found that individuals with a tightly woven network of supportive family and friends are less bothered by stress and have lower instances of depression, eating-related disorders, body-image disorders, and common infectious illnesses.

Enjoy yourself

It's important to put aside time each week for doing what pleases you – be it a candlelit dinner, playing the trombone, or window shopping with friends. Spending time on yourself not only makes you happy, it can reduce stress – both of which will give you inner radiance.

Watch what you say to yourself

If you're aiming for a relaxing life, watch what you say to yourself. You can make a stressful situation worse by describing yourself as stupid, ugly, slow, or untalented. Negative self-talk does nothing to resolve the pressure you're feeling, and makes you feel worse and in less control of yourself – all of which will increase your tension.

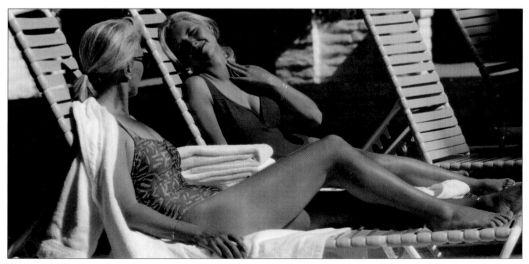

■ **In order to reduce your stress levels,** *it's important to be able to enjoy yourself. And if you are suffering from stress, confiding in friends or family can help you get a perspective on a problem.*

Adopt a pet

Numerous studies have shown that pet owners not only have lower stress levels, but experience fewer bouts of anxiety and depression. Before you start looking at puppies (or kittens or whatever), be aware that there is a staggering number of unwanted cats, dogs, and other animals, in the United States. Hundreds of thousands of these animals, abandoned by owners, are put to sleep in overcrowded shelters each day. Thus, if you are not an animal lover – or if you feel you cannot adequately care for a pet – do not even consider bringing an animal into your life. For those who can't keep a pet, volunteering for a local no-kill animal adoption organization – which are appearing all over – can serve a similar purpose.

Next time you're feeling stressed, think of the color pink. Pink has been found to ease tension by relaxing the muscles and soothing violent or aggressive tendencies.

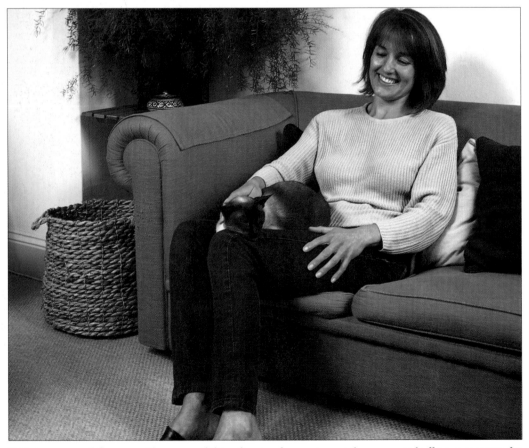

■ **Pets are good for you:** *The responsibility of caring for a pet can take your mind off your anxieties for a while. Relaxing at home with your pet is also proven to be a great tension reliever.*

MASSAGE MELTS STRESS

Massage is a terrific way to create a feeling of calm. It has a sedative effect upon the nervous system, promotes voluntary muscle relaxation, can relieve muscle pain, and helps increase blood circulation. Next time you're feeling frazzled, why not make an appointment with a licensed massage practitioner for one of the following types of massage:

 Craniosacral therapy: Through gentle manipulation of the bones of the skull and neck, this massage promotes relaxation and is used to treat conditions such as headaches.

Reflexology: This is more than a very relaxing foot rub! The method is based on the belief that internal organs and glands, as well as the body's muscles, can be treated by stimulating specific points of the feet and hands.

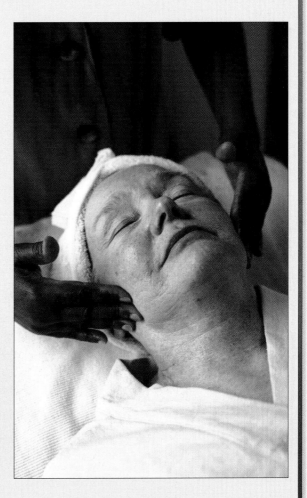

Shiatsu: Meaning "finger work" in Japanese, this technique uses a sequence of rhythmic pressure at specific body points.

Swedish massage: This technique uses stroking and kneading movements and is the method most of us are familiar with.

■ **Facial treatments** *are just as relaxing as body treatments, and help eliminate tension in the temples and jaw.*

Breathe deeply

A good way to reduce stress and relax is to breathe deeply. Deep breathing pulls your attention away from a given stressor and refocuses it on your breath. This type of breathing is not only comforting (thanks to its rhythmic quality), but it has also been shown to lower rapid pulse and shallow respiration – two temporary symptoms of stress. Whenever you're faced with an aggravating situation – or whenever you want to feel calmer – inhale deeply through your nose. Hold your breath for up to 3 seconds, then exhale through your mouth. Continue as needed.

If the stress in your life seems just too much for you to handle – even with these stress diminishing tips – consider seeking help from a professional therapist.

Try aromatherapy

Sedative essential oils such as lavender are heavily prescribed by aromatherapists to help lower stress levels and make you feel calm. Get your aromatherapy fix with a portable inhaler (available at aromatherapy boutiques and some natural food stores), use a scented candle, try an aromatherapy infuser, or mist the room with a spray.

BREATHING EXERCISES

If you are susceptible to shallow or rapid breathing when you're stressed, you may get some benefit from developing your own breathing routine. This can help you deal with stressful situations, and can also help some people who are prone to panicky feelings – often the symptom of an underlying anxiety. Take a few minutes out each day to practice these breathing exercises until they become part of your routine.

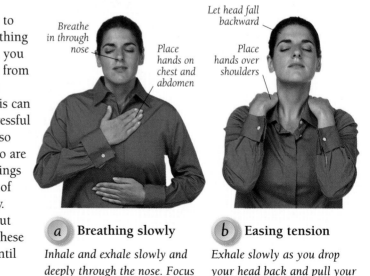

Breathe in through nose

Place hands on chest and abdomen

Let head fall backward

Place hands over shoulders

a **Breathing slowly**

Inhale and exhale slowly and deeply through the nose. Focus on the rhythm of your breath.

b **Easing tension**

Exhale slowly as you drop your head back and pull your shoulders gently forwards.

Try the relaxation response

Many experts recommend regular use of progressive muscle relaxation as a way to help reduce stress. Lie comfortably on the bed or floor, palms facing upward. Close your eyes and visualize a ray of light entering your head. As it fills your skull, feel the light warming your eyes, your face, your jaw. Then notice the light moving down and gradually filling your whole body with its warmth. Allow this same feeling to encompass the rest of your body, literally "melting" into the surface you're lying on.

This is a form of meditation that was created by Harvard University physician and researcher, Herbert Benson, M.D. Benson's research found that the relaxation response creates a physical state of deep rest that changes the physical and emotional responses to stress (e.g., decrease in heart rate, blood pressure, and muscle tension). To try a simple version of the relaxation response, repeat a sound or a one-syllable word (such as one, om, God, oh). If other thoughts creep into your head, passively ignore them and continue to repeat your sound or word. Continue for up to 20 minutes. Repeat several times a day or as needed.

Joining a local relaxation class is a great way to learn about the basic techniques of breathing and calming your mind and body.

A simple summary

✓ Fitness is essential to a healthy, strong, gorgeous body.

✓ Flexibility is an important characteristic of a youthful-acting body.

✓ Diet goes beyond keeping a fit figure – it's essential to all aspects of beauty.

✓ Without rest, your cells don't renew themselves.

✓ Sleeplessness affects many people at some time in their lives and can destroy a sense of well-being.

✓ Calm is beautiful, kindness is beautiful, and you are beautiful.

✓ Stress ruins your health, your personality, and your looks.

✓ You can't get rid of what's stressing you? Then learn how to stay calm!

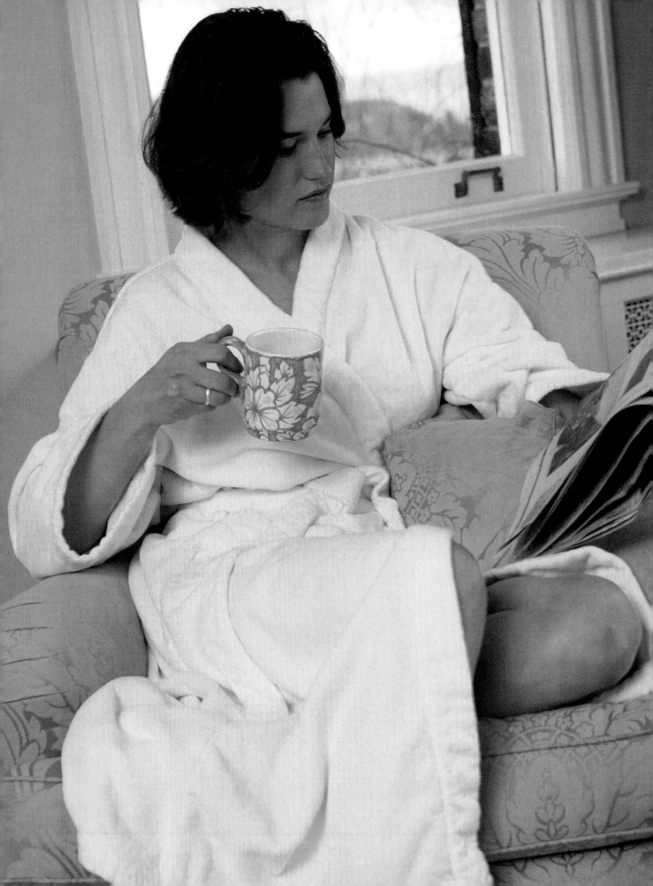

Chapter 19

Bringing It All Home

YOU'RE BUSY. YOU'VE GOT WORK TO DO, kids to raise, classes to attend, a gym to get to, a dog to walk, dinner to fix, a floor to vacuum. With so much to do it's easy to ignore your own needs. Yet if you neglect yourself long enough, you risk growing cranky, feeling rundown, and looking haggard. Obviously, none of these are good things. Avoid becoming bedraggled, and give yourself a weekly pampering. You don't need a lot of time and money to coddle yourself with a do-it-yourself spa ritual. The only essentials are a bathroom, a quiet hour or two, and a few ingredients. Go ahead, indulge a little!

In this chapter...

✓ Creating an at-home spa ritual

✓ All about massage

✓ Last words

TAKE THE TIME TO RELAX AND HAVE SOME QUALITY TIME TO YOURSELF

Creating an at-home spa ritual

BATHS HAVE EXISTED in one form or
another since the beginning of time. The pre- and
post-biblical Greeks, Turks, and Romans loved their
spas. Today's French use the same ocean-water
therapy centers as their ancestors, and 21st century
Californians enjoy Calistoga mud treatments.

DEFINITION

The word spa, which entered
the English language around
1610, was taken from the
famous mineral springs
in the resort town of Spa,
Belgium. Today, the term
refers to a health or beauty
resort that offers water-based
treatments; it is also used
loosely to describe any
establishment offering beauty
or wellness therapies.

Even if the closest you've come to a spa experience is the mask-and-makeover parties of
your teen years, you know how refreshing it feels to step away from life's cares and into
a world of self-directed hedonism. But spa time is about more than luxury, it's about
self-care: when you don't make time for yourself, your mood suffers, as do your well-
being, your looks, and even your health. Fortunately, you don't need to travel to some
fancy, faraway spa to unwind. An easier, more doable option is to bring the spa home
by turning your bathroom into a pampering center.

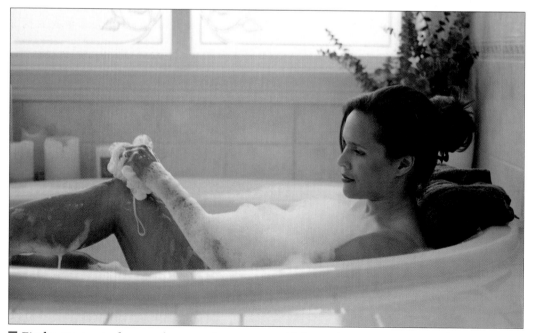

■ **Find a moment when** *you have your home to yourself, forget about commitments and worries, and
treat your body to the peaceful, tranquil spa it deserves.*

The spa routine

Choose a time when you have a few uninterrupted hours. Evening is ideal; after your spa time, you can simply crawl into bed with a book or slip into your favorite party dress for a night out. Follow these simple steps:

(1) Select soft music: New Age, classical, or jazz are ideal. If your stereo is in another room, turn its volume to a level that is audible in the bathroom, or place a portable CD player in a dry corner of the bathroom.

Do not bring homework, office work, newspapers, a radio, or any other potential irritants into your self-made spa sanctuary. In order to recharge your spirit, you must truly "get away from it all."

(2) Position a glass of drinking water next to the tub; it's easy to feel dehydrated in a steamy bathroom.

(3) Get a bottle of massage oil, almond oil, or sesame oil; or try an *essential oil*.

(4) Place facial cleanser, toner, and moisturizer within easy reach. You may choose to have a large bowl to hand, ready for facial steaming.

(5) Get out a comfortable robe and find two or three plush towels. If your bathroom is not equipped with a clock, place a watch in an easily visible position.

(6) Secure one or more scented candles in spots where they cannot be knocked over; dim or switch off the lights.

■ **In your at-home spa,** *soft candlelight and scented flowers can add to the relaxing atmosphere of the surroundings.*

> ### DEFINITION
>
> **Essential oils** *are concentrated extracts, derived from the roots, bark, stalks, flowers, leaves, and/or fruit of plants. Because each essential oil boasts specific pharmaceutical properties – such as antiseptic, anti-inflammatory, analgesic, or antiviral – these oils are popular herbal remedies. In the beauty realm, however, it is the oils' seductive scents that are most prized. Popular scents include lavender, orange, and bergamot.*

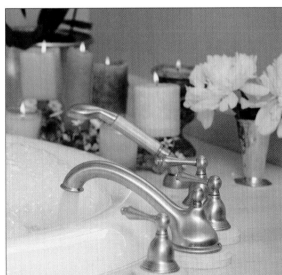

(7) Fill the bath with warm water. Add your favorite bath oil, Epsom salts, bubble bath, or four drops of an essential oil.

Avoid hot water when bathing. Not only does it dry your skin, but overly hot water can make you feel sluggish.

(8) Lower yourself into the water, lie back, and relax. Refrain from thinking about your day, your debt, your hips, your in-laws, or anything else that makes you crazy. Keep your mind clear and breathe deeply. Continue thinking of nothing and breathing deeply for up to 20 minutes; any longer than this and you risk drying out your skin.

Face first

Facials make skin glow by temporarily increasing blood circulation to the face. Giving yourself an at-home version of this spa treat is easy. After washing your face, fill up a large bowl or your bathroom sink with very hot water. If you'd like, add one or two drops of essential oil to the water.

ESSENTIAL HOW-TO'S

Scented essential oils can help transform your bathroom from an everyday room to a luxurious retreat. Two to four drops of essential oil can be added directly to foot baths, the bathtub, a nail-soaking liquid, or a facial sauna. Essential oil can also be added to an aromatherapy diffuser to scent the room. In addition to your favorite fragranced oils, look for scented candles, bath pillows, and body-care products to pamper yourself with.

Essential oils – known also as aromatherapy oils – fall into two categories: relaxing or rejuvenating. Soothing aromas include lavender, chamomile, sandalwood, and ylang ylang. Energizing fragrances are lemon, grapefruit, any of the mints, and eucalyptus.

■ **Choose a scented oil** *that suits your mood, so that you achieve just the right ambience.*

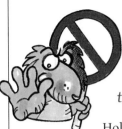

If you suffer from broken capillaries, steam's heat can make these small, distended blood vessels worse; better to skip the steaming step.

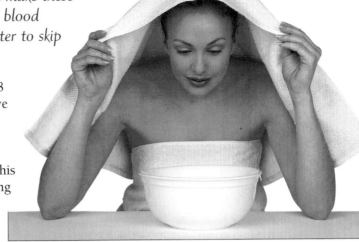

Hold your head 12 to 18 inches (30 to 45 cm) above the water, and then create a tent by draping a large towel over your head, neck, shoulders, and the bowl or the sink. Remain in this position for 5 to 10 minutes, being careful to keep the towel draped securely around the bowl or sink. Take away the towel and then tone your skin thoroughly.

■ **Steaming liquifies** *the impurities trapped within your pores, helping your skin rid itself of this unwanted material.*

All about massage

MASSAGE IS THE ULTIMATE *feel-good spa service. In addition to relieving stress, loosening tight muscles, and calming the spirit, massage improves circulation, creating a gorgeous all-over glow.*

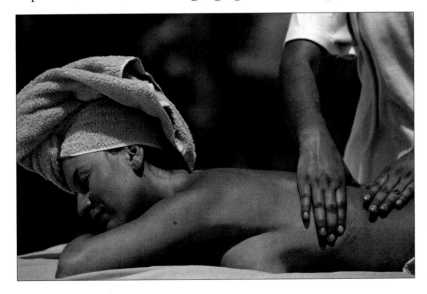

■ **Treat yourself** *to a massage while on vacation. You might learn some techniques that can help you perfect your self-massage skills.*

HOW TO GIVE YOURSELF A FACE MASSAGE

A facial massage helps temporarily boost circulation to the face and this gives the complexion a firm, rosy finish. The best time to try one is straight after a bath, when you are relaxed and warm, and your skin is supple. Better still, try giving yourself a facial massage just after steaming your face.

Massage techniques

When you give yourself a facial massage, remember that the skin on your face is fragile. To ensure a soft touch, try and use only one or two fingers at once. Stroke your face gently – be careful not to pull your skin. Motions should be upward and outward, following the natural contours of your face. Start by applying your favorite facial moisturizer, and then repeat the following moves three times each. The steps are easy to learn and will leave your skin feeling revitalized – you'll be tempted to try it again and again.

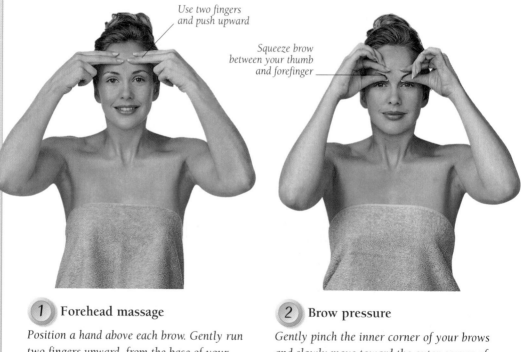

Use two fingers and push upward

Squeeze brow between your thumb and forefinger

1 **Forehead massage**

Position a hand above each brow. Gently run two fingers upward, from the base of your brows toward the middle of the forehead.

2 **Brow pressure**

Gently pinch the inner corner of your brows and slowly move toward the outer corner of each brow. Release and then repeat.

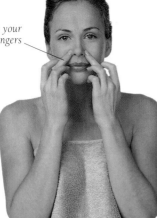

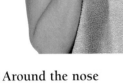

Use your middle fingers

Follow the line of your cheek bones

③ Around the nose

Apply pressure to the area next to your nostrils, using one finger only, so that the pressure is gentle. Hold for 3 seconds before releasing.

④ Cheek focus

Using your fingers, gently massage from the outer mouth to the ears. Move in an upward direction using a light spiral motion.

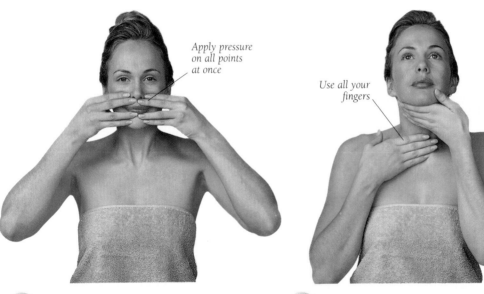

Apply pressure on all points at once

Use all your fingers

⑤ Looking at lips

Apply gentle pressure between the nose and mouth, below the mouth, and above the base of the chin. Hold for 3 seconds before releasing.

⑥ Working on your neck

Using circular, firm motions, gently massage upward from the base of your neck to your chin.

Do-it-yourself body massage

Now you have concentrated on your face, your body deserves a turn! Here are some hints and tips on how to do your own body massage. It really is simple and will leave your skin feeling glowing and supple. Make sure you're warm and comfortable. Sit on a stool, or, if you prefer, a bath mat or a plush towel. Pour a small amount of massage, almond, or sesame oil into the palm of one hand. Add a drop of essential oil if desired. Rub your hands together to distribute the oil and place one hand on each side of your left ankle. With relaxed hands and small, circular motions, move up the calf. Pour more oil (and essential oil, if you're using it) into your palm as needed throughout the massage. Repeat the steps with the right leg.

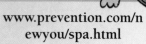

INTERNET

www.prevention.com/n
ewyou/spa.html

Part of a magazine's web site, this virtual spa helps you devise your own beauty and wellness rituals.

Starting above your left knee, work oil into your thigh using circular motions. Move up and down the thigh twice before repeating the procedure on your right thigh. Then, using your right hand, stroke firmly up and then down the length of your left arm. Using a kneading movement, massage the upper left arm; and then repeat the steps on your right arm.

Around your hips

Stand up. Massage your hips and buttocks using a two-handed kneading motion. Begin with the left side, starting at the base of the hip and moving up to the waist. Continue this bottom-to-top motion and move toward, then across the buttock. Repeat on your right side.

If you have a bit more time, recreate a spa "day of beauty" package by adding a manicure, pedicure, full-body exfoliation, and a scalp treatment.

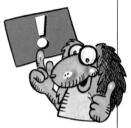

■ **When giving yourself** *a body massage, apply enough pressure to be effective, but make sure that you are gentle with your skin — don't pull at it.*

SPAS AWAY FROM HOME

An at-home, do-it-yourself spa is a terrific way to pamper yourself. For deeper relaxation and rejuvenation, however, it pays to visit a professional spa.

Different spas

There are a number of different types of spa. Generally speaking, health spas are where people go to lose weight. These spas can be Spartan or lushly appointed, and usually feature a personalized program of body analysis, aerobic exercise, weight training, stretching, low-calorie meals, cooking classes, and nutritional counseling. Health spa stays generally stretch from a weekend to several weeks.

Wellness spas aim to treat the entire person – body and spirit. Most offer classes on "lifestyle issues" including stress management, smoking cessation, goal-setting, and spirituality, as well as movement systems such as yoga and tai chi. Many also feature healthy cooking instruction and various types of massage services. Wellness spa visits run from 2 days to several weeks.

A day spa is a salon-like facility that offers beauty and wellness services. These are in-and-out places where guests spend an hour to an entire day.

Resort spas combine entertainment with relaxation. Visitors can engage in activities such as horseback riding, hiking, or water sports. Or guests can relax with various types of massages and water therapies. Resort spas also feature beauty services, including scalp massages, manicures, and facials.

Destination spa is a general term for a facility where guests stay several nights. They can be health-oriented, wellness-oriented, entertainment-oriented, beauty-oriented, or a combination. In Europe, the term still describes a resort that offers water therapies.

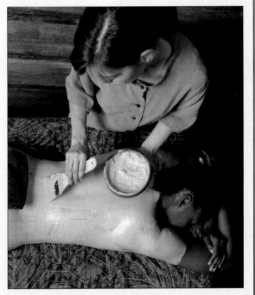

■ **A variety of health, beauty,** *and relaxation services, such as body wraps, mud treatments, and water therapies are offered at most spas.*

Last words

YOU'VE MADE IT! DO YOU FEEL MORE BEAUTIFUL? *You should. After all, you are now an official expert on your skin, your hair, your makeup, your nails, your body care, your health, and your relaxation – in short, you are an expert on all those things that contribute to personal beauty. In my opinion, this is the only kind of beauty.*

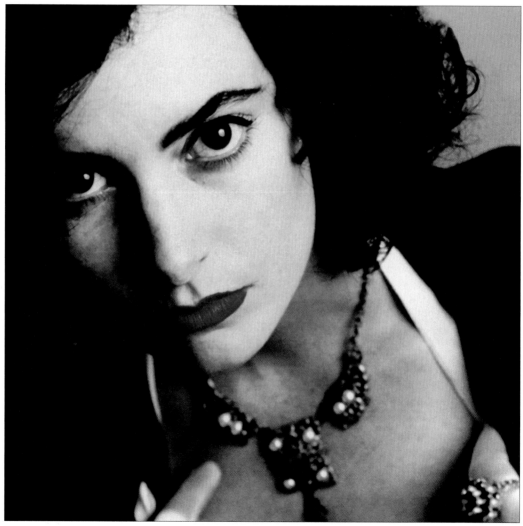

■ **Show yourself off:** *If you're confident about the way you look, you'll not only feel beautiful, but your inner radiance will shine through and you will look beautiful too.*

Looking good

Of course, you won't always have the time to pamper yourself and spend hours on your makeup and hair, or have the luxury of an at-home spa treatment. But you can adopt the simple daily habits that enhance your natural looks and make the real you shine. And once you have adopted good habits, it's easy to maintain the look you want.

When you really think about what beauty is, you realize that the world's greatest beauties are not those that prescribe to some cookie cutter standard of attractiveness. Rather, they are women who celebrate their unique physical features and their unique spirits. There is no reason why you cannot be one of them.

> Trivia...
> During the 1980s and 1990s, in the New England and Atlantic seaboard region of the United States, soda fountains were often referred to as "spas." Why? This was a reference to the carbonated soda water that was used to make the fizzy concoctions served at fashionable health spa establishments.

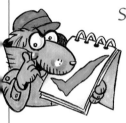

Stop trying to emulate models and celebrities, and don't be intimidated by their seemingly perfect looks. Focus on all your positive features and get out there and show yourself off! Enjoy!

A simple summary

✔ You don't need a lot of time or money to recharge with a simple at-home spa treatment.

✔ Taking care of yourself is an essential part of feeling good and looking attractive.

✔ You should make the time to pamper yourself once in a while – get the house to yourself.

✔ A bathroom and plenty of water are essential to creating a home-spa.

✔ A good facial requires a light touch – be gentle on your skin and don't use too much pressure.

✔ Self-massage is an easy way to stimulate blood flow, loosen tight muscles, and promote relaxation.

Homemade Beauty Products

SOME BEAUTY PRODUCTS are not only expensive, they may contain ingredients you wish to avoid. But don't despair. Why don't you try making your own? Using ingredients that you may already have in your cabinet, or combining natural ingredients with your favorite beauty product, you can produce nourishing hair, skin, and nail treatments within minutes. The following recipes feature in this book, with a few added extra ones too; they have been collected together so that you can refer to them at a glance. Have fun!

Hair recipes

Pre-shampoo treatment

- 2 to 4 tablespoons of almond or sesame oil

Warm oil in a small pot over a gentle heat. Apply to dry hair and allow to remain for 20 minutes to an hour. Shampoo hair and follow with your regular rinse-out conditioner. (If your hair is fine, thin, or oily, you may not need the regular after-shampoo conditioner.)

Semi-homemade shampoo

- 2 teaspoons of almond, sesame, avocado, or macadamia nut oil
- 1 tablespoon of coconut milk or dairy milk
- ¼ cup of a shampoo of your choice

Combine the ingredients in a bowl and whisk them together for 2 or 3 minutes. The quantity is enough for two shampoos. Cover and store the mixture in a refrigerator and use it within 2 days. You will find that the oil will give your hair a lovely shine and manageability.

Semi-homemade spray-on conditioner

- 1 tablespoon of your favorite conditioner
- 8-ounce (227-gram) spray bottle
- Water

Place a tablespoon of your favorite conditioner in the spray bottle and then fill it up with water. Shake the bottle well before using. The spray is excellent for controlling frizzy hair, conditioning dry hair, or treating dehydrated hair. There is no need to rinse your hair after spraying.

Homemade deep conditioner

- 4 teaspoons of almond, sesame, or avocado oil
- 2 teaspoons of coconut oil
- 3 teaspoons of honey
- 1 teaspoon of cider vinegar

This recipe is perfect for people with dry or damaged hair, because it is a fairly rich conditioner. Slowly heat all the ingredients in a saucepan, except for the honey and vinegar. Remove the pan from the heat and then stir in the honey and vinegar. Use this mixture on your hair after your normal shampooing routine. Leave it on for 15 minutes, before rinsing it off with warm water. The result? Smooth, and well-conditioned hair.

Hair gel

- 2 tablespoons of flax seeds
- 1 cup of water
- The oil from one vitamin E capsule (optional, good for dry hair)
- 1 tablespoon of rosewater or 3 drops of your favorite essential oil

Unlike the commercial varieties, this styling gel also acts as a conditioner, so it is particularly good for dry hair. Combine the flax seeds and water. Bring the mixture to a boil, and then allow the mixture to cool for 20 to 30 minutes. Strain out the seeds and stir in the vitamin E oil if you're using it and the rosewater or essential oil. Pour the mixture into a jar and store it in the refrigerator. It will keep for up to 1 month.

Skin recipes

Chamomile toner

- ½ cup of distilled witch hazel
- 1 cup of strong chamomile tea

Combine the ingredients in a glass jar or a plastic container and store it in the refrigerator. The mixture can be used in exactly the same way as an ordinary toner; use it to remove grime or oil from your complexion on a hot day, or apply it as part of your normal skin-care routine – after cleansing and before you moisturize.

Sage-vodka astringent

- ⅓ cup of dried sage leaves
- 1 cup of water
- ½ cup of unflavored vodka

Astringents help remove excess sebum from oily complexions – the alcohol ingredient is very drying, so this recipe is best avoided if you have a normal to dry complexion. Mix the water and the sage leaves in a small pot. Bring the mixture to a rolling boil and boil for 5 minutes. Allow it to cool thoroughly, and then strain the leaves and combine the liquid and vodka in a glass jar or plastic container.

Blemish treatments

Some of the best treatments for spots can be made at home. Here are three you can try:

- ½ teaspoon of yeast
- Warm water

Mix the yeast with a few drops of warm water, to form a paste. This can be smoothed over a pimple, left to dry, and then rinsed off after 20 to 60 minutes. It can be used once a day.

- ½ teaspoon of baking soda
- Warm water

Mix the baking soda with a few drops of warm water to form a paste. Use it to smooth over a pimple and rinse off after 20 to 60 minutes. This can be used once a day.

- Tea-tree oil

Dab spots with tea-tree oil, up to twice a day. (Test a small patch on your forearm, 48 hours previously, to make sure it does not irritate your skin.)

Oatmeal mask

- ½ cup of water
- 1 teaspoon of dried rosemary or sage
- 1 ½ tablespoons of oatmeal
- 10 raw almonds

This mask is best for normal to oily complexions. Bring the water and dried rosemary or sage leaves to the boil and simmer for 5 minutes. Allow the mixture to cool. In the meantime, grind the oatmeal and almonds in a blender until they are a fine powder. Add some of the herb mixture to the thick paste. Gently spread the mixture onto clean skin, avoiding the eyes and mouth, and allow the mask to dry completely. Leave on for 15 to 30 minutes and then remove with a damp washcloth and warm water.

Avocado mask

- ½ an avocado, mashed
- 2 tablespoons of plain yoghurt

This mask is best for dry or normal complexions. Combine avocado pulp with plain yoghurt. Apply it to your clean face and neck and leave it on for 20 to 30 minutes. Wipe the mask off with dry tissues.

Kitchen scrub

- ½ tablespoon of your favorite cleanser
- 1 tablespoon of coarse-grind cornmeal, coarse Kosher or sea salt, or coarsely ground almonds

This is a really easy-to-make mechanical exfoliant. Use it on your face and body – be gentle – and after scrubbing, rinse well with lukewarm water.

Fruit exfoliator

- Papaya

One of nature's most effective chemical exfoliants is papaya fruit. It contains a strong enzyme called *papain* that dissolves excess sebum as well as dead skin cells. Smooth mashed papaya onto your face and allow to sit for up to 5 minutes. Remove with a damp washcloth and a few splashes of water. Other enzyme-rich fruit you may want to try includes ripe tomatoes and pineapple.

Nail recipes

Cuticle oil

- One or two drops of massage oil, almond oil, olive oil, or sesame oil per nail

Place a small drop or two of massage oil, almond oil, olive oil, or sesame oil at the base of the nail, and rub into the cuticle, up the nail folds, and onto the nail plate itself. Repeat with your remaining nails. This can be done daily to moisturize the nails, cuticles, and surrounding skin so that nails stay strong and flexible enough to fend off breaks and skin remains supple and hang-nail free.

Nail mask

- 2 tablespoons of almond, olive, or sesame oil

Warm oil in a small pot over a gentle heat. Massage onto clean nails and allow to sit for at least an hour.

Nail antiseptic

- Rubbing alcohol or witch hazel

Before applying base coat or nail polish, saturate a cotton ball with rubbing alcohol or witch hazel and swipe over nails to remove dirt and oils.

Other Resources

Books

If there is a particular aspect of beauty that you want to delve into further – such as learning how to look after aging skin, styling curly hair, dealing with hair loss, or living a less stressful life – there are plenty of books out there on the market. Here are just a few that you could refer to:

General beauty

Beauty, The New Basics
Rona Berg, Workman, 2001

Beauty Secrets of India
Monisha Bharadwaj, Ulysses Press, 2000

Beauty Wisdom
Bharti Vyas and Claire Haggard, HarperCollins UK, 1998

Make Your Own Cosmetics: Neal's Yard Remedies
Neal's Yard Remedies, Aurum Press UK, 1997

The Natural Beauty & Bath Book
Casey Kellar, Lark Books, 2000

Woman's Face: Skin Care and Makeup
Kim Johnson, Knopf, 1997

Skin

Beautiful Skin: Every Woman's Guide to Looking Her Best at Any Age
David E. Bank and Estelle Sobel, Adams Media Corporation, 2000

Naturally Healthy Skin: Tips and Techniques for a Lifetime of Radiant Skin
Stephanie Tourles, Storey Books, 1999

The Skin Care Book: Simple Herbal Recipes
Kathlyn Quatrochi, Interweave Press, 1997

Skin Secrets: The Medical Facts Versus the Beauty Fiction
Nicholas Lowe and Polly Sellar, Collins & Brown, 1999

Solving Skin Problems
Ricki Ostrov, Marshall Editions, 1999

Total Skin: The Definitive Guide to Whole Skin Care for Life
David Leffell, Hyperion, 2000

The Wrinkle Cure: Unlock the Power of Cosmeceuticals for Supple, Youthful Skin
Nicholas Perricone, Rodale Press, 2000

Hair

The Bald Truth: The First Complete Guide To Preventing And Treating Hair Loss
Diane B. Eisman and Eugene H. Eisman, Pocket Books UK, 2000

Curly Gurl
Lorraine Massey, Workman Publishing, 2000

Hair Secrets
Maggie Jones and Marilyn Sherlock, Collins & Brown, 2000

Hair Savers for Women: A Complete Guide to Preventing and Treating Hair Loss
Maggie Greenwood-Robinson, Three Rivers Press, 2000

Naturally Healthy Hair: Herbal Treatments And Daily Care for Fabulous Hair
Mary Beth Janssen, Storey Books, 1999

Makeup

The Art of Makeup
Kevyn Aucoin, HarperCollins, 1995

Classic Makeup And Beauty
Mary Quant, DK Publishing, 1996

Face Forward
Kevyn Aucoin, Little Brown and Company, 2000

Making Faces
Kevyn Aucoin, Little Brown and Company, 1999

Style

Carol Spenser's Style Directions for Women
Carol Spenser, Piatkus Books UK, 1999

Health and wellness

Aromatherapy for Dummies
Kathi Keville, IDG Books, 1999

The Art of Happiness: A Handbook for Living
The Dalai Lama and Howard C. Cutler, Riverhead Books, 1998

Bharti Vyas's Two-day Treat
Bharti Vyas, HarperCollins, 2000

The British Medical Association Family Doctor Guide to Stress
Greg Wilkinson, Dorling Kindersley, UK, 1999

Choosing Simplicity: Real People Finding Peace and Fulfillment in a Complex World
Linda Breen, Gallagher Press, 2000

The Dark Side of the Light Chasers: Reclaiming Your Power, Creativity, Brilliance, and Dreams
Debbie Ford, Riverhead Books, 1999

Divine Intuition: Your Guide to Creating a Life You Love
Lynn A. Robinson, DK Publishing, 2001

Indulge Yourself with Aromatherapy
M. Lou Luchsinger, Sterling Publishing, 2000

Lit from Within: Tending Your Soul for Lifelong Beauty
Victoria Moran, Harper San Francisco, 2001

The Magic of Well-Being
Judith Jackson, DK Publishing, 1997

Planet Organic: Organic Beauty
Josephine Fairley, DK Publishing, 2001

The Simple Living Guide : A Sourcebook for Less Stressful, More Joyful Living
Janet Luhrs, Broadway Books, 1997

Simple Steps to Impossible Dreams
Steven K. Scott, Simon & Schuster UK, 1999

Swell: A Girl's Guide to the Good Life
Cynthia Rowley and Ilene Rosenzweig, Warner Books, 1999

Take Time for Your Life: A Personal Coach's Seven-Step Program for Creating the Life You Want
Cheryl Richardson, Broadway Books, 1999

Useful organizations

Where can you find a list of health spas in your area? Who can you ask for advice if you are contemplating something major, such as cosmetic surgery? Here are a number of specialist organizations that can supply you with information:

General Beauty

American Association of Cosmetology Schools
15825 N. 71st Street
Scottsdale, AZ 85254-1521
(800) 831-1086
www.beautyschools.org

American Beauty Organization
401 N. Michigan Avenue
Chicago, IL 60611
(800) 868-4265
Fax (312) 245-1080
www.salonprofessionals.org

Consumer Information Center
PO Box 100
Pueblo, CO 81002
(800) 8-PUEBLO
www.pueblo.gsa.gov

Hair

American Board of Certified Haircolorists
28132 Western Avenue
San Pedro, CA 90732
(310) 547-0814
www.haircolorist.com

American Hair Loss Council
100 Independence Place, Suite 207
Tyler, TX 75703
(888) 873-9719
www.ahlc.org

Intercoiffure America
540 Robert E. Lee Boulevard
New Orleans, LA 70124
(504) 288-9003
E-mail: johnjay@gs.net

International Haircolor Exchange
4515 Poplar Avenue, Suite 307
Memphis, TN 38117
(800) 265-6755
E-mail: shecolor@aol.com

The Salon Association
15825 N. 71st Street, Suite 100
Scottsdale, AZ 85254-1521
(800) 211-4TSA
www.salons.org

Makeup

Canadian Cosmetic Careers Association
309 Main Street
Unionville, ON
L3R 6A5
(416) 410-9175
www.ccccosmetics.com

Canadian Cosmetic, Toiletry and Fragrance Association
420 Britannia Road East, Suite 102
Mississauga, ON
L4Z 3L5
(905) 890-5161
www.cctfa.ca

Cosmetology Advancement Foundation
PMB 102, 4262 Northlake Boulevard
Palm Beach Gardens, FL 33410
(561) 630-7766
www.cosmetology.org

National Acrediting Commission of Cosmetology
Arts & Sciences
901 North Stuart Street, Suite 900
Arlington, VA 22203-1816
(703) 527-7600
www.naccas.org

National Cosmetology Association
401 N. Michigan Avenue
Chicago, IL 60611
(312) 527-6765
www.salonprofessionals.org

Skin

Canadian Dermatology Association
774 Echo Drive, Room 521
Ottawa, ON
K1S 5N8
(800) 267-3376
www.dermatology.ca

Skin Cancer Foundation
245 Fifth Avenue
New York, NY 10016
(212) 725-5176
www.skincancer.org

Health and wellness

American Herbalists Guild
1931 Gaddis Road
Canton, GA 30115
(770) 751-6021
www.americanherbalistsguild.com

American Massage Therapy Association
820 Davis Street, Suite 100
Evanston, IL 60201
(847) 864-0123
www.amtamassage.org

Centers for Disease Control and Prevention
1600 Clifton Road NE
Atlanta, GA 30333
(800) 311-3435
www.cdc.gov

The Day Spa Association
PO Box 5232
West New York, NJ 07093
(201) 865-2065
www.dayspaassociation.com

International SPA Association
546 E. Main Street
Lexington, KY 40508
(888) 651-4772
www.experienceispa.com

National Advisory Council on Aging
Health Canada
Postal Locator: 1908A1
Ottawa, ON
(613) 957-1968
www.hc-sc.gc.ca

National Association for Holistic Aromatherapy
PO Box 17622
Boulder, CO 80308
(800) 566-6734
www.naha.org

National Institute on Aging
US Department of Health & Human
Services
PO Box 8057
Gaithersburg, MD 20898
(800) 222-2225
www.nih.gov/nia

Spa Canada
Box 26, 108 Mile Ranch, BC
V0K 2Z0
(800)704-6393
www.spacanada.com

Beauty on the Web

THE INTERNET is a good place to browse for information on beauty products, techniques, and trends. So, whether you're thinking about a new hair style, you're worried about the ingredients of a cosmetic you use, or you want to find out more about a skin treatment, here are some sites that may be able to offer you the information or advice you're looking for:

General beauty

www.about-face.org

Created by the San Francisco-based organization About-Face, this site is dedicated to combating negative and distorted images of women and of female beauty. Must-see features include a gallery of demeaning or offensive advertisements (plus addresses where you can contact the perpetrators), resources for image disorders, and ten things you can do to empower yourself (because a powerful woman is a beautiful woman).

www.beautyengine.com

Searching for a beauty-related topic? This beauty-focused search engine can help.

www.beautify-tips.com

Plenty of beauty tips to help you with skin, hair, makeup, nails, fashion, fragrance, and more.

www.beautyworlds.com

An informative site that examines historical beauty icons, as well as looking at scientific studies on beauty, and information on how beauty affects self-esteem.

www.digitalbeauty.com

Makeup, surgical procedures, hair care, fashion trends, and cutting-edge beauty news are all discussed at this site.

www.free-beauty-tips.com

A web site devoted to beauty tips.

www.informedbeauty.com

A smart web site that espouses the beauty-building power of self-esteem, health, mental strength, and creativity.

www.lookgoodfeelbetter.org

A terrific site featuring health and beauty care for cancer patients.

www.pioneerthinking.com

This site features do-it-yourself ideas for health, beauty, and well-being.

www.womanht.com

This web site, titled A Woman's Heart, features information on make-it-yourself skin, hair, and body products, as well as instructions on do-it-yourself facials.

Skin

www.aad.org

This is the official web site for the American Academy of Dermatology. It has information on skin ailments and diseases, and explains why and how skin changes as we age. It also lists dermatologists in your area.

www.asds-net.org

As the homepage for the American Society for Dermatologic Surgery, this site features discussions of various dermatological procedures.

http://dermatology.about.com

You'll find study links, articles, product reviews, and treatment information at this site.

www.dermatology.ca

The web site for the Canadian Dermatology Association.

www.dermatologychannel.net

Look up medical information on skin disorders.

www.derm-info.net

This site supplies information on a range of skin ailments and diseases, and takes a look at treatments and products.

www.dermskin.com

This e-commerce site features articles on a variety of skin-care topics.

www.mustela.com

French-based international skin-care company Mustela offers skin-care advice and products for expectant mothers and infants.

www.nih.gov/nia

Run by the United States National Institute on Aging, this web site has plenty of information on, and advice about, how to care for aging skin.

www.oneskin.com

This site tells you all you want to know about skin ailments, as well as featuring message boards so that readers can share their own experiences and insights.

www.skinema.com

Produced by a dermatologist, this site takes a wry look at the skin conditions of the stars.

www.skinpatient.com

This thorough site features information on specific skin – as well as hair and nail – conditions, plus online patient support groups and ingredient information for a wide range of cosmetics.

www.totalskincare.com

This site takes a look at skin-care issues. It also has information on skin-care products, as well as examining a variety of treatments.

Hair

www.clairol.com

This site offers heaps of advice on coloring your hair, how to avoid hair-color problems, and how to look after treated hair.

www.goblonde.com

If being blonde is important to you, check out Go Blonde, a site that features how-to information, makeover pictures, and general adventures in blonding.

www.hairboutique.com

This informative site has lots of articles, and information on a range of topics, from hair thinning and aging, to hair styles and products.

www.haircare4men.com

This man-friendly site features male-oriented advice and hair-care products.

www.hairdos.com

This site features a hairstyle-selector, hair-color information, and a selection of hair photos.

www.hairdresseruk.com

Featuring a selection of hairstyles to peruse, this site offers information about styling, celebrity styles, and virtual makeovers.

www.hairnet.com

This site is aimed at professional stylists, but it is also full of hairstyle critiques, step-by-step hair looks, and the lastest news on chemical hair treatments and services.

www.hair-news.com

Dedicated to "the art and science of hair," this site features hair-care help, an updated newsletter, and information on hair-care products.

www.hairstylist.com

This site includes a hair-style search, a hair-product finder, advice on hair color, and a questions and answers section.

www.helenecurtis.com

Choosing a hip new hair style? Try this web site. It also takes a look at how hair ages.

www.keratin.com

If you want to know all about hair, what it's made of, how it grows, take a look at this informative web site. It has all the latest news from the hair world.

www.morehair.com

If you suffer from hair loss or unwanted hair growth, you're not alone. This site takes a look at how to deal with the problem; examines hair loss products and treatments; and offers advice about hairpieces.

www.naturallycurly.com

If you have natural curls, waves, or ringlets, this site has lots of suggestions about how to style and care for them.

www.redandproud.com

Celebrating that rare phenomenon – red hair.

www.shampoo4me.com

If you're having problems finding the shampoo that suits your tresses, browse here. The site also includes information on perming, coloring, and hair care.

www.supercuts.com

This is the official site for Supercuts salons. It tells you how to choose hair-care products that are right for you, and lists product ingredients.

www.visual-makeover.com

This amusing site looks at hair care, hair styles, and how to do a complete hair make-over.

Makeup

www.aavs.org

If you're interested in compassionate cosmetic shopping, the American Anti-Vivesection Society publishes a useful guide.

www.allergymakeup.com

A must-see for allergy sufferers, this site features information on applying makeup while suffering from allergies, and how to camouflage allergy signs.

www.beautybuzz.com

Here you'll find articles on makeup, fragrance, and fitness, as well as professional beauty advice, copious product reviews, and trend reports.

www.beautynewsletter.gq.nu

This web site features product reviews, quizzes, and the lastest news on beauty and cosmetics. It also includes information for professional makeup artists.

www.ebeauty.com

There's plenty of advice on cosmetics and make-overs at this helpful web site.

www.emakeup.com

Peruse cosmetic reviews, makeup chats, beauty articles, tips, and web-site links.

www.eyebrowz.com

Take a look at celebrity brows, get the low-down on styling your own brows, and look at pictures of brow make-overs.

www.hsus.org/programs/research/cc-brochure

This site for the Humane Society of the United States gives lots of information on how cosmetics are tested on animals.

www.intomakeup.com

This site looks at home-made cosmetics, and has a run-down of the best cosmetics available on the market.

www.makeupmania.com

A professional makeup artist's store that features difficult-to-obtain professional cosmetics and special-effects makeup.

Nails

www.1st-spot.com/topic_nailcare.html

Packed with information about nail care and nail products.

www.cir-safety.org

If you're concerned about the ingredients in nail products and treatments, visit this web site. It lists cosmetic ingredients, and gives advice on possible allergic reactions or signs of poisoning.

www.epa.gov

The United States Environmental Protection Agency's web site includes information and regulations about nail salon standards and hygiene practices.

www.feetforlife.org

Maintain healthy feet and toenails with the information found at this site.

www.hooked-on-nails.com

At this site you can learn about nail growth, health, care, and types of manicures and pedicures, as well as nail maintenance.

www.international-foot-and-shoe.com.au

All about keeping feet healthy and beautiful.

www.sechevite.com

There's product information, nail-care tips, and help with finding a nail salon near you at this web site for Seche International nailcare.

www.stepwise-uk.com

A site that shows you how to maintain healthy toenails and feet.

www.waningmoon.com

Includes information on how to remove polish stains from nails, details about acrylic nails, and useful information on nail care for men.

Spas

www.clubspausa.com

At this site, maintained by The Day Spa Association, you can brush up on your spa etiquette, learn spa terms, and find day spas near you.

www.journeywoman.com/herspastop

This site contains reviews of numerous destination spas throughout the world.

www.phys.com/health/spa

Create a home health spa with information from this Conde Net web page.

www.women.com/travel/spas/getaways

Here you'll find reviews of day spas and destination spas. There are also numerous home-spa how-to's.

Body care

www.celluliteexpert.com

If you want to know about cellulite, this web site has plenty of information about what causes cellulite, and how to help reduce it.

www.prevention.com/newyou/spa.html

This web site gives advice on beauty and wellness rituals.

www.healthwell.com

You'll find heaps of advice on lifestyle, aging, fitness, and nutrition here.

Fragrance

www.fragrance.org
The official web site of The Fragrance Foundation, this educational site is all about fragrance.

Cosmetic surgery

www.bodylanguage.net
The official web site for Body Language Magazine, a British publication that offers reports on new surgical procedures and surgeons worldwide.

www.cosmeticsupport.com
Billing itself as the international "cosmetic surgery and body transformation support site," this web site features surgery facts, online support groups, chats, before-and-after photos, and help in selecting a surgeon.

www.cosmeticsurgery-news.com
Find late-breaking news on procedures, surgeons, and surgery trends.

www.cosmeticsurgeryinamerica.com
This site acts as a resource to teach you about plastic surgery, specific procedures, and terminology.

www.lipoinfo.com
All about liposuction, including answers to frequently asked questions and before-and-after photographs.

www.plasticsurgery.org
Run by the American Society of Plastic Surgeons, this site gives information on different procedures, after-surgery care, and features a physician referral service.

www.yestheyrefake.net
This pro-surgery site has heaps of information on the various cosmetic procedures available; it also includes a message board, so that readers can share their own experiences and insights.

Health and wellness

www.aromaweb.com
Aromatherapy information, including how to choose essential oils, recipes, worthwhile books, web links and more.

www.dr.weil.com
This is the official web site of Dr. Andrew Weil, an American medical doctor who is well known for fusing traditional and alternative therapies.

www.fitnessonline.com
A regularly updated site that features a bevy of fitness tools, expert advice columns, fitness-related articles, and exercise plans.

www.healthy.net
Health-care advice for the entire family.

www.holisticonline.com
Find out about insomnia, stress reduction, and more, all with a friendly, New Age bent.

www.onebody.com
This site brings together alternative, complementary, and traditional medicine for a holistic look at wellness.

www.queendom.com
This entertaining site features a variety of personality, intelligence, and health-related tests, as well as articles on physical and mental health, women's issues, and expert advice columns.

www.selfgrowth.com
This comprehensive site features a large selection of articles and links on a vast range of topics, including stress reduction, physical fitness, and creativity.

www.wholehealthmd.com
This site features health-care information from an integrated alternative medicine, nutrition, and traditional medicine approach.

A simple glossary

Accutane A strong, synthetic form of vitamin A, taken orally to suppress sebum production and to treat severe cystic acne.

Acetone An ingredient in some nail-polish removers. It is a colorless liquid that evaporates quickly, is flammable, and dissolves in water.

Acne Often used as a general term to describe any group of recurring blemishes, acne is a chronic skin disease, common during adolescence – it involves inflammation of the skin's sebaceous glands.

Active ingredient The ingredient(s) in a formula that helps the product achieve its stated purpose.

Aerobic Any exercise that uses large muscle groups and is maintained for longer than 15-minute periods is known as aerobic exercise – jogging and walking are good examples.

Aestheticians Trained beauty professionals who specialize in skin care, often practicing at skin-care salons, spas, and in dermatologists' offices.

Age spots Known as liver spots or senile lentigines in dermatologist-speak, they are harmless dark tan or brown patches – similar to oversized freckles. Most often seen on hands, forearms, and face.

Alpha hydroxy acids These are naturally occurring substances that break down the dead cells that sit on skin's surface, dulling the complexion and clogging pores. Alpha hydroxy acids also stimulate new collagen growth, giving users a slightly tighter, more youthful complexion, and the acids' light bleaching effect helps treat discoloration, freckles, and acne scars.

Antioxidants Naturally occurring substances, including certain vitamins and plant extracts, which fight off free radicals – the unstable compounds that are thought to attack and injure cells.

Ashy Hair with cool, almost grayish, tones.

Astringent A type of toner – usually formulated with alcohol or some equally drying substance – used on oily complexions to draw out and remove excess sebum.

Backcombed This is done by holding your hair upright and combing toward the roots. It makes hair stand up, giving it a fuller look – however, it can damage hair strands.

Balneotherapy Generally refers to therapeutic baths in natural mineral spring waters.

Beauty According to *Webster's Collegiate Dictionary*, "the quality or aggregate of qualities in a person or thing that gives pleasures to the senses or pleasurably exalts the mind or spirit."

Bilateral symmetry In beauty talk, this refers to balanced, left-to-right symmetry, for example, evenly shaped eyes.

Botox A muscle-paralyzing substance that is injected into muscles – usually in the upper third of the face – to eliminate or prevent crow's feet, between-brow furrows, and horizontal creases on the forehead.

Chemical exfoliants Ingredients such as enzymes or alpha hydroxy acids that you can apply to your body, to loosen and slough off dead and old skin cells, debris, and excess sebum. The exfoliation takes no physical work on one's part – no rubbing, and no rinsing.

Chemical sunscreens Sunscreens that use chemicals to absorb UVA and UVB light, preventing the sun from damaging skin cells.

Circadian rhythm This is a synonym for the bodies' internal clock.

Clarifying Cleaning hair of residues from shampoo, conditioners, or styling products.

Cold cream A thick, luxurious cream that melts makeup, excess sebum, and dirt. Because of its heavy, oily nature, cold cream is always best-suited to dry skin.

Collagen A fiber found in the dermis that helps give skin its structure.

Combination skin Skin that features patches of oily and dry, or oily and normal skin.

Complexion bars Mild cleansers in bar form that look like soap.

Cranial molding An ancient form of head binding; an infant's head is bound between two boards, so that as the child grows the head shape is molded and permanently changed.

Cuticles In hair, the outermost layer of the hair strand. In nails, the thin tissue that grows from the finger to overlap the nail plate and rim the base of the nail.

Cystic acne Acne featuring a scattering of scarlet, nodular blemishes on the face, neck, shoulders, or back. Dermatologists also call this severe or nodular acne.

Décolletage A French word used to describe the skin of the chest and breasts.

Demi-permanent hair color Hair color that lasts from 12 to 24 shampoos.

Dermabrasion A process that uses a small rotating abrasive brush to sand away the top layers of skin.

Dermis Skin's middle layer, directly under the epidermis, where skin's collagen and elastin fibers are located.

Double-process color A two-step process for lightening medium or dark hair, it involves first bleaching and then treating with a semi-permanent or permanent hair color in the blonde shade of one's choice.

Dry skin Skin that doesn't produce enough sebum to keep the epidermis moist.

Elastic A fiber found in the dermis – it helps give the skin structure.

Endomologie® A patented technique involving a mechanized device with motorized rollers and suction devices. Used on certain areas of the body, it is said to increase circulation, which in turn boosts skin's firmness and helps eliminate the appearance of cellulite.

Epidermis The top layer of skin, which measures less than 1 millimeter in thickness over most of the body.

Essential oil Concentrated extract of plants, bark, roots, flowers – each oil has a specific pharmaceutical property.

Eumalin A type of melanin responsible for darker hair shades, including chestnut, coffee, and black.

Exfoliate To remove the surface, in this case, the skin's surface layer, where dead skin cells and dirt reside.

Eye makeup remover A special type of makeup remover made to melt budge-proof eye makeup such as waterproof mascara, water-resistant eyeliner, and false-eyelash glue.

Feldenkrais method Usually carried out in two to five 1-hour sessions, the technique involves discovering improper posture habits, and replacing them with correct ones.

Fight or flight response A kind of temporary power surge designed to help the body in times of real or perceived danger.

Free radicals Unstable compounds that attack and injure vital cell structures. They are blamed not only for premature aging, but also for damaging DNA and suppressing the immune system.

Glycolic acid An alpha hydroxy acid derived from sugar cane.

Hair clarifying treatments Pre-shampoo formulas or clarifying shampoos that dissolve styling product remnants, allowing vestiges of hairspray, gel, mousse, and more to be rinsed from strands. Also helpful for people who live with deposit-causing, mineral-rich water. Overuse of clarifying products can strip necessary sebum from the hair.

Hair shaft The visible part of the hair. It is also a synonym for hair strand – the individual hairs that grace most of our heads.

Hangnail A snag of skin near the cuticle or at the sides of the nails. Occurs most often in dry, flaking, or cracked skin.

Henna A natural vegetable tannin that stains hair.

Highlights Stripes of brighter or lighter color that are painted onto hair.

Histamines Chemicals found in your body's tissues, which are released when you have an allergic reaction – your body's way of scaring off a perceived invader.

Humectants Used in skin-care and hair-care products to attract and retain water.

Inner cortex The fragile portion of the hair strand that is under the cuticle layer, comprised of keratin; the place where melanin – hair's natural pigment – is located.

Jessner's peel A form of skin peel, it consists of salicylic acid, lactic acid, and resorcinol.

Keratin A tough protein that makes up nails and human hair.

Kinerase Also known as furfuryl adenine, kinerase is a natural plant-derived ingredient that has been shown in clinical studies to retard the aging process by reducing discoloration, fine lines, and rough texture.

Laser resurfacing A procedure that removes skin's outer layer with a cosmetic laser. It can lighten or banish discoloration, scars, and fine and moderate wrinkles, as well as tighten slack skin, giving the face a firmer, younger appearance.

L-cysteine Also known as L-cysteine hydrochloride, or HCL. A popular food additive that can be made from petroleum, but is much more commonly made from human hair.

Lifting This refers to a nail enhancement – such as an acrylic tip, or a false nail – coming loose from the nail, creating a gap where moisture and bacteria can enter.

Lip color Includes lipstick, lip pencils, colored lip gloss – anything that adds color to your lips.

Lowlights Stripes of darker color that are painted into hair to create contrast.

Low maintenance These are cuts that suit your hair's texture, type, and wave, and are therefore easier to maintain because hair falls into place naturally.

Lunula The whitish, half-moon area visible at the base of the nail.

Makeup remover A product designed to break down makeup for easy removal.

Matrix Also known as the nail root, this is the area hidden beneath the cuticle where nail keratin is created.

Mechanical When referring to hair care, this includes brushing, twirling your hair between your fingers, and backcombing.

Mechanical exfoliants Hair removers that one physically controls, such as a razor.

Melanin The pigment that gives skin its color.

Melasma Also known as the mask of pregnancy. Caused by hormone-activated melasma, it is a condition consisting of brown patches on the forehead, cheeks, or above the lip. Most commonly occurs during the second trimester of pregnancy.

Microdermabrasion facial A facial that uses a small tubelike device to spray aluminum crystals, diamond dust, or salt across the skin to lift off dead skin cells and the outermost layer of the epidermis. A suctioning action simultaneously sweeps away exfoliated skin cells and used abrasive material.

Mind-body workouts Workouts that exercise both mind and body, such as tai chi, the various forms of yoga, and Pilates. The exercise requires training one's thoughts on breath, posture, individual moves, and how one's body feels as it makes each individual move.

Mousy This term refers to hair the color of mouse fur.

Nail bed The finger tissue directly under the nail plate whose network of small blood vessels provides nutrition for the nail.

Nail folds The folds of skin at the nail's base and sides that frame and support the nails.

Nail plate The hard, smooth, slightly convex, rectangular sheath that is a nail.

Normal skin Skin that produces enough sebum to keep itself supple, but not so much that the complexion looks slick.

Oily skin Skin that has too much sebum.

One-feature rule Playing up one facial feature and leaving the remaining features subdued.

Overwashing This is when you wash your hair more regularly than necessary. How much is too much? It varies between individuals.

Peel A rejuvenating skin-care procedure performed by an aesthetician or dermatologist. An acid solution, comprising of alpha hydroxy acid, beta hydroxy acid, resorcinol, or other ingredients, is painted on the skin and then rinsed off.

Permanent color Hair color that stays on hair permanently.

Permanent wave A hair service that creates permanent curl, waves, or body.

Phaeomelanin A type of melanin in hair that contributes to light and reddish tones such as blonde, caramel, ginger, and auburn.

Phytonutrients These are chemicals found in plants – they help plants ward off infections and bugs, and help protect them from ultraviolet light and toxins.

Pilates A form of exercise, similar to yoga, using simple stretch and calisthetic movements to stretch, lengthen, and strengthen muscles.

PhotoFacial® Developed by Californian dermatologist Patrick Bitter, Sr., this is a non-invasive facial that uses intense, non-laser light to treat pigmentation problems, broken and enlarged capillaries, fine lines, scarring, and the flushing associated with rosacea.

Pollywog brow See tadpole brow.

Relaxers Hair process that straightens hair, but not all the way – just enough so that tightly wound coils of hair look like soft curls or even loose waves.

Resorcinol This is a vitamin-A-based exfoliating agent, often used as part of a Jessner peel.

Rhinoplasty The medical name for a nose job.

Rolfing Usually carried out in ten, 1-hour sessions, the technique involves deeply massaging the connective tissues that enclose muscles, to provide the body with greater flexibility and mobility.

Rosacea Also called acne rosacea, an ongoing inflammation of the cheeks, nose, mid-forehead, and chin.

Royal jelly Made by bees to feed a hive's queen bee, it is a jelly-like substance that is thought to have healthy, rejuvenating properties.

Salicylic acid Also known as beta hydroxy acid, this relative of aspirin works by penetrating pores and loosening the impacted sebum and dirt that cause blackheads, whiteheads, and cystic pimples.

Sebum Dermatologist-speak for oil that is created in the skin and secreted through the pores to keep skin moist and supple.

Semi-permanent color Hair color that washes out in 6 to 12 shampoos.

Sensitive skin Not a true skin type, but skin – whether oily, normal, or dry – that reacts to more factors than others.

Setting In makeup, this refers to fixing something in place. For example, applying powder to foundation helps it "set," by absorbing excess sebum and moisture.

Signature scent A single scent worn exclusively.

Sleep hygiene A term used by doctors, this refers to routines that encourage good, nourishing sleep.

Smoker's face A face featuring fine lines around the mouth from puckering, lines near the eyes from squinting through smoke, a gray-tinged complexion caused by nicotine-slowed blood circulation, thin skin, slackness, and dryness.

Spa The term refers to a health and beauty establishment, offering water-based treatments, or beauty and wellness therapies.

Subcutis Skin's bottom layer; acts as a reservoir for water and fat cells and serves as a cushion between the upper layers of skin and the body's bones and muscles.

Sunblocks Physical sunscreens, such as titanium dioxide and zinc oxide, which form a barrier to block the entry of UVA and UVB light.

SPF Sun Protection Factor. This is the amount of UVB rays a sunscreen protects you from. An SPF of 20 would allow you to stay in the sun 20 times longer than if you were not wearing sun protection.

Surfactants Detergents used in hair care and some skin cleansers that cleanse and create lather.

Symmetry Balanced, equal.

Tadpole brow Brow shape featuring a thick teardrop or wedge shape at its inner corner, which resembles a tadpole head and is connected to an overly plucked, wispy "tail."

Temporary hair color Hair color that stays in the hair only until the next shampoo.

Thalassotherapy A treatment that uses seawater and seaweed to promote beauty and nourish health.

Thermal formula A conditioner that contains ingredients that stay on the hair even after rinsing. It is used to help protect hair from high temperatures during heat-styling.

Threading An ancient form of hair removal originating in Israel and the Middle East. It is performed by a skilled practitioner who uses a length of thread to quickly lasso and pull individual brow or facial hairs.

Toner A general term for the skin-care step that comes between cleansing and moisturizing. Also, a particular kind of toner formulated without alcohol and used by those with normal to dry skin.

Trentinoin A vitamin-A derivative and one of the few skin-care ingredients proven in medical studies to reverse some signs of sun damage and aging, such as fine lines, discoloration, rough texture, and dullness. Because trentinoin works to keep pores clear, when used on a regular basis it also helps prevent pimples. *Retin-A®* and *Renova®* are two examples of products containing trentinoin.

UVA rays Long-length sun waves that can penetrate cloud cover and glass, UVA rays are present in the same intensity throughout the day, remain strong even in winter, and are responsible for skin cancer and creating the skin changes – like blotchiness and collagen breakdown – often associated with aging skin.

UVB rays Short-length sun waves responsible for tanning, burning, and skin cancer, UVB rays are at their strongest during late spring, summer, and early fall, at locations near the equator, and at higher altitudes. UVB rays are most intense from the hours of 10 a.m. and 3 p.m.

Waist-to-hip ratio This is the ratio you get when you measure your waist and hips, and then divide your waist measurement by your hip measurement.

Weight-bearing exercise This refers to any exercise that allows your body to come into direct contact with the ground, for example, jogging. Weight-bearing exercise helps you develop strong bones.

Wood's lamp Type of light projecting a long wavelength of blue light deeper into the skin than visible light and used by aestheticians and dermatologists to assess a patient's sun damage, which shows up as dark, mottled areas.

Index

Acknowledgments

Author's Acknowledgments

The author would like to thank the following people for help with this project: Richard Demler for simply "being there," LaVonne Carlson for hiring me, Jennifer Williams for being the most patient, saintlike editor this slow-writing author has ever known, Lisa Lenard and Joy Dickinson for ensuring this book reads smoothly, Caroline Hunt and the team at Studio Cactus – Laura Watson, Kate Hayward, Jane Baldock, and Sharon Moore – for good cheer and their role in creating this gorgeous book.

Publisher's Acknowledgments

Dorling Kindersley would like to thank the following people for their contributions to this project: Neal Cobourne for designing the jacket and Melanie Simmonds for picture research.

Packager's Acknowledgments

Studio Cactus would like to thank Dr David Harris FRCP (Consultant Dermatologist, The London Clinic of Dermatology at the Hospital of St John and St Elizabeth, 60 Grove End Road, London, NW8 9NH) for his advice on the chapters relating to skin care and skin treatments. Studio Cactus would also like to thank Damien Moore for photography, Jane Baldock and Kerry O' Sullivan for modeling, and Barry Robson for the dog illustrations. Thanks also to Polly Boyd for proofreading, and to Hilary Bird for compiling the index.

Picture Credits

t = top, b = bottom, c = center, r = right, l = left

John Bulmer: 207, 209
Tracy Morgan: 310
Stephen Oliver: 8br, 105
Studio Cactus: 106br, 119tr, 196, 197, 199, 233, 243, 244, 249, 250, 251, 258
Photodisc: 2, 5, 11, 12, 14, 16, 20, 21, 22, 30, 36, 41, 43, 44, 47, 53, 54, 58, 60, 62, 67, 69, 74, 83, 84, 89, 90tr, 91, 92, 96, 98tr, 101, 102, 111, 112, 125, 170, 171, 172, 174, 178br, 183, 186, 192, 193, 202, 205, 206bl, 216, 218, 221, 224, 225, 226, 230, 232, 234, 236, 240, 252, 254, 256, 260, 261, 262, 264, 266, 269, 271, 273, 274, 276, 278, 284, 288, 291, 292, 294, 296, 298, 300, 301, 302, 304, 306, 309, 311, 314, 316, 317, 319bl, 323, 324
Laura Watson: 24

Jacket

Photodisc: back jacket, cl
Studio Cactus: back jacket, tl
Richard Mitchell: author photograph

Further picture credits

Studio Cactus would like to thank Caroline at Transform Cosmetic Surgery Ltd and Sharon Dobbs at The Laser Clinic, and also Catalyst PR and Storm Hairdressing for their help in supplying images:

25: Hair by **Pierre Alexander Art Team, Manchester, for Goldwell**
Photography by Ian Lee
Makeup by Collette
Styling by Amechi London

141, 160: Hair by **Pierre Alexander, for Goldwell**
Photography by Bruce Smith
Makeup by Gemma Smith

131: Hair by **Donna Allen, Smiths, Soho London, for Goldwell**

130, 165: Hair by **Errol Douglas, London, for Goldwell**

133: Hair by **Errol Douglas Hairdressing, for Goldwell**
Photography by Simon Bottomley
Styling by, Pippa Holt

129, 144: Hair by **Keith Francis, for Goldwell**
Photography by Mike Balfre
Makeup by Karen Lockyer

138, 149: **Goldwell**

80tl, 80tr: **The Laser Clinic (www.laserclinic.co.uk)**

147bl, 148: Hair by **Natasha Grocutt, Hair Ott, Portsmouth, for Goldwell**
Photography by David Hindley
Makeup by Karen Lockyer

142: Hair by **Hammonds, 2 Walker Lane, Killamarsh, Sheffield, S21 8ER, for Goldwell**

168: Hair by **Allan Henry & Sandra Webb at Hype Coiffure, London, for Goldwell**
Photography by David Hindley
Makeup by Caroline O'Donnelly

156: Hair by **Terry Jacques, Terry Jacques Hair Salon, London, for Goldwell**
Photography by Richard Barnes

154: Hair by **JR's Hairdressing, Glasgow, for Goldwell**

208: Hair by **JR's Artistic Team, Glasgow, for Goldwell**
Photography by Jack Harper
Makeup by Terri Craig
Styling by Fiona Black

162: Hair by **Mo & Margaret Nabbach, M&M Academy, London, for Goldwell**

109, 122: Hair by **Ott Artistic Team, Portsmouth, for Goldwell**
Photography by Mike Balfre

90bl, 110: Hair by **Rush Artistic Team, South London, for Goldwell**
Photography by Mike Balfre
Makeup by Karen Lockyer

135: Hair by **Rush, London, for Goldwell**

283: Photography by Scott Michael-Carroll
Makeup by **Christine Cohen at Errol Douglas**

9, 127cl, 127br, 150, 155, 164, 204cr, 204br: Hair by **Carl Shaw, for Goldwell**
Photography by Mike Balfre
Makeup by Virginia Nichols

146: Hair by **Jamie Smith, Smith's Salon, London, for Goldwell**
Photography by Mike Balfre
Makeup by Karen Lockyer

117, 147tr, 190: **Storm Hairdressing**

76, 268, 272, 280bl, 280br, 281bl, 281br, 282bl, 282br, 285bl, 285br, 286bl, 286br: **Transform Cosmetic Surgery Ltd (0500 595959 transforminglives.co.uk)**

The people illustrated in this book are models. Images are used for illustrative purposes only and do not imply endorsement, use of, or a connection to any product, service, or subject.

All other images © Dorling Kindersley
For further information see: www.dkimages.com